ORTHOPEDIC NURSING SECRETS

Michael E. Zychowicz, RN, MS, NP-C
Assistant Professor, Division of Nursing
Mount Saint Mary College
Newburgh, New York

Nursing Secrets Series Editor

Linda J. Scheetz, EdD, RN, CS, CEN
Assistant Professor, College of Nursing
Rutgers, The State University of New Jersey
Newark, New Jersey

HANLEY & BELFUS, INC.
An Imprint of Elsevier

HANLEY & BELFUS, INC.
An Imprint of Elsevier

The Curtis Center
Independence Square West
Philadelphia, Pennsylvania 19106

Library of Congress Control Number: 2003101037

ORTHOPEDIC NURSING SECRETS

ISBN 1-56053-530-X

Printed in the United States

Last digit is the print number: 9   8   7   6   5   4   3   2   1

CONTENTS

CONTRIBUTORS

Andrea Dodge Ackermann, RN, MS, CCRN
Instructor, Division of Nursing, Mount Saint Mary College, Newburgh, New York

Valerie V. Armstrong, RN, MA, NP-C, CCRN, MSCN
Department of Neurology, Mayo Clinic Jacksonville, and St. Luke's Hospital, Jacksonville, Florida

Pamela Bilyeu, RN, BSN, CNOR, CURN, ONC
Operating Room, Saint Vincent Healthcare, Billings, Montana

Jill Brennan-Cook, RN, MS, CEN
Instructor, Division of Nursing, Mount Saint Mary College, Newburgh, New York

Tom Bush, MSN, RN, CS, FNP
Assistant Professor, Department of Orthopaedic Surgery, University of North Carolina School of Medicine, Chapel Hill, North Carolina

Brandi L. Handel, RN, MSN, APN
Clinical Nurse Specialist, Department of Orthopaedics, Robert Wood Johnson University Hospital, New Brunswick, New Jersey

Barbara J. Heckman, MSN, RN, ANP-C
Nurse Practitioner, Neurological and Spine Surgery, P.C., Hawthorne, New York

Amy L. Hite, MSN, FNP-C, ONC
Orthopedic Nurse Practitioner, New Century Orthopedic Surgery and Sports Medicine, Pittsburg, Kansas

Cindy Jo Horrell, RN, MS, AOCN
Oncology Nurse Practitioner, Great Lakes Hematology Associates at the Regional Cancer Center, Erie, Pennsylvania

Debra A. Hrelic, RNC, PhD(c)
Instructor, Division of Nursing, Mount Saint Mary College, Newburgh, New York

Barbara Krajewski, RNC, MS, FNP-C
Adjunct Professor, Graduate School of Nursing, College of New Rochelle, New Rochelle, New York; Westchester Medical Center, Valhalla, New York

Linda LaRocco, RN, MS, ANP-C
Instructor, Division of Nursing, Mount Saint Mary College, Newburgh, New York

Dianne Murphy, RN, MS, CCRN
Instructor, Division of Nursing, Mount Saint Mary College, Newburgh, New York; Staff Nurse, Critical Care Unit, Orange Regional Medical Center, Middletown, New York

Dottie Roberts, MSU, MACI, RN, BC, ONC
Clinical Nurse Specialist, Rehabilitative and Medical Services, Palmetto Baptist Medical Center, Columbia, South Carolina

Sandra Van Dyke, RN, MS
Assistant Professor, Division of Nursing, Mount Saint Mary College, Newburgh, New York

Suzanne H. Waters, RN, MS, FNP, C-S
Director of Staff Development, Vassar Brothers Medical Center, Poughkeepsie, New York; Family Nurse Practitioner, Wound Care Center, Poughkeepsie, New York; Family Nurse Practitioner, First Care Family Practice Physicians Association, Monroe, New York

Michael E. Zychowicz, RN, MS, ANP-C
Assistant Professor, Division of Nursing, Mount Saint Mary College, Newburgh, New York; Nurse Practitioner, Orthopedics and Sports Medicine, P.C., New Windsor, New York

PREFACE

Of all clinical specialties in which I have practiced as a nurse and nurse practitioner, orthopedics has been the most exciting and the most rewarding. During our careers most of us have had excellent opportunities to learn from many exceptional mentors. In return, we have an obligation to share with future nurses as well as our peers the knowledge that we have acquired during our professional development. It is a great pleasure to share this knowledge in *Orthopedic Nursing Secrets*, another entry in the highly successful Nursing Secrets Series®.

The purpose of this book is to share pearls of knowledge with nursing students as well as established nurses who provide care to patients with orthopedic disorders. It is designed to be a useful reference for students in the classroom as well as nurses in both inpatient and outpatient settings, including those who work in the emergency department, operating room, intensive care unit, medical and surgical units, student health services, sports medicine offices, physiatry practices, rehabilitation facilities, and pain management centers. The text discusses essential nursing considerations in a wide variety of orthopedic areas. Each chapter consists of thought-provoking questions and straightforward answers. Authors have focused on applying their clinical expertise to each topic. Any nurse who provides care to patients with musculoskeletal conditions should find this book useful, informative, and enjoyable to read.

Special gratitude is due to Linda Scheetz, the Nursing Secrets Series® Editor, who has become a valued role model and mentor in the short time that I have known her. I am grateful for the numerous opportunities for professional growth and development that she has made available to me.

Michael E. Zychowicz, RN, MS, NP-C

DEDICATION

To my dogs, Sam and Fred, who unconditionally sacrificed hours of playtime during the development of this book.

1. PHYSICAL EXAMINATION

Michael E. Zychowicz, RN, MS, NP-C

1. What are the components of the musculoskeletal examination?

The components of the musculoskeletal physical examination include inspection, palpation, range of motion, muscle testing, neurovascular testing, deep tendon reflexes, and special tests.

2. During the inspection component, what should the examiner note?

The examiner inspects the joint(s) for shape and contour as well as the surrounding muscle for size and shape. The examiner should inspect the surrounding skin and subcutaneous tissues for edema, erythema, nodules, ecchymosis, obvious deformities, and other abnormalities. Be sure to compare both sides of the body throughout the physical exam.

3. What should be palpated during the exam?

Perform palpation of the skin and muscle as well as the major ligamentous, tendinous, and skeletal anatomic landmarks at each joint or region being examined. While palpating, feel for warmth, edema, crepitus, nodules, abnormal movement, abnormal underlying tissue contour, and joint effusion. Another reason for palpation is to elicit tenderness at specific structures to confirm a diagnosis. The examiner may also palpate the joint while performing range of motion (ROM) to feel for crepitus.

4. When are active and passive ROM performed?

Active ROM should be performed for each joint examined. Passive range of motion should be performed if active ROM is limited.

5. How is strength testing graded?

Strength is graded on a scale of 0–5. If no muscular contraction is noted, strength is graded as 0. It is graded as 1 if there is a slight muscle contraction but no movement at the joint. If the patient is able to move the joint without gravity, strength is graded as 2. Strength is graded as 3 if the patient is able to move the joint against gravity but not against resistance. If the patient has some weakness against resistance, strength is graded as 4. Strength is graded as 5 if the patient is able to move the joint against resistance.

6. How are deep tendon reflexes graded?

Reflexes are graded on a 4-point scale. Absent reflexes are graded as 0. Reflexes are graded as 1+ if they are sluggish or slightly diminished. "Normal" reflexes are graded as 2+. When reflexes are brisk or slightly hyperactive they are graded as 3+. Reflexes that are hyperactive and extremely brisk with clonus are graded as 4+.

7. How does the examiner elicit deep tendon reflexes in the upper extremities?

Cradling the patient's forearm with the examiner's forearm or simply having the arm relax in the patient's lap is the first step to elicit the **biceps reflex**. The patient's elbow should be flexed between 45° and 90°. The examiner places pressure on the patient's biceps tendon at the elbow with a finger, then taps the finger with the reflex hammer, indirectly hitting the biceps tendon. The biceps should contract, causing flexion at the elbow.

For the **triceps tendon reflex**, the examiner again cradles the patient's arm while it is flexed at the elbow between 45° and 90°. The examiner identifies the triceps tendon proximal to the olecranon, then gently taps the tendon with the reflex hammer. The triceps muscle should contract, causing extension at the elbow.

Striking the brachioradialis tendon with the reflex hammer approximately 1 inch proximal and lateral to the distal radius elicits the **brachioradialis tendon reflex**. In eliciting this reflex, the forearm is positioned in a neutral position with slight flexion at the elbow. With a normal response, the patient's forearm should supinate slightly with slight flexion at the elbow.

8. How does the examiner elicit deep tendon reflexes in the lower extremities?

The **patellar reflex** is tested by first identifying the patellar tendon between the patella and the insertion at the tibial tubercle. The examiner flexes the patient's knee to 90° and taps the tendon with the reflex hammer. The normal reaction is contraction of the quadriceps muscle group with extension at the knee.

The **Achilles tendon reflex** is elicited by tapping the tendon proximal to the calcaneal insertion at the heel. The examiner should gently, passively dorsiflex the patient's ankle to place gentle tension on the Achilles tendon. The response should be plantarflexion at the ankle.

9. How is range of motion at a joint measured?

ROM at joints can be accurately measured by using a goniometer. The pivot point of the goniometer should be aligned with the joint being measured. In addition, the arms of the goniometer should be aligned with the bones proximal and distal to the joint. Starting in the neutral position, active and/or passive ROM at the specific joint is performed in all of the planes being measured. The examiner takes note of the degrees of movement of the goniometer corresponding to the end ROM in each plane of the joint.

10. Why should the examiner compare both sides of the patient's body even though the patient complains of unilateral symptoms?

If the patient has a complaint involving only one body part, the examiner should check both sides of the body to assess how the findings of the part in question compare with the "normal" part. This approach helps the examiner determine whether the exam findings are "normal" for the patient and helps to identify a diagnosis.

11. How can the nurse assess nerve function during the examination?

Nerve testing is performed to assess injury or dysfunction of the spinal and peripheral nerves. The spinal and peripheral nerves have a typical reflex, motor, and sensory distribution. These can be tested with deep tendon reflexes, strength testing, and sensation over the distribution of the nerve. The sensory distribution of individual spinal nerves to an area of the skin is called a **dermatome**. Peripheral nerves also have a typical distribution. A patient may have decreased or absent reflexes, decreased or absent strength, and/or altered sensation along the distribution of a nerve. Such findings may correlate with the patient's complaint and history. They assist the examiner in diagnosing the complaint and help guide appropriate treatment or further diagnostic testing.

12. What is the difference between varus and valgus?

Varus refers to a joint or portion of the body that is angled toward the midline of the body. For example, a patient with significant degenerative arthritis of the knees may develop a bow-legged appearance of the knees. In the varus deformity the lower leg is angled at the knee toward the midline of the body. **Valgus** refers to a portion of the body that is angled away from the midline. The knock-kneed patient is a good example of a valgus deformity. The lower leg is angled laterally at the knee away from the midline of the body.

13. What is the normal ROM of the cervical spine?

Normal cervical flexion is to 45°, with hyperextension to 55°, lateral bending to 40° bilaterally, and rotation to 70° bilaterally.

14. Describe the significant areas to palpate at the cervical spine.

The bony landmarks to palpate at the cervical spine include the spinous processes, the mastoid process, and the cervical facet joints. The major soft tissue landmarks to palpate include the paraspinal, trapezius, and sternocleidomastoid muscles.

15. What spinal nerves are assessed during examination of the cervical spine and upper extremities? List their corresponding sensory, motor, and reflex components.

The spinal nerves assessed during an exam of the cervical spine and upper extremities include C5, C6, C7, C8, and T1.

Spinal Nerve	Sensory Component	Motor Component	Deep Tendon Reflex
C5	Lateral upper arm	Shoulder abduction and biceps contraction	Biceps and brachioradialis
C6	Lateral forearm and 1st, 2nd, lateral side of the 3rd finger	Wrist extension and biceps contraction	Biceps and brachioradialis
C7	Middle finger	Elbow extension, wrist flexion and finger extension	Triceps
C8	Distal-medial border of the forearm and 4th and 5th fingers	Finger flexion, abduction and adduction	None
T1	Proximal medial forearm and medial side of upper arm	Finger abduction and adduction	None

16. What peripheral nerves should be assessed? List their sensory distribution and motor innervation.

The major peripheral nerves that supply the upper extremities are the musculocutaneous, axillary, median, ulnar, and radial nerves Their sensory distribution and motor innervation are outlined below.

Peripheral Nerve	Sensory Component	Motor Component
Musculocutaneous	Lateral surface of the forearm	Biceps contraction
Axillary	Lateral upper arm over the deltoid patch	Deltoid contraction

(Table continued on next page)

Peripheral Nerve	Sensory Component	Motor Component
Median	2nd finger along the distal radial border	Thumb abduction and pinch mechanism, and thumb/little finger opposition
Ulnar	5th finger along the distal ulnar border	5th finger abduction
Radial	Dorsal surface of 1st and 2nd finger web space	Thumb and wrist extension

17. How is the patient assessed for meningitis?

Two tests can be performed to assess for meningeal irritation: the Kernig and Brudzinski signs. Both are performed with the patient in a supine position. In attempting to elicit the Kernig's sign, the patient should tell the examiner whether neck and back pain is present with flexion of the neck. The Brudzinski sign is positive if the patient flexes one or both legs while the examiner flexes the patient's neck.

18. What is the significance of the Spurling maneuver?

A positive Spurling maneuver can be present in patients with cervical neuroforaminal stenosis from cervical disk herniation or arthritic spurring that irritates the cervical spinal nerve(s). The patient performs hyperextension and rotation of the cervical spine as the examiner applies slight axial compression to the cervical spine.

19. How is Chvostek's sign elicited?

Chvostek's sign may be present in a patient with hypocalcemia due to hypoparathyroidism. To elicit the sign, tap the facial nerve of one side of the patient's face slightly anterior to the ear. If the test is positive, the patient's facial muscles will contract on the ipsilateral side.

20. Describe the normal ROM of the lumbar spine.

Normal lumbar range of motion is to 90° of flexion, 30° of hyperextension, 35° of lateral bending, and 30° of rotation.

21. What are the significant areas to palpate at the lumbar spine?

In the area of the lumbar spine, the examiner should palpate the spinous processes, the supraspinous and interspinous ligaments, and the paraspinal muscles.

22. In assessing the lumbar spine and lower extremities, which spinal nerves should be assessed? List their corresponding sensory, motor, and reflex components.

The spinal nerves to examine in assessing the lumbar spine, hip, pelvis, and the lower extremities include T10–T12, L1–L5, and S1–S4.

Spinal Nerve	Sensory Component	Motor Component	Deep Tendon Reflex
T10	Abdomen at the level of the umbilicus	None	None

(Table continued on next page)

Spinal Nerve	Sensory Component	Motor Component	Deep Tendon Reflex
T11	Abdomen slightly below the umbilicus and above the inguinal ligament	None	None
T12	Abdomen just above the inguinal ligament	Iliopsoas	None
L1	Upper anterior thigh below the inguinal ligament	Iliopsoas	None
L2	Anterior middle thigh	Iliopsoas, quadriceps	None
L3	Lower anterior thigh above the knee	Iliopsoas, quadriceps	None
L4	Anterior knee and medial side of the calf, ankle, and foot	Quadriceps, tibialis anterior	Patellar
L5	Lateral knee and calf. Dorsum of the foot	Extensor hallucis longus, gluteus medius	None
S1	Lateral ankle, lateral and plantar surface of the foot	Peroneus longus and brevis, gastrocnemius and soleus	Achilles
S2	Posterior thigh and popliteal fossa	Bladder muscles	None
S2, S3, S4	Three concentric perianal sensory rings. S4 is the inner-most while S2 is the outermost.	Bladder muscles	None

23. List the sensory and motor components of the major peripheral nerves of the lower extremities.

Peripheral Nerve	Sensory Component	Motor Component
Anterior femoral cutaneous	Anterior thigh	
Lateral femoral cutaneous	Lateral thigh	
Posterior femoral cutaneous	Posterior thigh	
Femoral nerve	Anterior middle thigh	Hip flexion, knee extension
Inferior gluteal nerve		Hip extension
Superior gluteal nerve		Hip abduction
Obturator nerve	Medial thigh	Hip adduction
Tibial nerve	Medial and lateral foot	Knee flexion, ankle plantarflexion
Long saphenous	Medial foot	Abducts great toe
Sural	Lateral foot	Abduction of the 5th toe
Superficial peroneal	Dorsal foot	Foot eversion, ankle plantar-flexion
Deep peroneal	1st/2nd toe web space	Foot dorsiflexion, ankle inversion, extends toes

24. What test is used to assess whether low back pain is due to the sacroiliac joint?

The **Patrick test** is used to assess for sacroiliac (SI) pathology. This test, also known as the Faber test, is performed with the patient in the supine position. First, place the foot of the side to be examined on the knee of the opposite leg. While keeping this foot in place, fully externally rotate the examined hip, providing slight additional pressure. SI dysfunction is indicated if the patient develops increased low back pain with this test.

The **Gaenslen test** can also be used to assess for SI dysfunction. The patient lies supine on the exam table, positioned to the side of the table with one leg and buttock off the table. Have the patient pull the legs to the chest by flexing both knees and hips. Next, have the patient fully extend the leg that is off the side of the table while the other leg remains flexed. If the patient complains of increased pain, the patient may have SI dysfunction.

25. What physical tests can be performed to assess for a herniated lumbar disc?

The **Milgram test** is performed with the patient in the supine position with both legs extended. The patient is asked to lift both extended legs 2 inches above the exam table and hold that position for up to 30 seconds. If the patient is unable to hold this position for the full 30 seconds, a lumbar disc herniation is suggested.

The **Valsalva maneuver** is performed by asking the patient to "bear down" in a sitting position. If the patient develops new or increased pain in the back and/or leg, a lumbar disc herniation is suggested.

The positive **straight leg raise, or Lasegue's test,** is also indicative of a lumbar disc herniation. The test is performed with the patient lying supine on the exam table with both legs fully extended. The examiner attempts to flex one leg at the hip up to 90° while the knee remains straight. The patient may develop tightness in the posterior thigh that may be indicative of tight hamstring muscles. If the test is positive, the patient will complain of increased pain into the leg and/or back. This pain is increased if dorsiflexion is applied to the ankle during the straight leg raise.

26. What is the normal Babinski's reflex?

To elicit the Babinski's reflex, the examiner strokes the lateral plantar surface of the foot from the heel to toes with the handle of the reflex hammer. With a normal Babinski's reflex in the adult, the toes may flex and adduct or simply have no reaction. The positive Babinski test in the adult displays extension of the first toe with abduction and flexion of the other toes. This test is indicative of an upper motor neuron lesion from a tumor or trauma. The Babinski test is normally present with newborn children.

27. What is the normal ROM for the shoulder?

Normal shoulder ROM includes 180° of forward flexion, 50° of hyperextension, 180° of abduction, 50° of adduction, and 90° of internal and external rotation.

28. What are the significant areas to palpate at the shoulder?

During a complete exam of the shoulder, the examiner should palpate the suprasternal notch, clavicle, acromioclavicular joint, acromion, spine of the scapula, proximal humerus at the greater tuberosity and bicipital groove, and coracoid process. The examiner should also palpate the accessible rotator cuff muscles (supraspinatus, infraspinatus, and teres minor), subacromial bursa, subdeltoid bursa, axilla, biceps, deltoid, and trapezius.

29. What does the drop arm test assess?

The drop arm test assesses the rotator cuff muscles. The test is performed by passively abducting the patient's arm. The patient is then asked to actively adduct the arm at a slow rate with the elbow in extension. Normally, the patient should be able to adduct the arm at a steady rate through the entire arc. A rotator cuff tear should be suspected if the arm falls to the side with the patient unable to perform the motion slowly. The arm typically drops at approximately 90° of abduction.

30. What other tests can be performed to assess the rotator cuff?

The **supraspinatus test** is simple to perform and is used to assess for tears of the supraspinatus, one of the rotator cuff muscles. The patient abducts both arms with the elbows extended and the thumbs pointed down. The examiner provides downward pressure, attempting to adduct the arms, while the patient resists, attempting to abduct the arms at the shoulder. If the patient is unable to resist the examiner's downward pressure or if notable weakness is present, there may be a partial or complete tear of the supraspinatus muscle.

The patient may have a **painful arc with abduction at the shoulder** if the rotator cuff is injured or inflamed. The pain usually presents as the patient's arm actively abducts between approximately 60° and 120°. The discomfort is due to impingement of the rotator cuff muscles between the acromion and the humerus.

Another test for rotator cuff inflammation is the **impingement sign**. The shoulder is passively flexed and abducted. Pain at the end range of movement is positive for impingement of the rotator cuff at the shoulder.

31. A patient who has had a shoulder subluxation or dislocation may have an apprehension sign. What does this mean?

The apprehension test is used to assess for instability at the shoulder after acute subluxation or to assess for chronic instability at the glenohumoral joint. The examiner asks the patient to abduct the arm at the shoulder with the elbow flexed and to externally rotate the arm at the shoulder. The examiner then places one hand on the patient's shoulder at the acromion and applies gentle anterior pressure. With the other hand, the examiner passively externally rotates the arm at the shoulder. If the test is positive, the patient becomes "apprehensive" because the shoulder has the feeling that it may dislocate during this maneuver.

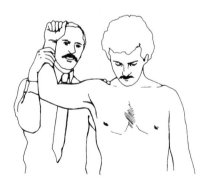

Apprehension test. (From Mellion MB: Office Sports Medicine, 2nd ed. Philadelphia, Hanley & Belfus, 1996, with permission.)

32. In addition to palpation, what other test assesses the biceps tendon?

The **Speed test** is performed with the patient's arms extended at the elbow, supinated, and flexed at the shoulder to approximately 90°. The examiner applies downward force on the patient's arms with the patient resisting. Discomfort over the anterior shoulder in the area of the bicipital groove is indicative of biceps tendinitis.

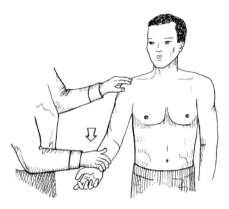

Demonstration of the Speed test for bicipital tendinitis. (From Frontera WR, Silver JK (eds): Essentials of Physical Medicine and Rehabilitation. Philadelphia, Hanley & Belfus, 2002, with permission.)

The **Yergason maneuver** assesses for instability of the biceps tendon at the bicipital groove. The patient flexes the arm at the elbow to 90°. The examiner holds the patient's wrist with one hand and the elbow with the other hand, providing downward pull of the arm. The patient should resist the examiner while the examined arm is externally rotated at the shoulder.

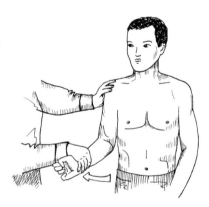

Demonstration of the Yergason test. (From Frontera WR, Silver JK (eds): Essentials of Physical Medicine and Rehabilitation. Philadelphia, Hanley & Belfus, 2002, with permission.)

33. Aside from the structures of the shoulder, what problems can produce left shoulder pain?

First and foremost, the heart can cause referred pain to the left shoulder with angina or myocardial infarction. The left shoulder can be painful with cervical disc herniation, cervical fracture, and diaphragmatic irritation.

34. What is the significance of scapular winging?

Scapular winging is present if the patient has weakness or injury to the serratus anterior muscle. As the name implies, the patient develops a winged appearance to the scapula. To assess for winging, observe the scapula posteriorly as the patient pushes against a wall while standing or performs a push-up. Serratus anterior weakness can be due to multiple causes, including damage to the C5, C6, and/or C7 nerve root, brachial plexus injury, and long thoracic nerve injury.

35. What tests can be performed to assess for thoracic outlet syndrome?

The **Allen maneuver** is performed by abducting the arm and flexing the elbow of the arm to be examined. The examiner palpates the radial pulse of the arm, then has the patient rotate the head toward the opposite shoulder. Thoracic outlet syndrome may be present if the pulse is obliterated with rotation of the head.

The **Adson maneuver** is performed again with the examiner palpating the radial pulse of the arm to be assessed. The patient's arm is extended and externally rotated at the shoulder. The patient then rotates the head toward the arm being tested and takes a deep breath. If the pulse is obliterated, thoracic outlet syndrome is indicated.

36. What is the normal ROM for the elbow?

Normal ROM at the elbow shows 180° of flexion, 0° of extension, and 90° of supination and pronation of the forearm.

37. What are the significant areas to palpate at the elbow?

The examiner should palpate the olecranon, medial and lateral epicondyle, and radial head. Soft tissues to palpate include the ulnar nerve, flexor and extensor mass of the forearm, triceps, biceps, olecranon bursa, and epitrochlear lymph nodes.

38. What is the carrying angle?

The carrying angle is the angle made at the elbow between the humerus and the forearm. There should be a slight valgus angle with the elbow extended, palm facing forward, and arm at the patient's side. For women, the carrying angle is approximately 10°–15°; men typically have a 5° carrying angle.

39. How does the examiner assess for ulnar nerve irritation?

Patients with ulnar nerve irritation typically complain of numbness, tingling, and/or pain into the medial forearm, medial fourth finger and entire fifth finger. These symptoms can be exacerbated with a Tinel test at the elbow of the affected arm. To elicit the Tinel sign, the examiner taps over the ulnar nerve at the elbow as it passes between the medial epicondyle and the olecranon. If the patient's usual symptoms are reproduced, the test is considered positive.

40. How do the exam findings differ in golfer's elbow and tennis elbow?

The patient with tennis elbow (lateral epicondylitis) complains of elbow discomfort in the area of the lateral epicondyle and forearm extensor mass, whereas the patient with golfer's elbow (medial epicondylitis) has discomfort at the forearm flexor mass and medial epicondyle. The patient with lateral epicondylitis has increased discomfort with palpation over the lateral epicondyle and the extensor mass of the forearm.

Another test for lateral epicondylitis is resisted extension of the wrist. During this maneuver the patient pronates the hand, makes a fist, and extends the wrist with slight radial deviation while the examiner provides resistance to the movement. The patient experiences increased elbow pain if lateral epicondylitis is present. The patient also complains of increased pain at the elbow if the examiner provides stretch of the extensor mass while passively stretching the wrist of the affected arm.

The examiner should perform the exact opposite tests for medial epicondylitis. There will be pain on palpation over the medial epicondyle. Passive extension and resisted flexion of the wrist of the affected arm increase elbow pain if medial epicondylitis is present.

41. How does the examiner assess for instability of the elbow?

In examining the elbow for stability, the examiner is assessing for increased pain and/ or movement while providing varus and valgus stress to elbow. To assess the medial collateral ligaments, the examiner stabilizes and holds the upper arm at the elbow with one hand while the patient slightly flexes the elbow. With the other hand holding the patient's forearm, the examiner exerts valgus stress by attempting to bend the forearm laterally at the elbow. The examiner should inspect the elbow for an increase in the valgus angle. Palpation of the medial elbow with the hand stabilizing the elbow also verifies increased gapping at the medial elbow.

To assess the lateral collateral ligament of the elbow, the examiner provides varus stress to the elbow while stabilizing the elbow with one hand and attempting to bend the forearm medially. Again, the examiner inspects for increased angulation and palpates for gapping at the lateral elbow. The examiner should compare the joint of the opposite side of the body. If the patient has increased gapping at the elbow compared with the opposite side, the collateral ligament may be completely torn. The patient may have simply sprained the ligament if only discomfort is present.

42. Describe the normal ROM at the hand and wrist.

Normal ROM at the wrist shows 90° of flexion, 70° of hyperextension, 55° of ulnar deviation, and 20° of radial deviation. At the metacarpophalangeal (MCP) joint there should be 90° of flexion with 30° of hyperextension at the fingers and 50° of flexion with 0° of extension at the thumb. At the proximal interphalangeal joint there should be flexion to 100° with extension to 0°. At the distal interphalangeal joint there should be flexion to 90° and hyperextension to 20°. The interphalangeal joint of the thumb should flex to 90° and extend to 20°. The fingers should abduct 20° with thumb abduction of 70° and adduction of all digits to neutral.

43. What are the significant areas to palpate at the hand and wrist?

The examiner should palpate the phalanges, interphalangeal joints, metacarpals, metacarpophalangeal joints, carpals, carpometacarpal joints, distal radius, radiocarpal joint, distal ulna, and distal radioulnar joint. The radial pulse, tufts of the fingers, flexor and extensors of the wrist and fingers, the thenar and hypothenar eminences, and the palm of the hand should also be palpated.

44. What are the physical exam tests for carpal tunnel syndrome?

Patients with carpal tunnel syndrome usually have complaints of pain, numbness, or tingling of the radial border of the affected hand into the first, second, and third fingers as well as the radial border of the fourth finger. These symptoms may wake patients from sleep, become aggravated with activities, or be continuous.

The two tests for carpal tunnel syndrome are the Tinel and Phalen tests. Both attempt to cause irritation to the medial nerve and reproduce the patient's typical carpal tunnel symptoms. To perform the Tinel test, tap the patient's wrist in the center of the volar surface. To perform the Phalen test, have the patient flex the wrists to 90°, placing the dorsal surface of the hands together. The patient should hold this position for up to 1 minute in an attempt to reproduce the symptoms. Both tests are positive if the patient's symptoms are aggravated.

45. What information does the Allen test give?

The Allen test is useful to assess blood flow to the hand by way of the radial and ulnar arteries. The first step is to identify the radial and ulnar arteries. After the arteries have been identified, have the patient clench the fist tightly, squeezing the blood from the hand. Next, grasp the patient's wrist with both hands, squeezing one thumb against the radial artery and the other against the ulnar artery to occlude blood flow. Have the patient open the hand while the arteries are still occluded. The palm should remain pale. Pressure should be released from one of the arteries, allowing the palm to become pink immediately. This procedure is repeated from the beginning, releasing the pressure on the other artery. If the palm remains pale or is slow to pink when blood flow through one of the arteries is released, that artery may be completely or partially occluded.

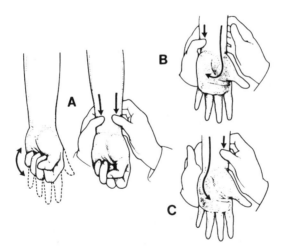

The Allen test. (From James EC, Corry RJ, Perry JF: Principles of Basic Surgical Practice. Philadelphia, Hanley & Belfus, 1987, with permission.)

46. How can blood flow of an individual finger be assessed?

A modified Allen test can be performed to assess blood flow through the digital arteries of an individual finger. The patient clenches the fist to evacuate blood from the finger. While the patient's fist is clenched, the examined finger is pinched laterally at the base with the examiner's first and second finger. This maneuver occludes the digital arteries. The patient extends the fingers while the artery remains occluded, leaving the finger pale. The examiner releases one of the arteries, allowing the finger to become pink. The test is performed from the beginning while releasing the opposite digital artery. If the finger remains pale or slowly becomes pink after the artery is released, the examined artery is partially or completely occluded.

47. How is the Trousseau sign elicited? What may it indicate?

The Trousseau sign is elicited by applying the blood pressure cuff to the patient's upper arm and inflating the cuff to occlude blood flow. The cuff should remain in place for 3–5 minutes. The test is positive if the patient develops carpal spasm or twitching of the hand. A positive Trousseau sign may be indicative of hypocalcemia.

48. How is the Finkelstein test performed? What does a positive test indicate?

Have the patient place the thumb into the palm of the hand, closing the other fingers and making a fist. The patient then performs ulnar deviation of the hand and wrist. If the patient has no pain or only slight discomfort, the test is negative. The test is positive if pain is produced along the radial border of the wrist over the extensor pollicis brevis and abductor pollicis longus. A positive test is indicative of de Quervain's tenosynovitis.

49. What is the normal ROM of the hip?

The normal hip range of motion should be 15° of hyperextension, 120° of flexion with the knee flexed, 90° of flexion with the knee extended, 40° of internal rotation, 45° of external rotation, 45° of abduction, and 30° of adduction.

50. What are the significant areas to palpate at the hip?

The major bony landmarks to palpate at the hip include the anterior superior iliac spine, iliac crest, greater trochanter, ischial tuberosity, sacrum, and sacroiliac joint. Soft tissue palpation at the hip should include the femoral artery, inguinal ligament, trochanteric bursa, inguinal lymph nodes, and the flexor, extensor, adductor, and abductor muscle groups surrounding the hip.

51. What tests can be performed to assess infants for congenital dislocation of the hip?

The Barlow maneuver, Ortolani test, Allis test, Galeazzi test, and telescoping test.

52. How is the Barlow test performed?

The Barlow test is performed by applying gentle downward pressure to the femur while the hip is flexed and slightly adducted. This is an attempt to dislocate the hip of the examined leg. The examiner then applies gentle traction to the thigh as the leg is abducted, attempting to relocate the hip if it is dislocated. The dislocation/relocation of the hip is palpated by the examiner.

53. What is found with a positive Ortolani test?

With a positive Ortolani test, the examiner feels a click at the infant's hip as the femoral head reduces over the rim of the acetabulum. The maneuver is similar to the Barlow test and is performed by flexing the hips and the knees while the child is lying supine. The examiner then abducts and lifts the thighs at the hip, feeling and listening for the click at the hip.

54. How does the Allis test indicate hip dislocation of the child's hip?

To perform the Allis test, have the child lie in the supine position. Flex the hips and knees, place both feet on the table, and inspect the position of both knees. Hip dislocation is possible if one of the knees is significantly higher or lower than the other.

55. How is the Galeazzi test performed?

The Galeazzi test is essentially the same as the Allis test. The only difference is that the knee position is also assessed with the hip in adduction and abduction.

56. What is found with the telescoping test?

During the telescoping test for congenital hip dislocation, the examiner may feel excessive movement at the child's hip as the femoral head dislocates and relocates at the acetabulum. The test is performed with the patient lying supine as the examiner grasps the thigh with one hand and stabilizes the hip with the other hand. The examiner then provides gentle traction to the thigh, attempting to dislocate the hip, followed by gentle pressure to the thigh, attempting to relocate the hip.

57. What information is gathered with the Trendelenburg test?

The Trendelenburg test is used to assess the gluteus medius muscle and a possible pathologic process at the hip. The gluteus medius is a primary abductor of the hip and is innervated by the L5 nerve root. The test is performed by first having the patient stand on both feet. The patient then lifts one leg to stand on only one foot. The examiner takes note of the pelvis, inspecting to ensure that the pelvis remains level and the patient retains balance. If the pelvis dips toward the non-weight-bearing leg, injury or weakness of the gluteus medius is indicated.

58. Why is the Thomas test performed?

To assess for a flexion contracture at the hip. The patient is examined in a supine position. The examiner asks the patient to flex one leg at the hip and knee, pulling that leg to the chest. If the opposite leg is lifted from the exam table in addition to the tested leg, there is a possibility of a hip flexion contracture.

59. What is normal ROM of the knee?

Normal knee ROM is 130° of flexion and 15° of hyperextension.

60. What are the significant areas to palpate at the knee?

At the knee the examiner should palpate the medial and lateral tibial plateaus, medial and lateral femoral condyles, adductor tubercle of the femur, head of the fibula, tibial tubercle, and patella. Soft tissues to be palpated include the quadriceps muscle, quadriceps tendon, infrapatellar tendon, medial and lateral menisci, medial and lateral collateral ligaments, hamstring muscles, popliteal fossa, popliteal artery, and iliotibial band. Bursae to palpate at the knee include the pes anserinus, prepatellar, and superficial infrapatellar. A Baker's cyst in the popliteal fossa may also be palpable.

61. What are the major tests to assess the anterior and posterior cruciate ligaments?

The Lachman and anterior drawer tests assess stability of the anterior cruciate ligament. The posterior drawer test assesses the posterior cruciate ligament.

The **Lachman test** is performed while the patient is lying supine with the knee flexed to approximately 30°. With one of the examiner's hands stabilizing the thigh and the other hand applying forward traction on the tibia, the examiner inspects and feels for forward translation of the tibia.

The **anterior drawer test** is performed with the patient lying supine on the exam table. The hip is flexed slightly with the knee flexed to approximately 90° while the foot remains flat on the table. The examiner can sit on the foot to stabilize the lower extremity.

The examiner grasps the proximal tibia with both hands, palpating the joint line with the fingers and applying traction to the tibia. An anterior cruciate ligament tear may be present if translation at the tibia is present during the Lachman and/or the anterior drawer.

The **posterior drawer** is performed in much the same fashion as the anterior drawer. However, the examiner pushes posteriorly against the tibia instead of pulling anteriorly. A posterior cruciate ligament tear is suspected if the tibia translates posteriorly.

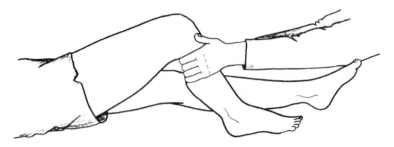

Position for the anterior drawer test. The hip is flexed 45°, and the knee is flexed 90°. The tibia is in neutral rotation. Anterior pull can be applied to the proximal tibia with both hands. (From Frontera WR, Silver JK (eds): Essentials of Physical Medicine and Rehabilitation. Philadelphia, Hanley & Belfus, 2002, with permission.)

62. How are the medial and lateral collateral ligaments assessed?

Applying varus and valgus stress to the knee tests the collateral ligaments. If excessive movement at the knee is observed or palpated, the corresponding collateral ligament is possibly torn. If the patient has no movement with varus and valgus stress but has tenderness with palpation over the ligaments, the ligaments may be sprained.

63. What would an examiner find if a patient has an effusion of the knee?

The first step in the **bulge sign test** is to milk the fluid from the medial aspect of the knee laterally and into the suprapatellar pouch while the knee. The examiner then places gentle pressure with the fingers on the lateral aspect of the knee. If a bulge is noted at the knee medially in the hollow area created by milking the fluid, the test is positive for an effusion.

To perform the **ballottement test**, have the patient extend the knee. If the knee is painful, have the patient extend it as far as possible. The examiner places pressure on the suprapatellar pouch with the palm of one hand while pushing the patella down into the trochlear groove of the femur. Normally, the patella rests in the trochlear groove against the femur. A large effusion with fluid between the femur and patella lifts the patella out of the trochlear groove. If the examiner feels a click as the patella taps against the femur, an effusion of the knee is present.

64. What are the various physical assessment findings with a meniscus tear of the knee?

Many findings can be present with a torn meniscus. The classic signs are pain with palpation of the corresponding joint line, pain with end-range flexion of the knee, and pain at the knee with rotatory stress applied to the knee. To apply rotatory stress to the knee, the examiner grasps the calf and cups the heel while the examined knee is flexed to approximately 90°. The examiner then gently internally and externally rotates the calf, foot, and ankle at the knee. Patients may also have positive findings with an Apley grind test and the McMurray test. They may complain of bucking, catching, giving out or locking, and decreased ROM with either flexion or extension.

65. How are the Apley grind and McMurray test performed?

The **Apley grind test** is performed with the patient in the prone position and the examined leg flexed to 90° at the knee. The examiner grasps the heel and exerts downward force as the tibia is internally and externally rotated at the knee. This maneuver places compressive force on the menisci. If a torn meniscus is present, the patient may complain of pain at the joint line corresponding to the tear, or the examiner may feel or hear a click at the knee.

The **McMurray test** is performed with the patient lying supine. While standing on the side of the patient to be examined, the examiner holds the patient's leg with one hand at the ankle and the other at the anterior knee joint. The knee and hip are flexed to approximately 90°. To assess the medial meniscus, the lower leg is rotated internally at the knee, varus stress is applied to the knee, and the leg is passively brought to full extension. To assess the lateral meniscus, the lower leg is rotated externally at the knee, valgus stress is applied to the knee, and the leg is passively brought to full extension. The test is positive for a suspected torn meniscus if the patient complains of pain, has an audible or palpable click, or is unable to completely extend the knee.

66. How can the patella be assessed?

One of the tests for assessing the patella is the patella grind. The patient lies supine with the leg extended at the knee and the quadriceps muscles relaxed. With the examiner's fingers on the patella, force is applied to distract the patella distally. The patient is asked to contract the quadriceps muscles while the examiner provides slight resistance to the patella. The patella should slide under the examiner's fingers in the trochlear groove without pain. Pain may be indicative of chondromalacia patella or degenerative disease.

67. What is normal ROM for the ankle and foot?

Normal foot and ankle ROM is 20° of dorsiflexion, 45° of plantarflexion, 20° of eversion, and 30° of inversion

68. What are the significant areas to palpate at the foot and ankle?

The examiner should be sure to palpate the plantar fascia, deltoid ligament, talofibular ligament, calcaneofibular ligament, tibiofibular ligament, and collateral ligaments. Palpate the distal fibula, distal tibia, talus, calcaneus, metatarsals, and phalanges. Tendons to palpate include the tibialis anterior and posterior, Achilles, peroneus longus and brevis, flexor digitorum longus, extensor and flexor hallucis longus

69. What is the maneuver to assess for deep venous thrombosis (DVT) in the calf? How is it performed?

Homan's sign is used to assess for DVT of the calf. This test is performed with the patient lying supine on the exam table. The examiner dorsiflexes the ankle of the calf to be tested. If the patient develops pain in the calf, DVT is suggested.

70. What test can be used to assess for an Achilles tendon tear?

The Thompson test can be performed to assess for a complete rupture of the Achilles tendon. Have the patient lie prone on the exam table with the knee of the examined leg flexed to 90°. The examiner then squeezes the calf and watches for plantarflexion of the foot. If there is no movement of the foot after the calf is squeezed, the Achilles tendon may be completely ruptured. If the foot does plantarflex with this maneuver, this finding does not exclude a partial tear or strain of the Achilles tendon.

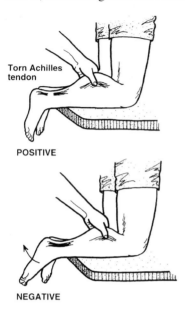

Torn Achilles tendon

POSITIVE

NEGATIVE

Thompson's test is a reliable clinical test to identify the presence of a complete tear in the Achilles tendon. (From Frontera WR, Silver JK (eds): Essentials of Physical Medicine and Rehabilitation. Philadelphia, Hanley & Belfus, 2002, with permission.)

71. How does the examiner perform the drawer test for the ankle?

The drawer test for the ankle is used to assess the stability of the ankle joint after an ankle injury. Specifically, this test assesses the anterior talofibular ligament for complete tear. The examiner cups the patient's heel with one hand and stabilizes the tibia with the other hand. The examiner then applies traction to the foot with the hand that is holding the heel in an attempt to translate the foot forward at the ankle. If the ankle is unstable and the test is positive, the foot will translate forward at the ankle.

BIBLIOGRAPHY

1. Apley AG, Solomon L: Concise System of Orthopaedics and Fractures, 2nd ed. London, Reed Educational and Professional Publishing, 1996.
2. Bickley LS, Hoekelman RA: Bates' Guide to Physical Examination and History Taking, 7th ed. Philadelphia, Lippincott Williams & Wilkins, 1999.
3. Estes MEZ: Health Assessment and Physical Examination, 2nd ed. Albany, NY, Delmar, 2002.
4. Hoppenfeld S: Physical Assessment of the Spine and Extremities. East Norwalk, CT, Appleton-Century-Crofts, 1976.
5. Jarvis C (ed): Physical Examination and Health Assessment, 3rd ed. Philadelphia, W.B. Saunders, 2000.
6. Lewis SM, Heitkemper MM, Dirksen SR (eds): Medical-Surgical Nursing: Assessment and Management of Clinical Problems, 5th ed. St. Louis, Mosby, 2000.
7. Maher AB, Salmond SW, Pellino TA (eds): Orthopaedic Nursing. Philadelphia, W.B. Saunders, 1994.
8. Mourad LA: Orthopedic Disorders. St. Louis, Mosby, 1991.
9. Schoen DC: NAON Core Curriculum for Orthopaedic Nursing, 4th ed. Pittman, NJ, Anthony J. Jannetti, 2001.

2. DIAGNOSTIC TESTS, MODALITIES, AND PROCEDURES

Michael E. Zychowicz, RN, MS, NP-C

1. What information can be gathered about a patient's condition by performing a bone scan?

The information obtained by performing a bone scan is valuable in diagnosing and evaluating a variety of musculoskeletal disorders. Diagnosis of primary malignant bone tumors or malignant tumors with bony metastasis can be made by bone scan. A bone scan is useful in evaluating for osteomyelitis, occult fractures, unexplained joint or bone pain, prosthetic joint problems (e.g., infection or loosening), or the response of a tumor to chemotherapy or radiation. Metabolic bone diseases, avascular necrosis, and arthritis are other conditions that can be assessed by bone scans. The major benefit of performing a bone scan is that many abnormal findings, including metastatic bone disease, appear on the bone scan 3–6 months earlier than on plain x-rays.

2. For which patients is a bone scan contraindicated?

A bone scan is contraindicated for pregnant women and patients who have had a prior allergic reaction. Because the bone scan is a nuclear medicine study using radionuclides, there is a significant risk in exposing the unborn fetus to ionizing radiation. In certain instances, however, the benefits of the test may outweigh the risk to the fetus.

3. How should the nurse educate the patient before a bone scan is performed?

The nurse should explain the procedure and its purpose to the patient. Ensure that the patient knows that an injection of radionuclide will be given approximately 2–3 hours before the actual scan and that the test is painless. Depending on the body part(s) to be evaluated, the test may last up to 1 hour. The nurse should encourage the patient to drink plenty of fluids to assist in the excretion of the isotope by the kidneys. In addition, fluids decrease the radiation exposure to the urinary bladder. The patient should be reminded to empty the bladder just before the scan because a full bladder may interfere with the test as well as make the patient uncomfortable.

4. After a bone scan, how long until the radionuclide is excreted from the body?

Typically, the radionuclide is completely excreted by the body over 6–12 hours. The patient should be encouraged to increase fluid intake to assist with the elimination of the isotope.

5. Should the patient avoid other people after a bone scan?

No. The patient can resume activities as usual after the bone scan. The small amount of radionuclide in the body is not harmful to others. However, the patient should not have another nuclear medicine study until 24-48 hours after the bone scan. The results of such tests may be altered by residual radiation.

6. A patient's report states that "hot spots" were noted on the bone scan. What do they mean?

The bones take up the radionuclide that is injected into the circulation. Areas of increased bone turnover have an increased concentration of the radionuclide. The radioactivity that is emitted is noted on the bone scan. A "hot spot" is an area of increased uptake of the radionuclide, corresponding with increased bony blood flow, bone metabolism, and bone turnover. The hot spot is seen on the bone scan as a concentrated area of radioactivity. Such areas may indicate fractures, metastatic malignant bone disease, or osteomyelitis, amomg other conditions. In contrast, "cold spots" are areas with little or no bone activity, such as avascular necrosis.

7. How does magnetic resonance imaging (MRI) use a magnet to gain an image of the body?

When a magnetic force is applied to the body, the nuclei of the cells begin to resonate. When the magnetic force is discontinued, energy is released from the cell nuclei. The sensory equipment of the MRI senses this release of energy as radio waves and converts it to an image. The image can subsequently be seen on a monitor, printed on film, or captured electronically on a computer or CD-ROM.

8. What are some indications for obtaining an MRI

An MRI can be obtained to assess tissues, including blood vessels, muscles, ligaments, cartilage, fat, and bones. An MRI can also be used to assess tumors.

9. What is the difference between the open and closed MRI?

For a closed MRI, the patient lies on an exam table and is passed through a tube at the center of the magnet. For an open MRI, the patient does not need to pass through the chamber of the magnet. The current technology of open MRI does not provide as clear an image as closed MRI.

10. If the image from a closed MRI is clearer than the image of an open MRI, why would a patient have an open MRI?

The patient who is claustrophobic may choose to have an open MRI. The clinician also may offer the claustrophobic patient an anti-anxiety medication before the procedure, allowing the patient to follow through with a closed MRI. The open MRI is also indicated for patients who are obese and/ or have a large chest or abdomen that may not fit into the closed MRI.

11. How much time is needed to complete an MRI study?

Depending on the body part being examined and the speed of the machine, the test may take 30–60 minutes to complete.

12. What is gadolinium?

Gadolinium is a contrast media that may be injected intravenously to increase visualization of the tissues during an MRI study.

13. How can the nurse help prepare the patient who is anxious about having an MRI?

The first action is to determine whether the patient has a specific concern or issue. If the patient is claustrophobic, the nurse can instruct the patient in relaxation techniques. The patient may be able to obtain a prescription (e.g., diazepam) to decrease anxiety during the test. Reassure the patient that there is no radiation or pain during the MRI. Fully explaining the procedure and answering questions may also alleviate some anxiety. An open MRI is an option if the patient is claustrophobic (see question 10).

14. What contraindications or precautions apply to performing an MRI?

Ensure that all metallic objects are removed before the MRI, including jewelry, credit cards, clothing with metallic snaps, pins, watches, hearing aids, and dentures. Patients with internal metallic items (e.g., metallic clips, pacemaker, metallic foreign body) that can dysfunction or become dislodged during the MRI should not undergo the test. Pregnant patients are usually not tested because of possible fetal damage. Additional contraindications include medical instability, extreme obesity, confusion, combativeness, claustrophobia, and inability to remain still for the length of the procedure. The patient should be reminded to remove any credit are ID cards with a magnetic strip because the magnet field from the MRI will desensitize the cards.

15. What information does computed tomography (CT) provide?

Information provided by the CT scan includes the structure of the bone, fractures, soft tissue tumors, and bony metastases. The CT scan can provide information about a joint, including evaluation for loose bodies within the joint space. The CT scan can provide valuable information in evaluating certain spinal conditions, including tumors, stenosis, fractures and disc herniation.

16. Describe the nurse's role in obtaining a CT scan.

The nurse should absolutely be sure there are no allergies if a CT with contract is ordered. The nurse should ensure that the patient understands the procedure as well as ensuring the consent is completed and all metal is removed. A pregnancy history should be obtained in addition to carrying out any pre-procedure orders such as medications, enema, or avoidance of oral ingestion (NPO).

17. What should the nurse teach the patient about the CT scan?

As usual, the nurse educates the patient about the actual procedure, including possible side effects and allergic reaction to the contrast dye. The patient should be made aware that the test may take up to 1 hour and that the machine may make a loud clicking noise as it works. Inform patients that they will be lying on a narrow table in the CT machine and should tell the clinician if they are claustrophobic.

18. What is the purpose of using contrast dye?

The contrast dye enables the examiner to detect and visualize lesions more clearly.

19. What are the symptoms of an allergic reaction to the contrast?

The patient may develop typical allergic symptoms, such as urticaria, hives, rash, generalized or localized angioedema, shortness of breath, palpitations, hypotension, nausea, and vomiting.

20. What are some of the typical, nonallergic side effects of IV contrast injection?

Patients may report a salty or metallic taste in the mouth. They may also vomit or complain of nausea. Patients also report a flushed or warm sensation.

21. Why would a patient with a musculoskeletal problem have a CT scan rather than an MRI?

A patient who is unable to have an MRI because of metal in the body can certainly have a CT scan, if indicated. A CT scan is useful in assessing the cortex of bones as well as calcification and ossification.

22. What precautions and contraindications apply to CT scans?

A CT scan is performed with x-rays and has the same contraindications as plain radiographs, mainly pregnancy. If a patient has allergies to contrast dye, a CT scan with contrast should not be performed.

23. What information can be gathered from musculoskeletal x-rays?

Musculoskeletal x-rays are used for multiple reasons. With an x-ray, the examiner is able to assess for any fractures or bony abnormalities, including thickening and narrowing, of the bony cortex. In viewing the joint space, the examiner can assess degeneration, osteochondral defects, calcification of the cartilage or synovium, effusion, arthritic spurring, or loose bodies. The examiner may identify calcific tendinitis and bony tumors. The clinician may also assess abnormal position of one bone in relation to another, as in spondylolithesis or degenerative joint disease, or the presence of foreign bodies.

24. How does the density of body tissue correlate to the picture obtained from an x-ray?

The image on the x-ray film is reflective of the density of the body tissues. The image of tissues with increased density is whiter or light. As the density decreases, the image becomes darker or blacker. Bone has a high density and therefore is white on x-ray, whereas air has a low density and is dark on x-ray.

25. What precautions or contraindications apply to obtaining an x-ray?

Lead shielding should be used to protect the genital areas of patients in their reproductive years. In addition, pregnant women should have x-rays only in an emergency situation with a lead apron covering the abdomen and pelvis. The nurse should also ensure that radiopaque objects that may interfere with the x-ray picture, such as jewelry or clothing with buttons, are removed from the region being x-rayed.

26. What information can be gathered from performing thermography?

Thermography can give information about the amount of heat radiating from a particular part of the body surface. Compared with the surrounding body surface as well as the corresponding body part on the opposite side of the body, the thermography gives an indication of localized increased or decreased skin temperature. This information may be useful in assessing many musculoskeletal disorders, including tumors, epicondylitis, bursitis, reflex sympathetic dystrophy, carpal tunnel syndrome, and arthritis. Thermography may be useful in assessing the effectiveness of anti-inflammatory treatment or vascular disorders.

27. Should patients undergo any specific preparation for thermography?

There is no specific preparation for the procedure. The nurse should educate the patient about the test. The patient should be informed about specific restrictions that can interfere with its validity. The patient should avoid the following: (1) vasodilators, alcohol, caffeine, or smoking for 8–12 hours before the procedure; (2) topical preparations; and (3) injections or physical therapy for 1 day before the test.

28. Are there any precautions or contraindications to performing thermography?
No. The test involves no radiation, no dye, no injections, and no magnetic field.

29. Summarize the advantages and disadvantages of thermography.
The advantages of thermography are that the test is noninvasive, quick, and painless and does not expose the patient to radiation. A disadvantage to thermography is that the interpretation of the results is rather subjective.

30. How are electromyography (EMG) and nerve conduction studies (NCS) performed?
EMG and NCS are performed by placing an electrode needle into a select muscle group and then applying an electrical impulse to the patient.

31. What information can be gathered from performing EMG/NCS?
The NCS measures the speed of transmission of the electrical impulse over a distance. The EMG assesses the electrical activity of the tested muscle group during contraction and at rest. This test may assist in differentiating between myopathy and neuropathy. The EMG/ NCS can also assist in diagnosing specific peripheral nerve problems such as carpal tunnel syndrome or other neuromuscular disorders.

32. How long does the EMG/NCS study take to complete?
The clinician may need $^1/_2$ to 2 hours to complete the examination.

33. Can EMG/NCS have any complications?
Complications are extremely rare. A potential complication is bleeding after performing the test on a patient with a bleeding disorder. A patient may complain of soreness or pain after the procedure from the electrode and needle placement. A patient may develop an infection.

34. Aside from clarifying how and why the EMG/NCS study is performed, what other information may the nurse want to give the patient?
The patient may be restricted from having caffeinated beverages or nicotine products before the test. In addition, cholinergics, anticholinergics, and muscle relaxants may interfere with the results. The nurse should make the patient aware that the test may be somewhat uncomfortable because of the electrode needle insertion as well as the mild electrical stimulation during the procedure.

35. What can be done to decrease the patient's discomfort after the EMG/NCS study is complete?
The patient can simply take an over-the-counter anti-inflammatory pain medication and apply a warm or cold compress to the area for pain control.

36. What information can be gathered from a somatosensory evoked potential (SSEP)?
The SSEP is useful in evaluating nerve conduction, electrical activities of the muscles, peripheral neuropathies, and radiculopathies. In addition, SSEP is valuable in monitoring spinal nerves during spinal surgery.

37. How is SSEP different from EMG/NCS?

SSEP is noninvasive with electrodes placed on the skin, whereas EMG/NCS involve insertion of needles. The SSEP can also assess nerve conduction in a variety of areas that the EMG/ NCS study may not be able to access.

38. Although only electrodes are applied and no needles are inserted, is the SSEP test painful?

The test can be somewhat uncomfortable when electrical stimulation is applied. The nurse should make the patient aware that it is not a completely painless test.

39. How is an arthrography performed?

An arthrogram is an x-ray examination of a joint using air and/or radiopaque dye that is injected into the joint to be examined. After the joint is injected using sterile technique, the examiner may obtain plain x-rays, fluoroscopy, or tomograms with the joint in a variety of positions.

40. What is the advantage of an arthrogram over a plain x-ray?

With the arthrogram, the examiner is able to define the joint space and evaluate the joint for tears of the joint capsule. With arthrography, the examiner is also able to assess ligaments, tendons, menisci, joint pain from unknown cause, and congenital joint problems.

41. What are the possible complications of an arthrogram?

Because arthrography is an invasive procedure, the possibility of a joint infection does exist. In addition, the possibility of an allergic reaction to the radiopaque dye is present. The patient may feel crepitus of the evaluated joint for a few days after the procedure. If the crepitus does not dissipate after a few days of rest, the clinician should be notified.

42. Describe the nurse's role in obtaining the arthrogram.

Educating and supporting the patient are major roles for the nurse before and during the procedure. Consent for the procedure should be obtained. The nurse should ensure that the patient knows the signs and symptoms of an infection. It is the responsibility of the nurse to assess inpatients for signs of infection. The nurse should instruct the patient to apply ice and use anti-inflammatory pain medication after the procedure if pain persists.

43. What contraindications or precautions apply to obtaining an arthrogram?

The nurse should be aware if the patient has an allergy to radiopaque dye or if the patient is pregnant.

44. For what reasons is arthroscopy performed?

Arthroscopy can be performed to look into a joint for either diagnostic or treatment purposes. A clinician may perform an arthroscopy to remove loose bodies, repair an osteochondral lesion, perform a biopsy, address ligament or cartilage injury, or address impingement syndrome. A clinician may perform a diagnostic arthroscopy to develop a clear diagnosis of a joint problem, especially when other tests, such as MRI or arthrogram, are not helpful in determining a clear cause for the joint problem.

45. What are the nursing responsibilities with a patient undergoing diagnostic arthroscopy?

The nursing responsibilities are the same as with any other operative procedure. The patient should avoid oral ingestion (NPO status) for 8–12 hours before the procedure. The nurse should ensure that consent is obtained and that the patient understands the procedure. The nurse should check for any allergies, have the patient remove all jewelry and eyewear, and premedicate the patient as ordered. Postoperatively, the nurse should perform neurovascular checks and assess the operative site for bleeding and infection.

46. Arthroscopy is rather routine today. What are the potential complications?

Neurovascular injury, infection, bleeding, DVT, and thrombophlebitis.

47. When is joint aspiration appropriate?

One purpose for performing a joint aspiration is to relieve a painful effusion. When the patient has an inflamed, painful joint, the clinician may perform this procedure to obtain a sample of joint fluid for analysis to rule out such conditions as gout, hemarthrosis, and infection.

48. Describe the nurse's role in performing the joint aspiration.

The nurse should ensure that the patient understands the purpose for the procedure and how it is performed. The nurse should assist the clinician in gathering the equipment and preparing the patient. The nurse, as always, supports the patient during the procedure and applies pressure and a dressing after the procedure is complete. Assessment for infection and bleeding is important. The nurse is typically responsible for ensuring that the sample of joint aspirate is properly labeled, packaged, and sent to the lab for analysis.

49. Does the patient have to go to the operating room for joint aspiration?

No. Joint aspiration can be easily performed at the bedside or as an outpatient office procedure. Although it is not performed in the operating room, the clinician must use aseptic technique to avoid joint infection.

50. What are the characteristics of normal joint fluid?

Normal joint fluid should have a clear, light yellow appearance. Gram stain and culture should be negative and without growth; the viscosity is high; and the glucose content should be equal to the serum glucose. There should be no crystals, fat globules, or protein. White cell count is normally < 200 with polymorphonuclear neutrophils (PMNs) < 25%.

51. When can a person resume normal activities after arthrocentesis?

After an arthrocentesis, the patient may resume activities as tolerated. The patient may also require splinting after the arthrocentesis for protection of a painful joint due to underlying pathology.

52. What is the most concerning complication of joint aspiration?

After a joint aspiration, one of the complications of greatest concern is infection.

53. What does a myelogram assess?

A myelogram is performed to assess the spinal canal and structures within the canal. This test can help in diagnosing the cause for back and/ or leg pain of an undetermined origin. In addition, the myelogram can give information about tumors, cysts, intervertebral disk herniations, lesions in the spinal canal, and spinal stenosis.

54. How is a myelogram performed?

After cleaning and preparing the back in a fashion similar to that used for lumbar puncture, the clinician introduces a needle into the spine. With the needle in place, the clinician injects a contrast medium into the subarachnoid space. If the patient is allergic to the contrast medium, air can be injected in lieu of the contrast medium. After the dye is injected, the clinician positions the patient with the head slightly down. Fluoroscopy and x-ray evaluation are performed. In addition, a postmyelogram CT scan may be performed for further assessment of the spinal canal and structures.

55. What preparations should the patient undergo before myelography is performed?

The patient is typically on NPO status for 4 hours preceding the myelogram. The clinician performing the test may order an enema before the procedure. Ask the patient to void before the procedure, and administer any sedatives that may be ordered on an as-needed basis. The nurse should ensure that the patient understands the procedure and that consent is obtained. The nurse must check for allergies to the contrast medium used during the procedure. If the patient is taking medications that lower seizure threshold, they may need to be discontinued for up to 2 days before and 1 day after the procedure. Medications that decrease seizure threshold include tricyclic antidepressants, amphetamines, neuroleptics, phenothiazides, and central nervous system stimulants.

56. What are the considerations for patient positioning after myelography?

Patients generally are on bed rest for 8–12 hours following the procedure. If water-based contrast medium (metrizamide) was injected during the myelogram, the head of the bed should be elevated approximately 15°–40° for approximately 8 hours. This positioning enables the water-based medium to be reabsorbed by the body. After approximately 8 hours the water-based contrast is absorbed, and the patient can lie supine. If an oil-based contrast medium (iophendylate) was injected, the patient may be required to remain flat for up to 24 hours. After the procedure, the oil-based contrast is removed via syringe by the clinician because it is not readily absorbed by the body.

57. What are the possible side effects of a myelogram?

After the myelogram, patients may experience convulsions, fever, headache, nausea, and vomiting. Significant complications of which the nurse should be aware include brainstem herniation or compression, arachnoiditis, sterile meningitis, and paralysis.

58. What are the contraindications to performing a myelogram?

Evidence of increased intracranial pressure, pregnancy, and allergy to contrast dye.

59. When is bone marrow aspiration performed?

Bone marrow aspiration is performed to obtain a sample of the patient's bone marrow to rule out or confirm a diagnosis based on microscopic analysis of the sample. Some of the reasons for bone marrow aspiration include anemia of unknown etiology, osteoporosis, infection, tumor, bone marrow suppression, multiple myeloma, and metabolic bone disease.

60. On what part of the body may the clinician perform bone marrow aspiration?

A bone marrow aspiration may be performed at the sternum, spinus process of the vertebra, posterior superior iliac spine, anterior iliac crest, or proximal tibia.

61. Describe the nurse's role in performing bone marrow aspiration.

Before the procedure the nurse should be sure that consent is obtained and that the patient fully understands the procedure. The nurse may gather the necessary equipment as well as prepare and drape the patient. During the procedure, the nurse should support the patient as well as monitor vital signs. After the procedure, a sterile compression dressing is applied. In addition, the site should be monitored for bleeding as well as evidence of infection, including cellulitis and osteomyelitis. Evidence of a fracture should be assessed, especially at the sternum. The nurse can also label, package, and send the sample to the lab.

62. When is dual-energy x-ray absorptiometry (DEXA) performed?

A DEXA scan is the gold standard to assess bone mineral density. The test is useful in diagnosing osteoporosis or osteopenia. In addition, the DEXA scan is useful in assessing response to treatment for osteoporosis. By determining bone mineral density, the examiner can infer or predict the potential for sustaining future fractures.

63. How does the DEXA scan determine the density of the bones?

The actual examination takes approximately 20 minutes. The patient lies supine with the legs flexed at the knee and hip, resting on a foam block. While the patient remains still, the DEXA takes an x-ray of the hip and spine, which is analyzed by the computer. The computer determines the density of the bone at the hip and spine based on the absorption of the energy by the tissues during the test. The computer determines a T-score that corresponds to the number of standard deviations from "normal" bone mineral density. As the T-score becomes more negative, the patient is at increased risk for fracture. A T-score between -1 and -2.5 is considered osteopenia, whereas a T-score below -2.5 is considered osteoporosis.

64. What additional information should the nurse give the patient about the DEXA scan?

The patient should be told that the test will last at least 20 minutes in the supine position. All metal should be removed.

65. Do other tests exist to assess bone mineral density?

Currently, the gold standard for measuring bone mineral density is the DEXA scan. Other tests currently available include a variety of ultrasound machines that measure the density of the bones at the heel, wrist, or hand. Other tests include single-photon absorptiometry (SPA), radiodensitometry, and dual-photon absorptiometry.

66. What are the indications for discography?

Discography is used to identify intervertebral disc disruption. It is most useful in preoperative planning before a spinal fusion. Although an MRI can give a good indication of the level(s) at which disc degeneration or pathology exists, the discogram is used in conjunction with the MRI to determine which levels require fusion. Although a disc can look relatively good on MRI, the myelogram can better detect any subtle disruption of the disc, leading to a better postoperative outcome.

67. How is discography performed?

After the patient's skin is cleansed and prepared, a local anesthetic is infiltrated into the procedure area. The clinician inserts a needle into the nucleus of a selected intervertebral disc under fluoroscopic guidance. Radiopaque dye is then injected into the nucleus, followed by fluoroscopic and/or x-ray evaluation of the dye pattern within the disc. Leakage of dye from the disc is indicative of disc disruption or pathology.

68. What are the contraindications to discography?

Pregnant patients should not undergo discography because of the exposure to x-ray radiation. In addition, the procedure should not be performed if the patient has allergies to contrast medium, iodine, or seafood.

69. What is the nurse's role in discography?

The nurse must ensure that consent for the procedure is obtained and that the patient fully understands what the procedure entails. As with any other test involving dye and x-rays, the nurse should ensure that the patient is not pregnant or allergic to dye, iodine, or seafood. During the procedure, the nurse should support the patient and assist the clinician as needed. The nurse should observe the patient for any signs of anaphylaxis and perform neurologic assessments after the procedure.

70. What are the potential complications of discography?

Some of the significant adverse outcomes include infection, anaphylactic reaction, injury to a nerve root, or tear of the dura.

71. What do Bence-Jones proteins in the urine indicate?

Bence-Jones protein is present in the urine of patients with multiple myeloma, bony metastasis of a tumor, and macroglobinuria.

72. What is the significance of calcium levels in the urine?

An increased level of calcium found in the urine may indicate multiple myeloma, hyperparathyroidism, osteoporosis, Paget's disease, and bony metastasis of a tumor. Decreased urinary calcium is found in hypoparathyroidism, rickets, and osteomalacia.

73. In assessing inflammatory disorders, what lab tests may prove useful?

C-reactive protein (CRP), erythrocyte sedimentation rate (ESR), antinuclear antibody (ANA), and rheumatoid factor (RF) may provide useful information. CRP is normally not found in the serum but is present with infection, malignancy, and inflammatory diseases, including rheumatoid arthritis, rheumatic fever, and lupus erythematosus. ESR is a reflection of the speed at which a sample of unclotted red blood cells settles out over 1 hour. The red blood cells settle out faster in the presence of malignancy, necrosis, inflammatory disorder, or infection. The presence of RF in the serum is useful to differentiate rheumatoid arthritis from other inflammatory diseases. RF is also present in disease processes such as macroglobinuria, scleroderma, Sjögren's syndrome, and lupus erythematosus. ANA is present with disorders such as lupus, rheumatoid arthritis, scleroderma, Raynaud's disease, and Sjögren's syndrome.

74. What causes the ESR to increase in the presence of malignancy, necrosis, inflammation, and infection?

In the presence of malignancy, necrosis, inflammatory disorder, or infection, the red blood cells tend to aggregate and become heavier, settling at a faster rate as reflected in an increased ESR.

75. Do serum levels of alkaline phosphatase, serum calcium, or serum phosphorus increase with osteoporosis?

No. These lab studies can be within normal limits in people with primary osteoporosis.

76. How do metabolic bone disorders affect serum levels of calcium, phosphorus, and alkaline phosphatase?

The person with osteoporosis secondary to hyperparathyroidism has increased serum calcium, decreased serum phosphorus, and increased serum alkaline phosphatase. Hypoparathyroidism is associated with decreased serum calcium, increased serum phosphorus, and decreased serum alkaline phosphatase. The patient with osteomalacia has normal or decreased serum calcium, normal or decreased serum phosphorus, and increased serum alkaline phosphatase. In Paget's disease, lab work reflects normal serum calcium, normal serum phosphorus, and increased serum alkaline phosphatase. Patients with rickets have decreased serum calcium, decreased serum phosphorus, and increased serum alkaline phosphatase.

	Calcium	*Phosphorus*	*Alkaline phosphatase*
Hyperparathyroidism	Increased	Decreased	Increased
Hypoparathyroidism	Decreased	Increased	Decreased
Osteomalacia	Normal or decreased	Normal or decreased	Increased
Paget's disease	Normal	Normal	Increased
Rickets	Decreased	Decreased	Increased

77. What lab tests are useful in diagnosing systemic lupus erythematosus (SLE)?

Lupus erythematosus (LE) cells, antinuclear antibodies (ANA), anti-DNA antibodies, and serum complement are useful in the diagnosis of SLE. LE cells are not usually present in the blood unless SLE is present. LE cells are also related to the presence of scleroderma, rheumatoid arthritis, and hepatitis. ANA and anti-DNA antibodies measure the presence of antigen-antibody complexes in the blood that are associated with autoimmune disorders, including SLE. ANA may also be elevated with a variety of other disorders, including rheumatoid arthritis, scleroderma, Raynaud's disease, and Sjögren's syndrome. Serum complement is normally found in the blood but is diminished or absent with SLE. Complement is a normal protein involved with the inflammatory and immune process. Complement is depleted with a variety of conditions, such as SLE, rheumatoid arthritis, glomerulonephritis, Sjögren's syndrome, and disseminated intravascular coagulation (DIC).

78. Is an elevated level of serum uric acid specific for gout?

No. Uric acid is an end product of purine metabolism and is excreted in the urine. Elevated serum uric acid may be indicative of many disorders, including gout, chronic renal failure, congestive heart failure, psoriasis, myeloproliferative disorders, and glycogen storage disorders. When placed in context with the patient's history and physical exam, an increased level of uric acid can certainly assist in the diagnosis of gout.

BIBLIOGRAPHY

1. Detmer WM, McPhee SJ, Nicoll D, Chou TM: Pocket Guide to Diagnostic Tests. Norwalk, CT, Appleton & Lange, 1992.
2. Lewis SM, Heitkemper MM, Dirksen SR: Medical-Surgical Nursing: Assessment and Management of Clinical Problems, 5th ed. St. Louis, Mosby, 2000.
3. Maher AB, Salmond SW, Pellino TA: Orthopaedic Nursing, 3rd ed. Philadelphia, W.B. Saunders, 2002.
4. Mourad LA: Orthopedic Disorders. St. Louis, Mosby, 1991.
5. Schoen DC: NAON Core Curriculum for Orthopaedic Nursing, 4th ed. Pittman, NJ, Anthony J. Jannetti, 2001.

3. DEGENERATIVE DISEASE

Dottie Roberts, MSN, MACI, RN, BC, ONC, CNS

1. Why is osteoarthritis known as degenerative joint disease?

Osteoarthritis (OA) was previously known as degenerative joint disease because of the belief that the wear-and-tear of aging produced deterioration of articular cartilage. It is now identified as a process that involves new tissue proliferation in response to joint damage and cartilage destruction.

2. Describe the pathophysiology of osteoarthritis.

Healthy articular cartilage, which is smooth and glistening white in appearance, responds to the joint insult with enzymatic tissue breakdown at the cellular level. As the cartilage softens and loses its elasticity, chondrocytes begin to increase the synthesis of collagen and proteoglycans. This increase, however, is unable to keep pace with tissue destruction, and the compromised cartilage becomes more susceptible to friction. Structural changes cause cartilage fibers to rupture, and the subsequent fissuring and erosion give the cartilage a yellowish, dull, granular appearance. Eventually, the softened cartilage is abraded to subchondral bone in the center of the articular surface.

Concurrently, new bone formation at the joint margins causes bony outgrowth and spur development. The incongruity between the abraded central cartilage and the proliferating peripheral cartilage changes the normal stress distribution and results in restricted joint motion. Small pieces of cartilage and osteophytes also commonly break off the joint surfaces, causing pain and additional limitation in movement. Finally, the osteophytes attract phagocytic cells that attempt to cleanse the loose debris from the joint space. A secondary synovitis often results in a swollen joint capsule that further increases pain and restricts movement.

3. Can osteoarthritis result from strenuous exercise or accidental injury?

Although idiopathic (primary) OA occurs in people who have no history of joint injury of disease, secondary OA has an identifiable cause. Any condition that causes joint instability, directly injures articular cartilage, or subjects it to excessive force can lead to arthritic changes. Accidental injury of the joint or its supporting structures can contribute to development of posttraumatic OA. A greater incidence of osteoarthritis has also been associated with strenuous, repetitive, high-intensity exercise. Competitive sports such as running, soccer, and football expose joints of the lower extremity to both impact and torsional stress. Although the athlete may not have a history of specific joint injury, OA can develop from the cumulative effects of microtraumas that frequently go undetected.

4. Is any major nonmodifiable risk factor associated with OA?

No single cause has been linked to the development of OA, but numerous risk factors have been identified. Increased incidence of osteoarthritis in aging women is thought to be due to reduced estrogen levels that occur with menopause. Women are also more likely than men to develop osteoarthritis of the hands, with the characteristic appearance of Heberden's and Bouchard's nodes in the distal interphalangeal (DIP) and proximal interphalanageal (PIP) joints, respectively.

5. What are the major modifiable risk factors associated with osteoarthritis?

A major modifiable risk factor is excessive weight, which research has consistently linked to increased incidence of OA of the knee. The correlation between increased weight and hip OA is less positive. Hand OA is also weakly associated with obesity, indicating a possible connection between metabolic factors and disease development in overweight people.

Quadriceps weakness is commonly associated with OA of the knee. Slemenda et al. collected data from over 450 community-based arthritic volunteers, indicating that quadriceps weakness is a primary risk factor for knee pain, disability, and progressive joint damage.

6. What are the most common complaints in the nursing history of patients with osteoarthritis?

Pain is frequently the patient's dominant complaint and the reason for seeking medical attention. The patient often describes an "aching" localized pain that increases with joint use and improves with rest, especially during early OA. As the disease progresses, however, the patient may begin to complain additionally of night pain or pain at rest. Joint pain may also cause the patient to limp. Because the pain of osteoarthritis characteristically has an insidious onset, the patient is often unable to recall exactly when it began. Its intensity is more likely to be related to joint use and the patient's personal pain threshold than to disease severity.

Joint stiffness is another common complaint. The patient may describe symptoms that range from slow movement to pain with initial activity. Early morning stiffness is characteristic of OA, but it typically lasts less than 30 minutes, a point that differentiates OA from inflammatory joint disorders. Stiffness after rest or periods of inactivity, which is known as **articular gelling**, generally resolves within a few minutes. Joint symptoms often worsen in cool, damp, or rainy weather because increased intra-articular pressure may correlate with decreased atmospheric pressure. Along with joint stiffness, the patient may also describe grating or creaking with movement (crepitus) caused by loose cartilage pieces in the joint capsule.

7. How does the physical examination relate to the patient's history?

Physical findings are typically limited to symptomatic joints and vary based on OA severity. Painful joints are likely to be tender to palpation by the health care provider. Tenderness at the capsular or joint line is consistent with a diagnosis of OA, which has a capsular or intracapsular origin of pain. Tenderness away from the joint is more indicative of a periarticular condition, such as bursitis. Crepitation with passive joint movement by the health care provider is present in more than 90% of patients with OA of the knee and indicates loss of cartilage integrity. Reduced range of motion (ROM) is also a common physical finding that correlates to the patient's complaint of joint stiffness. Decreased ROM due to osteophyte infringement, joint remodeling, or capsular thickening may be exacerbated by mild joint and soft tissue edema.

8. What blood work is included in the diagnostic evaluation of the patient with suspected osteoarthritis?

The diagnosis of OA can almost always be made on the basis of history and physical examination. Thus, laboratory tests are used to screen for related conditions or to establish baseline values before initiating therapy. For example, in patients who are prescribed nonsteroidal anti-inflammatory drugs (NSAIDs) for arthritis treatment, a complete blood count (CBC) should be performed to establish baseline values. After therapy has started, a CBC should be ordered at regular intervals to screen for anemia related to occult gastrointestinal bleeding. The health care provider should also order renal and liver function tests for the elderly patient who takes aspirin or NSAIDs for symptom management. Rheumatoid factor (RF) and erythrocyte sedimentation rate (ESR) are often ordered for the patient with joint complaints, but they are not always diagnostic.

9. What radiographic findings may be seen in patients with arthritis?

Radiographic studies of affected joints are helpful in confirming the diagnosis of OA, but findings do not always correlate with the severity of the patient's symptoms. Asymmetric joint space narrowing becomes apparent as the disease progresses, reflecting the loss of articular cartilage or the progression of bone remodeling. The presence of subchondral cysts and an altered shape of the bone ends provide additional evidence of bone remodeling.

10. Is synovial fluid analysis useful in the patient with suspected OA?

Synovial fluid analysis offers a reliable method to differentiate suspected OA from other forms of arthritis. Fluid in the osteoarthritic joint is clear yellow and shows high viscosity due to a normal amount of hyaluronic acid. The white blood cell count (WBC) is low. The inflamed joint of a rheumatoid patient has cloudy fluid with an elevated WBC.

11. How is osteoarthritis managed conservatively?

Patient education is a cornerstone of successful OA management. Self-management programs, such as the Arthritis Self-Help Course administered by local chapters of the Arthritis Foundation, are ideal to assist the patient in understanding the disease and coping with its effects. The patient also needs to understand other tenets of conservative disease management, such as physical therapy and other nonpharmacologic interventions, pharmacologic treatment, and self-care modifications.

12. What self-care modifications are appropriate for patients with arthritis?

For the patient who needs to lose weight in order to lessen arthritis symptoms and slow disease progression, nutritional counseling may be critical. The health care provider should help the overweight patient to evaluate the current diet and to make appropriate reduced calorie changes. Related influences should be addressed, including finances, dentition, and age-related changes in taste and smell.

The American College of Rheumatology has identified exercise as another important contributor to successful OA management. Joint mobilization aids in maintenance of articular cartilage integrity, and regular exercise decreases quadriceps muscle weakness, which can contribute to progressive joint damage. The health care provider should contact the patient regularly to encourage adherence to an activity plan that focuses on cardiovascular conditioning, strength and flexibility, and joint mobility. The patient should also be urged to progress the exercise program gradually, starting at the current level of performance and increasing exercise repetitions as he or she is able. Education about timed analgesic administration helps the patient to participate more comfortably in exercise sessions.

13. What nonpharmacologic interventions can the patient perform?

Joint protection through a balance of rest and activity can be effective in relieving pain and improving joint biomechanics. The affected joint should be rested during periods of acute inflammation and maintained in a functional position through the use of splints or braces as needed. Lower extremities can be rested through restricted weight-bearing, but joint immobility should be limited to 1 week to avoid increased stiffness. Occupational and recreational activity may also need to be modified to protect affected joints from stress.

Applications of heat and cold may help decrease joint pain and stiffness. Ice can be helpful during periods of acute inflammation, and heat therapy may increase joint flexibility. Heat can be provided through various modalities, such as hot packs, ultrasound, paraffin wax, and whirlpool.

14. What is the typical pharmacologic treatment for osteoarthritis?

Acetaminophen or NSAIDs may be used for initial treatment of symptomatic OA. Up to 1000 mg of acetaminophen can be taken 4 times daily and supplemented briefly during exacerbations with opioids such as propoxyphene, codeine, or oxycodone. Health care providers also frequently recommend low-dose OTC ibuprofen (up to 400 mg 4 times daily) or aspirin for the patient who has normal renal function and no history of gastrointestinal problems. Persistent pain may require prescriptive doses of NSAIDs. Traditional NSAIDs such as ibuprofen or naproxen sodium may increase the risk for gastric ulceration or renal impairment because of their effects on prostaglandin levels through inhibition of the cyclooxygenase enzyme known as COX-1. Newer NSAIDS with COX-2 selectivity may be prescribed because of their decreased gastrointestinal toxicity. The health care provider must examine all NSAIDs, however, for the potential of interaction with other medications that the patient may be taking (e.g., methotrexate, lithium, angiotensin-converting enzyme inhibitors, warfarin).

15. What factors affect the treatment regimen for osteoarthritis in elderly patients?

Pharmacologic interventions provide an important supplement to other approaches to arthritis management. However, health care providers must be conscious of factors that affect the success of drug therapy in the elderly. Elderly patients with arthritis are likely to receive health care for other chronic conditions from multiple providers, increasing the chances that they will receive duplicate medications or experience the phenomenon of polypharmacy. The patient may also self-medicate with over-the-counter (OTC) agents that can adversely interact with the recommended treatment. Finally, the health care provider must consider changes in body composition and function that occur with normal aging and can affect the way in which medications are absorbed and metabolized in elderly patients.

16. What nonprescription supplements are often used to treat osteoarthritis?

The popularity of biologic agents such as glucosamine sulfate and chondroitin sulfate stems from interest in cartilage regeneration. Glucosamine is considered a building block for glycosaminoglycans in the articular cartilage, whereas chondroitin serves as a connecting matrix between protein filaments in the cartilage. The rapid onset of action for both agents suggests an anti-inflammatory effect. Research with chondroitin has led to controversial findings about its role in arthritis management. Glucosamine studies have had more promising results, with several short-term European trials demonstrating better relief of both OA pain and inflammation (Rehman and Lane). Routine use of glucosamine or other supplements as a principal treatment for OA should not be recommended until well-designed studies consistently prove their effectiveness and safety.

S-adenosyl-methionine (SAM-e) became available in the U.S. in 1999 after several decades of use in Europe. SAM-e is neither an herb nor a hormone. Instead, it is a naturally occurring substance believed to play a role in biochemical reactions that help the body grow and repair cells. The Arthritis Foundation reported that "there is sufficient information to support the claim that SAM-e provides pain relief for osteoarthritis." However, the Foundation cited no scientific evidence to support manufacturers' claims that SAM-e contributes to "joint health." The evidence supporting the benefits of SAM-e appears to be extensive compared with other supplements, but its risks, benefits, and costs must be carefully examined before long-term therapy can be recommended.

In clinical studies, all of these supplements had to be taken for 3–4 weeks before the patient noted any pain relief. Because of the delayed effect, the health care provider must urge the OA patient to continue conventional pharmacologic interventions for at least a month before trying to decrease their usage. Any changes should only be attempted with medical recommendation.

17. Is hyaluronic acid injection effective?

Viscosupplementation with hyaluronic acid (HA) has been used to treat OA of the knee. The viscoelasticity of HA contributes to its ability to supplement joint lubrication by synovial fluid. Some anti-inflammatory effects are also possible. A weekly dose is injected intra-articularly into the affected knee. The medication manufacturer or the clinical protocol determines the number of injections. Most patients do not realize therapeutic effects until several weeks after the last dose has been administered. Some patients have reported sustained relief of 3–5 months, but clinical studies have shown mixed effects for this costly treatment. Additional long-term studies are needed to confirm the efficacy of HA.

18. What complementary therapies are appropriate for osteoarthritis treatment?

Complementary treatment options have become increasingly popular for OA. Modalities such as copper or magnetic bracelets, which are supported only by anecdotal evidence, appear to be harmless and possibly worthless. Treatments such as bee stings, however, may cause severe toxicity. A few therapies have been shown to be modestly beneficial. For example, randomized clinical trials have determined that acupuncture is a safe and useful method for arthritis pain management. T'ai chi has been embraced as a low-impact form of exercise for arthritis. It combines a choreographed series of slow movements with coordinated breathing exercises and mental concentration.

19. Herbal supplements are popular, but are they effective?

Herbal supplements have become one of the most popular modalities for arthritis treatment. The Arthritis Foundation has identified a number of products that may be potentially useful for the pain or inflammation of arthritis.

Ginger inhibits production of prostaglandins and leukotrienes that contribute to pain and swelling, creating a potential analgesic effect. It is also believed to have anti-inflammatory characteristics.

Turmeric, a root similar to ginger, has been used for arthritis treatment in both ayurvedic and Chinese medicine. Its active ingredient is curcumin, which is believed to inhibit prostaglandin production and stimulate production of cortisol.

Cayenne red pepper (*Capsicum* species) contains capsaicin, which stimulates the release of pain-relieving endorphins. It also blocks pain by interfering with substance P, which is responsible for transmission of pain impulses. The American College of Rheumatology recommends capsaicin as a topical cream for treatment of OA of the knee.

20. What surgical treatments may be indicated for osteoarthritis?

Surgical treatment is considered when conservative measures have failed to control pain and when arthritis has impaired the patient's quality of life. Total joint arthroplasty (TJA) is a popular intervention, but the surgeon and patient may first consider other procedures such as debridement, cartilage transplant, osteotomy, or arthrodesis (fusion). For example, the younger patient with OA of the knee may be a candidate for a wedge osteotomy to alleviate arthritis symptoms in the short term. TJA has traditionally been performed in older patients, who generally place fewer demands on the prosthesis, thus decreasing the likelihood of loosening or breakage.

21. What preoperative education is needed before total joint arthroplasty?

Preoperative education may occur in the surgeon's office, where the nurse reviews information about joint anatomy and surgical instrumentation. Many hospitals or large orthopedic practices also offer a class for TJA patients to discuss preadmission testing and personal preparation. Information is typically offered about postoperative pain management, the possibility of transfusion, presence of drains, use of devices such as the continuous passive motion (CPM) machine or the abductor wedge, and strategies to meet the patient's elimination needs. The patient should also receive directions about cessation of NSAIDs, aspirin, or anticoagulants at a prescribed preoperative date. A discussion of expected hospital length of stay and discharge needs helps the patient plan transportation and family support.

22. What postoperative interventions are needed after total joint arthroplasty?

The general postoperative plan of care is based on the patient's overall health, including the presence of other chronic conditions. Attention to postoperative pain, pulmonary hygiene, skin and wound care, fluid balance, and vital signs is similar to provider responsibilities after any surgery. The orthopedic patient also requires regular assessment of neurovascular status to identify developing deficits that may affect function. After total hip arthroplasty, the patient may have activity restrictions based on the surgical approach. Referral to a physical therapist provides instruction in exercise and mobility. Weight-bearing limitations due to the use of a noncemented prosthesis may also be necessary. An occupational therapist offers the patient assistance in self-care activities, such as dressing and bathing, that may be affected by postoperative limitations.

23. What postoperative complications are possible after total joint arthroplasty?

Postoperative complications occur in approximately 25% of elderly TJA patients, but the in-hospital mortality rate is less than 1%. Most complications are transient, reversible conditions such as heart failure, atelectasis, and pneumonia. Infection and thromboembolic events continue to be the greatest threat to the TJA patient.

Deep vein thrombosis (DVT) and pulmonary embolism (PE) are the most common medical problems that develop after TJA. In the absence of prophylactic treatment, incidence of DVT may be as high as 57% after total hip arthroplasty and 84% after total knee arthroplasty. Early mobilization is one key to clot prevention. The patient may also be treated prophylactically with any combination of anticoagulants (low-dose heparin, warfarin, aspirin, or low-molecular-weight heparin), foot pumps or pneumatic compression stockings, and antiembolic stockings (TEDS). The patient should also be encouraged to perform ankle pumps by flexing and extending the feet and ankles at least 10 times every 1–2 hours while awake to prevent venous stasis.

Early infection, which can occur in the first 3 months after surgery, may be either superficial or deep. One sign of superficial infection is late wound healing. Early deep infection often results from intraoperative contamination, as does delayed infection, which occurs between 3 months and 1 year after surgery. With delayed infection, the patient complains of mild-to-moderate pain in the affected joint. The ESR may be elevated, but other signs of infection are often not apparent. Diagnosis must be made through joint aspiration followed by culture and sensitivity of the fluid. Finally, late infection occurs more than 1 year after surgery and appears to be due to hematogenous seeding. In all cases, treatment depends on the causative organism. Parenteral antibiotics are prescribed, and surgical debridement may be necessary. The joint prosthesis must often be removed. To minimize the risk of infection, the health care provider should perform all dressing changes using aseptic technique. The patient should also be assessed regularly for local and systemic signs of infection.

24. What is degenerative disc disease?

Degenerative disc disease (DDD), or osteoarthritis of the spine, is one of the most common spinal disorders. As a person ages, the discs that separate the vertebrae in the spine begin to dehydrate and lose their elasticity. The muscles and ligaments adjacent to the spine also become thicker and less pliable. Degeneration of intervertebral discs is an expected part of aging; problems develop if the discs begin to extrude from between the vertebrae and put pressure on nearby nerve roots or the spinal cord.

25. Describe the symptoms of degenerative disc disease.

Common symptoms include neck or back pain, pain that radiates down the back of the shoulder blades or into the arms, numbness and tingling, or possible difficulties with hand dexterity or walking. Muscle weakness occurs at a later stage in the degenerative process and indicates that the disease is more serious.

26. What should be included in a conservative treatment plan for the patient with degenerative disc disease?

Although DDD is relatively common, its effects are usually not profound enough to require medical attention. Approximately 80% of adults with DDD experience back pain, but only 1–2% ultimately require lumbar spine surgery. Bedrest is typically recommended only briefly during periods of acute pain. Medications that are commonly prescribed during the acute phase of back pain include NSAIDs, acetaminophen, and muscle relaxants. Opioid analgesics may be needed for breakthrough pain, and antidepressants can serve as adjunct analgesics and sleep aids. After resolution of the acute episode, experts often prescribe a therapeutic exercise program that includes stretching, flexion and extension, and no- or low-impact aerobics. DDD without nerve compression may also respond to manipulation by a chiropractor or physical therapist.

27. What are the more aggressive/invasive treatments for degenerative disc disease?

Intradiscal electrothermy (IDET) is performed through percutaneous insertion of a tiny needle that is followed by a small catheter. The catheter is placed into the disc, and the catheter tip is heated, causing disc shrinkage and deadening the nerve endings in the disc. This outpatient procedure is performed using conscious sedation. It typically allows the patient to return to a usual level of function on the following day.

Disc herniation is the most common indication for spinal surgery. Laminectomy and partial disc excision may be needed to decompress the nerve. Microdiscectomy is frequently preferred because the smaller incision results in less scarring and a more rapid recovery. The surgeon may choose to remove the entire disc and perform a fusion at the affected level.

28. What medical conditions are associated with Charcot joints?

Conditions that produce reduced pain sensation have been associated with the development of Charcot joints. Examples include diabetes mellitus, tertiary syphilis and tabes dorsalis, syringomyelia, multiple sclerosis, peripheral nerve lesions, and congenital insensitivity to pain. Neuropathic arthropathy occurs most commonly in diabetes, with an incidence as high as 2.5%

29. How does Charcot's neuropathy develop?

Charcot's neuropathy develops as a result of disruption in a joint's normal sensory innervation. Although the exact cause is not clear, development of Charcot joint is believed to require three types of neuropathy: autonomic, motor, and sensory. **Autonomic neuropathy** causes loss of vascular tone, which contributes to bone demineralization through vasodilation and increased perfusion. **Sensory neuropathy** results from loss of protopathic sensibility, which hampers the ability to detect a trauma that can precipitate the neuropathy. Because the person is unaware of injury and continues to bear weight on the affected joint, treatment is often delayed. Finally, **motor neuropathy** becomes worse through loss of proprioception. The person unconsciously places an increased load on the joints of the affected foot in an effort to get more information from the environment.

30. What features of the patient's history suggest a diagnosis of Charcot neuropathy?

With careful questioning, the health care provider typically learns of a longstanding decrease in sensitivity to heat and cold. Loss of sensation allows repeated joint injuries that contribute to bony deterioration and soft tissue laxity. Rapid destruction of an affected joint characteristically leads to swelling and deformity. Some pain occurs secondary to joint inflammation, but it is often less than expected based on the extent of destruction typically seen on x-rays. Awareness of light touch is generally preserved, and pulses in the affected extremity are palpable.

31. What are the key features of medical management for patients with Charcot neuropathy?

The primary focus is protecting the affected joint from additional injury. Casts, braces, or orthotics may be indicated to maintain proper alignment and to distribute stress appropriately across the joint. Although a cure is not currently available, several treatments have the potential to stop the bone and soft tissue destruction of Charcot neuropathy. Intravenous bisphosphonates such as pamidronate have been used to inhibit the characteristic bone resorption. Other promising treatments are under evaluation, including use of low-intensity ultrasound therapy or combined magnetic field (CMF) bone growth stimulation to enhance healing.

32. What surgical interventions may be used for the patient with Charcot neuropathy?

Fusion is often proposed for the unstable Charcot joint. Decreased sensation usually leads the patient to overuse the joint in the early postoperative period, however, and the fusion may be compromised. Amputation may be needed if other strategies fail.

33. Define chondromalacia patellae.

Chondromalacia patellae is a pain syndrome rather than a single diagnosis. Experienced by people of all ages, as early as adolescence, it involves patellofemoral joint pain that results from softening and fissuring on the articular surface of the patella. Chondromalacia patellae has also been identified as patellofemoral arthralgia or patellofemoral pain syndrome.

34. What causes chondromalacia patellae?

Some cases of chondromalacia patellae have no identifiable cause, but others are obviously the result of trauma. The repetitive injuries of long-distance running, for example, can lead to chronic inflammation. A chondral fracture can result from direct trauma to the patella and can lead to subsequent pain in the anterior knee. Other causes of patellofemoral pain may be related to malalignment of the knee, femoral neck, or tibia.

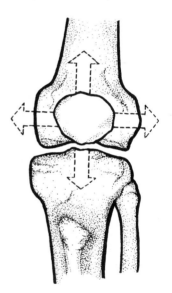

Forces on the patella in chondromalacia patellae. (From Frontera WR, Silver JK: Essentials of Physical Medicine and Rehabilitation. Philadelphia, Hanley & Belfus, 2002, with permission.)

35. What signs and symptoms are associated with chondromalacia patellae?

Common complaints include mild swelling and an aching pain in the knee after any activity that involves repeated knee flexion and extension. Sitting with the knee flexed at 90° can also lead to a dull pain that is referred to the popliteal fossa; the pain generally decreases after movement. On examination, the health care provider may notice lateral tracking of the patella during active knee extension. He or she may also observe that the patient bends forward excessively when rising from a chair because of knee pain. Painful crepitus is often associated with joint movement. Patellar subluxation may also be a contributing factor.

36. How is chondromalacia patellae managed?

Initial conservative management will probably include a progressive resistance exercise program. NSAIDs are prescribed for pain and inflammation, and ice is often useful for its local effects. After 6 months of treatment, persistent symptoms will probably prompt the health care provider to consider surgery. Patellar debridement brings good-to-excellent results in up to 60% of cases, although functional limitations may continue after surgery. Other procedures may be considered if the patient experiences repeated subluxation or dislocation.

37. How do bunions occur?

Bunions occur as a deformity of the first metatarsophalangeal (MTP) joint in the foot. The term *hallux valgus* is used to describe the characteristic lateral deviation of the great toe. Bunions may occur congenitally, or they may develop during periods of rapid growth such as adolescence. They may also be due to degenerative conditions within the MTP joint or to remodeling caused by local irritation from footwear.

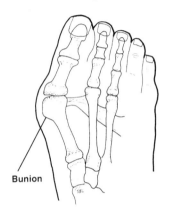

Anatomy of a bunion. (From Frontera WR, Silver JK: Essentials of Physical Medicine and Rehabilitation. Philadelphia, Hanley & Belfus, 2002, with permission.)

Bunion

38. How are bunions diagnosed?

The patient typically complains of pain related to irritation of the first metatarsal head as it rubs against the inside of a shoe. On examination, the health care provider notices enlargement of the dorsomedial area of the metatarsal head and may find calluses under the second and third metatarsal heads due to the patient's shift in weight-bearing. Standard anteroposterior (AP) and lateral x-rays are ordered; they commonly show exostosis of the first metatarsal head with subluxation or dislocation.

39. What are the treatment options for bunions?

Treatment may initially involve use of footwear with a wide toe box to allow enough room for the forefoot and to decrease pressure over the first metatarsal head. Orthotics and steroid injections of the MTP joint may be considered if the change in footwear does not provide adequate relief. If these conservative treatments fail or the patient desires cosmetic correction, surgical alignment of the affected toe will be necessary. The type of procedure is determined primarily by the amount of deformity and the severity of the valgus angle. Osteotomy of the metatarsal or fusion of the MTP joint may be chosen.

40. What is carpal tunnel syndrome?

Carpal tunnel syndrome (CTS) results from compression of the median nerve as it passes through the wrist to the hand. The nerve's pathway is called the carpal tunnel. It is bordered by the flexor retinaculum, a band of fibrous tissue that keeps the wrist tendons from bowing when the wrist is flexed. Compression of the median nerve in the carpal tunnel can cause sensory and motor changes in the thumb, index finger, and middle finger and on the medial surface of the ring finger.

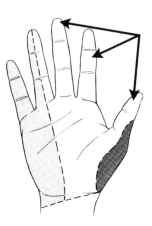

Patients with carpal tunnel syndrome complain of numbness or
paresthesia within the median nerve (white area, arrows).

41. What causes carpal tunnel syndrome?

CTS is an entrapment neuropathy that can develop spontaneously or as a result of
disease or injury. The most common cause is repetitive motion of the wrist that typically includes nearly constant flexion. A high incidence of CTS is reported among
cashiers, secretaries, computer operators, and factory workers. A number of health conditions are also associated with CTS, including pregnancy, hypothyroidism, gout, and
rheumatoid arthritis.

42. What are the treatment options for carpal tunnel syndrome?

Initial treatment involves splinting the wrist in a neutral position to prevent additional irritation of the median nerve. Injection of steroids into the flexor tendons was a
popular treatment that is now used less frequently because of reported problems with
scarring, infection, and median nerve damage. Gently manipulating the distal
metacarpal heads or stretching the involved digits may provide some pain relief.
Surgery is indicated for severe, longstanding symptoms; muscle atrophy; or progressive sensory loss in the fingers and hand. Carpal tunnel release involves dividing the
transverse ligament to relieve pressure on the median nerve; it can be performed endo-
scopically or through an incision in the wrist.

43. What is sciatic nerve dysfunction?

Sciatic nerve dysfunction is a form of peripheral neuropathy that results from
damage to the sciatic nerve. The sciatic nerve travels across the buttock to the leg, sup-
plying the muscles of the back of the knee and the lower leg. It also supplies sensation
to the back of the thigh, part of the lower leg, and the sole of the foot. The sciatic nerve
is often injured by fractures of the pelvis, trauma to the buttock or thigh, or pressure
from lesions or pelvic bleeding. The nerve may also be damaged during intramuscular
injections into the buttock or by prolonged sitting or lying with pressure on the buttock. The sciatic nerve is also commonly affected by diseases, such as diabetes mellitus, that cause polyneuropathy.

44. What are common symptoms of sciatic nerve dysfunction?

Both sensory and motor changes can be associated with sciatic nerve dysfunction.
Sensory changes, which may occur in the back of the calf or the sole of the foot, include numbness, decreased sensation, tingling, burning, pain, and abnormal sensations.

Weakness of the knee or foot is possible, leading to difficulty with walking. In severe cases, the person may be unable to move the foot or bend the knee.

45. How is sciatic nerve dysfunction diagnosed?

Neuromuscular examination typically reveals weakness with knee flexion, weakness of foot movements such as inversion or plantarflexion, and a weak or absent ankle-jerk reflex. An electromyogram (EMG) and nerve conduction test are useful in diagnosis.

46. What treatments are commonly recommended for sciatic nerve dysfunction?

Treatment for sciatic nerve dysfunction focuses on maximizing the patient's mobility and independence. The cause should be identified and treated, if possible; in some cases, spontaneous recovery follows removal of the cause. In the absence of a history of trauma, conservative treatment tries to control symptoms through use of analgesics and adjunctive medications. Physical therapy may be indicated to help the patient maintain muscle strength. Braces, splints, or orthotics may also be helpful. Surgery may be the treatment of choice to remove lesions that press on the nerve.

BIBLIOGRAPHY

1. American Association of Neurological Surgeons: The aging spine: Older doesn't have to mean more painful. 2000. Available at <http://www.spineuniverse.com/aans/aans_agingspine.html>.
2. Bayne O, Lu EJ: Diabetic Charcot's arthropathy of the wrist: Case report and literature review. Clin Orthop 357:122–126, 1998.
3. Borenstein D: Osteoarthritis: Clinical update. Medscape 2000. Available at <http://www.medscape.com/medscape/CNO/1999/ACR/ACR-05.html>.
4. Brander VA, Kaelin DL, Oh TH, Lim PAC: Rehabilitation of orthopaedic and rheumatologic disorders: Degenerative joint disease. Arch Phys Med Rehabil 81(3 Suppl 1):S67–S78, S78–S86, S101–S102, 2000.
5. Buckwalter JA, Lane NE: Athletics and osteoarthritis. Am J Sports Med 25:873-881, 1997.
6. Cooper SM: Improving outcomes in osteoarthritis: How to help patients stay a step ahead of the pain. Postgrad Med 105(6):29–38, 1999.
7. DiNubile NA: Osteoarthritis: How to make exercise part of your treatment plan. Physician Sports Med 25:47–57, 1997.
8. Federico DJ, Reider B: Results of isolated patellar debridement for patellofemoral pain in patients with normal patellar alignment. Am J Sports Med 25:663–669, 1997.
9. Frederich AMJ: Management of clients with peripheral nervous system disorders. In Black J, Hawks JH, Keene A (eds): Medical-Surgical Nursing: A Psychophysiologic Approach, 6th ed. Philadelphia, W.B. Saunders, 2001, pp 1983–2001.
10. Horstman J: The Arthritis Foundation's Guide to Alternative Therapies. Atlanta, Arthritis Foundation, 1999.
11. Hospital Extra: New drugs. Celecoxib (Celebrex): A new 'super NSAID.' Am J Nurs 99(4):24, 1999
12. Kee CC: Osteoarthritis: Manageable scourge of aging. Nurs Clin North Am 35(3):199–207, 2000.
13. Kuhn M: Complementary Therapies for Health Care Providers. Philadelphia, Lippincott Williams & Williams, 1999.
14. Ling SM, Bathon JB: Osteoarthritis in older adults. J Am Geriatr Soc 46:216–225, 1998.
15. Lowe TG: Degenerative disc disease and low back pain. 2001. Available at <http://www.spineuniverse.com/conditions/detail/tk_102900_ddd.html>.
16. Lumsden DB, Baccala A. Martire J: Tai-chi for osteoarthritis: An introduction for primary care physicians. Geriatrics 53(2):84, 87–88, 1998.
17. O'Koon M: Shopping for a "cure." Arthritis Today 1999. Available at <http://www.arthritis.org/ReadArthritis Today/1999_03_04.shopping.asp>.
18. Osteoarthritis. In Klippel JH (ed): Primer on the Rheumatic Diseases, 11th ed. Atlanta, Arthritis Foundation, 1997.

19. Ramos,L: Beyond the headlines. SAMe as a supplement: Can it really help treat depression and arthritis? J Am Diet Assoc 100:414, 2000.
20. Rehman Q, Lane NE: Getting control of osteoarthritis pain: An update on treatment options. Postgrad Med 106:127–134, 1999.
21. Roberts D: Arthritic and connective tissue disorders. In Schoen D (ed): Core Curriculum for Orthopaedic Nursing, 4 th ed. Pitman, NJ, National Association of Orthopaedic Nurses, 2001, pp 301–340.
22. Roberts D, Lappe J: Management of clients with musculoskeletal disorders. In Black J, Hawks JH, Keene A (eds): Medical-Surgical Nursing: A Psychophysiologic Approach, 6th ed. Philadelphia, W.B. Saunders, 2001, pp 551–586.
23. SAMm-e (S-adenosyl-methionine) (2000). Arthritis Foundation. Available at <http://www.arthritis.org/resource/statements/sam%5Fe.asp>.
24. Slemenda C, Brandt KD, Heilman DK, et al: Quadriceps weakness and osteoarthritis of the knee. Ann Intern Med 127(2):97–104, 1997.
25. University of Maryland Medicine: Sciatic nerve dysfunction. 2001. Available at <http://umm.drkoop.com/conditions/ency/article/000686.htm>.
26. University of Pittsburgh, Department of Neurological Surgery. Degenerative disc disease. 2001. Available at <http://www.neurosurgery.pitt.edu/spine/conditions/ddd.html>.

4. INFLAMMATORY DISEASES

Brandi L. Handel, RN

1. What is rheumatoid arthritis?

Rheumatoid arthritis (RA) is a chronic, autoimmune systemic disease that causes inflammation and deformities of connective tissue, mainly the joints. The synovial tissue becomes inflamed and forms pannus that damages cartilage, bone, and ligament and causes deformities. RA is characterized by periods of remissions and exacerbations and is progressive.

2. What is meant by autoimmune disease?

A normal, healthy immune system has the primary objective of differentiating tissues, cells, and organisms that are part of the body from tissue, cells, and organisms that are foreign or dangerous. After this differentiation, the immune system attacks any organisms that it sees as foreign or dangerous to the body. In autoimmune disease, the immune system is unable to differentiate correctly and instead begins to attack normal body tissue and cells.

3. What is meant by systemic?

Systemic disease refers to disease that affects various organs and systems throughout the body rather than a single system or organ.

4. What causes RA?

The cause is unknown, but genetics, autoimmunity, and environment seem to play a role in RA. Identical twins have a 32% rate of disease, whereas fraternal twins have a 9% rate. Ongoing research is examining various bacteria and viruses that are thought to be a potential cause of RA. There are no known risk factors for RA.

5. Describe the typical patient population diagnosed with RA.

RA is seen in women three times more often than in men. It can occur at any age but typically occurs in the fourth to sixth decade of life. It can occur in all races, but North American Indians have a higher prevalence.

6. What are the clinical manifestations of RA?

Patients have painful, red, swollen joints symmetrically, usually starting with the joints in the hands and wrists and progressing to any joint in the body. They may complain of morning stiffness lasting from 1 to 4 hours. They may also complain of hoarseness and difficulty with mobility and self-care activities. Affected areas may have obvious deformities and rheumatoid nodules, which are mobile, painless skin nodules anywhere on the body near a bony prominence. Typically patients look ill or anemic and complain of fatigue and lethargy. They are usually underweight and may have evidence of muscle wasting. Because RA is a systemic disease, patients may also have other systemic symptoms, such as vasculitis, neuropathy, pericarditis, lymphadenopathy, carpal tunnel syndrome, pulmonary nodules, pulmonary fibrosis, splenomegaly, and Sjögren's syndrome (salivary and lacrimal secretion decrease). RA symptoms go into remission, which is followed by an exacerbation. Exacerbations may be induced by physical or emotional stress.

7. How is RA diagnosed?

Diagnosis is usually based on patient history and physical exam. There is no specific laboratory diagnostic test, although the rheumatoid factor antibody test is positive in approximately 80% of patients with advanced RA. Other lab tests may reveal an elevated erythrocyte sedimentation rate (ESR), which is indicative of active inflammation, and an antinuclear antibody (ANA) titer, which is seen in 5–20% of patients with RA. Radiographs may be done but are not necessary for diagnosis. Results of x-rays usually reveal soft tissue swelling and joint effusion and, as the disease progresses, gradual lessening of joint space, inner joint margin fraying, subluxation, dislocation, and eventually bony ankyloses. Bone scans can also be used to identify early joint changes and to confirm the diagnosis.

8. What is rheumatoid factor?

Rheumatoid factor (RF) is an antibody directed against IgG. Two different lab tests can determine the presence of RF antibody in blood. In RA, 70–90% of patients test positive for RF, but a positive test is not required for the diagnosis of RA. People who test positive for RF may still be negative for RA. The RF test is positive in other inflammatory or connective tissue disorders, such as hepatitis, systemic lupus erythematosus, and Sjögren's syndrome.

9. How is RA treated?

There is still no known cure for this debilitating disease. Treatment is geared toward reducing the inflammatory process, alleviating pain, maintaining joint mobility, preventing deformities, and supporting the psychological needs of the patient. The general trend is aggressive early treatment to prevent deformity and loss of function. Disease-modifying antirheumatic drugs (DMARDs) are usually the first medications used. In addition to DMARDs, other medications such as nonsteroidal anti-inflammatory drugs (NSAIDs), high doses of enteric-coated aspirin, and low-dose corticosteroids are used to help relieve pain and decrease inflammation. Pain relief may also occur with the use of heat or cold therapy, massage therapy, and transcutaneous electrical nerve stimulation (TENS). Orthopedic appliances and prostheses may be used to help prevent deformities and to allow the patient to continue to walk. A physical therapy program is an important part of treatment because it allows patients to keep their joints mobile, maintain strength and function, and prevent muscle atrophy. Occasionally surgery is needed to help relieve pain and correct deformities, including osteotomy, synovectomy, arthrodesis, and arthroplasty.

10. Explain what is meant by DMARDs.

DMARDs are medications that have been shown to alter the course of RA for at least 1 year, as evidenced by a decrease in the inflammation of the synovium, a decrease in the damage of structural joints, and an improvement in physical function. Such medications include methotrexate, intramuscular and oral gold, hydroxychloroquine, sulfasalazine, leflunomide, and D-penicillamine.

11. As an orthopedic nurse, what should I teach my patients with RA?

Patients need to be instructed about the disease process, progression, and treatment. They also need to be educated about the importance of health maintenance, such as good nutrition, maintaining ideal body weight, getting adequate rest and exercise, avoiding periods of stress and illness, using relaxation techniques, and participating regularly in physical therapy using good body mechanics. They also need individualized instructions in home safety and lifestyle modifications.

12. What else can I do for patients with RA?

Patients need a strong psychological support system. RA is not only physically debilitating but also emotionally draining. Many patients experience bouts of frustration and depression over loss of strength and body deformities. Many different support groups have been set up to help patients deal with the psychological aspects of RA, such as the Arthritis Foundation. Psychological support needs to be stressed as much as physical treatment.

13. Where can patients get more information about RA?

The Arthritis Foundation has an informational website at http://www.arthritis.org. There are also local chapters throughout the United States.

14. What is epicondylitis?

Epicondylitis is a degenerative condition of the tendons of the elbow. It is also a common orthopedic sports injury. The many causes include local trauma and excessive, repetitive movements, as seen in activities such as tennis, golf, squash, badminton, and baseball pitching. This disease can affect any person of any race or age group. It may be a recurrent, chronic condition or a one-time acute episode.

15. What are the different types of epicondylitis?

There are two types of epicondylitis: lateral epicondylitis, also known as tennis elbow, and medial epicondylitis, also known as golfer's elbow. They are differentiated by the location of the injury.

16. How does lateral epicondylitis develop?

The large tendons of the elbow that attach the outside bony portion (lateral epicondyle) to the muscles of the forearm can be injured with excessive activity of the forearm (e.g., backhand strokes in tennis, knitting, or using a manual screwdriver). All of these activities involve a strong grasp during wrist extension and performance of a repetitive motion, which cause inflammation of the large tendons. This process results in pain on the outside of the elbow and pain that radiates up and down the lateral forearm. The pain intensifies with resisted wrist extension while the elbow is extended. The patient may also have warmth and swelling of the lateral aspect of the elbow.

17. How does medial epicondylitis develop?

The tendons of the elbow that attach the inner bony prominence (medial epicondyle) to the forearm can become strained with excessive activity of the forearm, as when golfers swing a club. This process causes inflammation of the tendons and results in pain and tenderness of the inner portion of the elbow, which increase with twisting, and straining of the forearm.

18. How is epicondylitis diagnosed?

The diagnosis is based on history and physical examination. Patients with lateral epicondylitis have pain with wrist extension, especially against resistance, and with palpation at the origin of the wrist extensors. Patients with medial epicondylitis have pain with wrist flexion, especially against resistance, and with palpation at the origin of the wrist flexors.

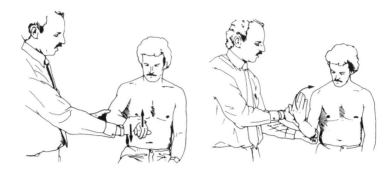

Testing for lateral epicondylitis (*left*) and medial epicondylitis (*right*). (From Mellion MB: Office Sports Medicine, 2nd ed. Philadelphia, Hanley & Belfus, 1996, with permission.]

19. What should I expect the x-rays of a patient with epicondylitis to reveal?

X-rays may be ordered but are usually not diagnostic because results are typically normal. If the epicondylitis has been chronic, x-rays may reveal calcium deposits in the tendon, but the elbow joint appears normal.

20. Describe the treatment for epicondylitis.

Treatment includes resting the elbow, ice in acute phases, heat in chronic phases, isometric exercises that strengthen the involved muscle, and anti-inflammatory medications, including aspirin and NSAIDs. Patients with severe inflammation and persistent pain may require local injections of cortisones. Even with these medications, it may take weeks for the pain to be completely relieved.

21. What other kinds of treatment may be used for epicondylitis?

A physical therapy program of exercise, massage, and icing after activity helps return the elbow to normal function. A brace for tennis elbow and a strap for golfer's elbow may be used to support the elbow and prevent reinjury, although these modalities have not been impressively effective. On rare occasions surgical treatment is necessary.

22. What do I need to teach patients about NSAIDs?

NSAIDs can cause serious side effects. Patients need to watch for signs of side effects and report them to a health care team. Gastrointestinal effects such as dyspepsia, nausea, vomiting, indigestion, gastric and peptic ulcers, gastroesophageal reflux, chronic diverticuli perforation, and GI bleed can occur. Patients should be instructed to take NSAIDs with food to avoid GI effects and to watch for signs such as stomach pain, rectal bleeding, and coffee-ground or bright red vomiting. NSAIDs can also cause bronchospasm, difficulty in breathing, hepatotoxicity, depressed renal function, hematologic problems, and headaches.

23. What is systemic lupus erythematosus (SLE)?

SLE is a systemic, inflammatory connective tissue disorder characterized by the presence of antinuclear antibodies in the blood that form lupus erythematosus cells and immune complexes that trigger inflammatory responses and subsequently cause tissue destruction. SLE is a chronic condition with periods of exacerbations and remissions.

24. What causes SLE?

SLE is considered an autoimmune disease, given the fact that so many immunologic abnormalities are present. Genetic factors are also thought to play a major role in SLE. There is a high prevalence of SLE in identical twins, and 5–12% of relatives of patients with SLE also develop the disease. Environmental factors are also thought to trigger SLE, such as sun exposure and burns, sulfa antibiotic drugs, and infectious agents.

25. Who is at risk for SLE?

SLE is typically seen in females between the ages of 15 and 45 years. The onset can range from infancy to old age; however, it is commonly seen during child-bearing years. There are not many cases of pediatric SLE. It affects women eight times more often than men. African Americans, Native Americans, and Asian Americans are diagnosed three times more often than white Americans.

26. What are the clinical manifestations of SLE?

There are no classic presentations of SLE, which can affect any organ system. Symptoms may develop gradually one at a time or suddenly with many symptoms at once. Patients must have 4 of the following 11 symptoms at the time of diagnosis: positive antinuclear antibody test (ANA), malar rash, discoid rash, photosensitivity, oral or nasopharyngeal ulceration, nonerosive arthritis, persistent proteinuria or casts, pericarditis or pleuritis, neurologic disorders (such as seizures or psychosis), hematologic disorders (such as leukopenia, thrombocytopenia, or hemolytic anemia), and immunologic disorder such as anti-DNA antibody, anti-Sm antibody, or false-positive serology test for syphilis.

27. Describe the rashes seen in SLE.

The **malar or butterfly rash** is seen on the face, covering the cheeks and nose. It is a fixed, erythematous rash that is raised with papules and/or plaques. It typically indicates that the patient has active disease.

The **discoid rash** can be found on the face, scalp, ears, neck, and arms. It begins as erythematous plaques or papules and progresses to larger, discoid lesions that scar, depigment, and cause alopecia.

The **photosensitive rash** occurs as an acute reaction to sun exposure. The rash may be found anywhere on the body and has characteristics similar to the malar rash.

The **subacute rash** is seen on any body part that has been exposed to sun, such as the chest, back, and arms. It is symmetric, raised, and erythematous and usually does not cause scarring.

28. What is the ANA test?

The antinuclear antibody test is a laboratory test that is usually ordered when clinical findings suggest evidence of autoimmune disease. It is done using fluorescence microscopy and measures gamma globulins that are produced by the body as a reaction to certain antigens. The ANA is considered the laboratory hallmark of SLE. Positive titers strongly suggest a positive diagnosis of SLE, although ANA is also positive in patients with systemic sclerosis, dermatomyositis, or Sjögren's syndrome and in a small population of healthy adults.

29. Describe the course of SLE.

SLE is characterized by periods of alternating exacerbations and remissions. It typically is highly active in the first few years of the disease and then gradually declines.

30. What is the prognosis of SLE?

SLE has a much better prognosis now than it did in the past. More than 85% of patients with SLE have a life expectancy greater than 15 years. The most common reasons for death in SLE are vascular events, infection, and active lupus nephritis.

31. How is SLE treated?

Treatment of SLE is geared toward suppressing manifestations, controlling inflammation, lifestyle modifications, coping with body image, and preventing long-term effects due to treatment. Conservative treatment for mild cases includes NSAIDS, rest, avoiding sun, using sunscreen, and topical steroids. DMARDs, such as hydroxychloroquine, are used for patients with polyarthritis, rash, photosensitivity, and arthralgias; they are generally quite safe. Corticosteroids and immunosuppressants are used less frequently now than in the past but are still used during severe, acute exacerbations. Other treatment includes healthy, balanced meals that are low in sodium, high in proteins and iron, and soft enough to swallow in patients with dysphagia and esophagitis.

32. What does the orthopedic nurse need to teach patients with SLE?

Patients need education about the disease process, symptoms, and treatment. They need to be instructed in the triggers for exacerbation and coached on how to avoid them. They need detailed teaching about medications, including administration, dosing, and side effects of each agent that they take, and they need to be warned against abruptly stopping medications. They also need to be instructed in skin protection through the use of sunscreen, avoidance of sun exposure, and avoidance of drying soaps, powders, and chemicals. The nurse can also give information about support groups such as the American Lupus Society.

33. What side effects of corticosteroids should the nurse discuss with patients?

- Truncal obesity
- Moon face
- Buffalo hump
- Bruising
- Hypokalemia
- Osteopenia
- Cataracts
- Mental disturbance
- Osteoporosis
- Renal failure
- Hypertension
- Adrenal suppression
- GI disturbances
- Hyperglycemia
- High sodium
- Infection
- Muscle weakness
- Hirsutism

34. What else should I teach patients about corticosteroids?

Explain to patients that they must always discontinue the corticosteroid gradually. Once they have reached remission, they are gradually weaned from steroids by 5 mg/week. If weaning is not possible, explain to patients that the dose may be gradually decreased until the lowest dose that provides relief of symptoms is reached.

35. Where else can patients get information about SLE?

The Lupus Foundation of America has a website that patients can access for information: <www.lupus.org>.

36. What is ankylosing spondylitis?

Ankylosing spondylitis (AS) is a chronic, progressive inflammation of the spine and sacroiliac joint. AS can result in complete cementing or fusion of vertebrae, which is known as ankylosing. AS is also a systemic rheumatic disease; it can cause inflammation in other joints distant from the spine as well as other organs, such as the heart, kidneys, lungs, and eyes.

37. What causes ankylosing spondylitis?

The cause of AS is unknown, but there is a strong familial tendency. Research has found a 60% rate of AS in monozygotic twins and a 20–25% rate in dizygotic twins. Environmental factors also are thought to play a role in AS. HLA-B27 is associated with AS and thought to play a role in its pathogenesis.

38. What is the HLA-B27 gene?

Human leukocyte antigen (HLA) -B27 is an antigen that is present in 90% of white patients with AS and 50–80% of nonwhite patients. The test for HLA-B27 is usually ordered to help confirm the diagnosis after clinical findings and positive radiologic findings of sacroiliitis suggest AS.

39. Is any age group or race more affected by AS?

No. All ages and races of people can be affected, including children. AS is more commonly diagnosed in early adulthood and is 3–4 times more common in males.

40. What are the signs and symptoms of AS?

Low back pain that radiates to the thighs; muscle spasms in the neck, back, and ribs; general malaise; morning stiffness; fatigue; and joint pain are common symptoms. Usually the pain is gradual and progressive over a few months, but occasionally it develops rapidly and intensely. Usually the pain is greater in the morning and decreases with heat and motion. Loss of spine mobility results when complete bony fusion occurs. Patients with fused spines are more susceptible to fractures because the spine is more brittle. AS can also cause a forward curvature in the upper torso, which limits breathing capacity and causes patients to cough and become short of breath with increased activity or infection. AS is a systemic disease and can also cause iritis, aortic valvular disease, pulmonary fibrosis, cauda equina syndrome with lower extremity weakness and bladder dysfunction, and discitis.

41. How is AS diagnosed?

Diagnosis is usually based on clinical and x-ray findings. Intervertebral bodies are fused on x-rays, and the spinal column reveals calcifications that suggest the classic "bamboo spine." In addition, 90% of patients with AS are born with the HLA-B27 gene, which can be detected by lab tests. Patients may also have an increase in ESR, alkaline phosphate, and creatinine phosphokinase.

42. Describe the treatment for AS.

The goals of treatment are to manage pain, relieve inflammation, and maintain mobility. These goals can be accomplished through the use of NSAIDs, salicylates, heat, and injectable corticosteroids. Indomethacin is the NSAID most commonly used for AS. DMARDs (e.g., methotrexate, sulfasalazine) are also used to manage AS and are often helpful early in the disease. Physical therapy is encouraged to maintain mobility and to prevent deformities. Patients are taught spine exercises that promote extension of the back and expansion of the chest. Occasionally surgery is needed, including total hip, total knee, and cervical or lumbar osteotomies.

43. What is the prognosis of AS?

AS is characterized by periods of remissions and exacerbations. Most patients are able to maintain functional capacity and continue to work. Patients with systemic manifestations, such as complete ankyloses, cardiac and pulmonary disease, iritis, and an affected hip joint, have a less favorable overall prognosis. Severe disease may cause a decreased lifespan, but most patients with mild AS have a normal life expectancy.

44. As an orthopedic nurse, what can I teach patients about AS?

Patients need to be encouraged to keep an erect posture, to sleep on their back with a flat pillow and a firm mattress, and to use chairs with high backs. They need to be taught deep breathing exercises, back extension exercises, and stretching exercises. Swimming and aerobics are good activities when the disease is not in an active phase. Patients can also be encouraged to wear an orthotic brace as needed, to adjust equipment and furniture (e.g., desks) to fit their posture, and to continue with activities of daily living in an effort to maintain mobility. They also need to be instructed to avoid smoking because AS leads to diminished expansion of the chest and pulmonary fibrosis.

45. What are bursae?

Bursae are sacs filled with synovial fluid; they are located in areas where tendons rub against bone, ligaments, or other tendons or where skin moves over a bony prominence. They minimize friction and pressure in such areas and allow better movement.

46. What is bursitis?

Bursitis is an inflammation of one or more of the bursae in response to excessive friction or pressure on the bursae (friction bursitis); chemicals, such as urate crystal deposits in gout (chemical bursitis); or infections (septic bursitis). Bursal irritation causes thickening of the bursa wall and effusion of the bursae, which result in bursitis.

47. Who is at risk for getting bursitis?

Bursitis is commonly seen in patients who are involved in activities that require a repetitive motion or who have experienced trauma to the bursae. Examples include the housewife who repetitively scrubs her kitchen floor on her knees, swimmers, baseball players, and tennis or other racquet sport athletes. Bursitis is also seen in patients with gout, diabetes, syphilis, tuberculosis, and rheumatoid arthritis.

48. What are the clinical symptoms of bursitis?

Patients usually complain of pain in a specific joint that sometimes radiates to an extremity. The pain can be sudden or gradual and usually intensifies with movement. Physical examination reveals that the affected joint (and possibly even the surrounding area) is red, tender, and swollen. Patients also may experience stiffness of the joint with limited range of motion.

49. How is bursitis treated?

Rest, ice therapy, heat therapy, and medication are usually effective interventions. NSAIDs, aspirin, and nonanalgesics can help manage the pain initially; if they are found to be ineffective, local joint injections of cortisone or anesthetic can be tried. Muscle strengthening and flexibility exercises are also beneficial.

50. Tell me more about local injections of cortisone.

Local injections of cortisone decrease inflammation in a specific bursa without causing systemic side affects. Usually a short- or long-acting cortisone is injected with a dose equivalent to 10–20 mg of prednisone.

51. What are the potential complications of cortisone injections?

Complications may include pain, infection, erythema, postinjection flare, tissue atrophy, and skin hypopigmentation.

52. What else can be done to treat bursitis?

You need to treat the underlying cause of the bursitis. If the cause is friction, the patient needs to avoid the repetitive motion that causes the friction or buy larger shoes. In some cases, excision of the bursa is necessary. In chemical bursitis the treatment is to eliminate the urate crystals or calcium deposits that irritate the bursa. Treatment of septic bursitis may require surgical incision and drainage of the infection or surgical excision of the bursa. The patient may also need to alter activities to avoid a recurrence or exacerbation of symptoms.

53. What does a Baker's cyst have to do with bursitis?

A Baker's cyst is a specific form of bursitis of the knee in which the bursa is distended and synovial fluid builds up behind the knee. The synovial membrane herniates through the posterior part of the knee capsule, and the synovial fluid leaks out the normal communication of the bursa with the knee. The cause is unknown. A chronic Baker's cyst causes only mild aching and stiffness, but trauma to the cyst may result in rupture and acute inflammation with severe pain, edema, and limited movement.

54. What is psoriatic arthritis?

Psoriatic arthritis (PA) is a chronic inflammatory disease that involves inflammation of the skin (psoriasis) and joints (arthritis).

55. What causes psoriatic arthritis?

PA is caused by a combination of genetics, immune factors (e.g., increased IgG and/or IgA titers and immune complexes), and questionable environmental factors, such as trauma and group A streptococci.

56. What patient population does PA affect?

PA affects men and women equally, although spinal involvement is more common in males (3:1 male-to-female ratio). PA usually occurs in patients who are in their mid-thirties to fifties.

57. Are patients with psoriasis more susceptible to PA?

Yes. PA occurs in 7% of people who have psoriasis vs. approximately 1% of the general population. Patients are usually diagnosed with psoriasis first, although this is not always the case.

58. What are the clinical symptoms of PA?

- Arthritis in the knee, ankle, and foot joints manifested by pain, stiffness, edema, warmth, and erythema
- Nail changes such as pitting, ridging, hyperkeratosis, onycholysis, and discoloration

- Sacroiliitis
- Pruritic silver scales on patches of bright red skin
- Tendinitis
- Swollen and painful fingers, commonly called "sausage digits"
- Conjunctivitis or iritis
- Acne
- Pleuritis, aortitis, loss of motion, and sleep disturbances with disease progression

59. How is psoriatic arthritis diagnosed?

Diagnosis is based on clinical findings of both psoriasis and arthritis. Most rheumatologists agree that there must be evidence of skin and nail changes before PA can be diagnosed. Patients may also have an increased ESR and a positive HLA-B27 test, and x-rays may reveal changes consistent with arthritis of the spine, sacrum, feet, and hand joints.

60. How is psoriatic arthritis treated?

The psoriasis and the arthritis are treated separately, but the goals of both treatments are to decrease pain, alleviate symptoms, suppress the disease, and rehabilitate the patient. Topical emollients and kerolytic agents are used initially for psoriasis; as the disease becomes more extensive, agents such as anthralin, corticosteroids, and vitamin D derivatives are used. Ultraviolet light therapy and methoxypsoralen are also used to control the symptoms of psoriasis. NSAIDs such as naproxen, indomethacin, piroxicam, and diclofenac are frequently used for pain. If they are not effective, DMARDS such as methotrexate, gold, azathioprine, and sulfasalazine are used most commonly. Joint replacement or synovectomy may be indicated if the patient has loss of joint function or intractable pain. Physical and occupational therapy are necessary to prevent joint contracture and to maintain strength and mobility. Exercise should include warm-up stretching, heat before exercise, and a hot shower afterward.

61. As an orthopedic nurse, what should I do for patients with PA?

Patients with PA need to be taught good skin and foot care. The nurse can teach patients how to apply the topical agents correctly in a thin layer and how to pat the skin dry after bathing rather than rubbing with a towel. The nurse can also stress the importance of inspecting feet and nails daily, wearing shoes that allow enough room for swollen toes, wearing cotton socks, and checking shoes for sharp edges before wearing. The nurse should also encourage patients to participate in routine range-of-motion exercises and to alternate rest and activity. Patients also need emotional support because many patients with PA have an altered body image.

62. What is systemic sclerosis?

Systemic sclerosis is a multisystem disease that affects connective tissue, causing thickening of skin. It also affects various internal organs and joints.

63. Is systemic sclerosis the same as scleroderma?

Yes. Systemic sclerosis was commonly called scleroderma in the past because of the skin involvement. The currently preferred name is systemic sclerosis because of the systemic affects.

64. What patient population develops systemic sclerosis?

Systemic sclerosis is 3 times more common in women than in men. It can occur in people of all races, but black women usually develop this disease more often than white women. It is usually diagnosed in early to middle adulthood, and the incidence increases with age.

65. What causes systemic sclerosis?

The cause is unknown, but risk factors associated with skin thickening have been identified, including environmental factors (working with plastics, coal, and silica dust), appetite suppressants, and conditions such as phenylketonuria, metabolic disorders, malignancies, infections, and neurologic disorders.

66. Name the two forms of systemic sclerosis.

Diffuse and limited.

67. What is the difference between the two forms?

Diffuse systemic sclerosis is more aggressive. Skin thickening occurs rapidly, affecting the skin of the elbows or knees and excluding the face. There is a rapid onset of kidney, lung, heart, and gastrointestinal involvement, usually within 1 year of diagnosis. Inflammation of the involved tissue causes fibrosis and collagen deposits in the tissue.

Limited systemic sclerosis is more gradual. Skin thickening affects the face, neck, hands, and feet. Patients may have these symptoms for years before other systemic symptoms appear. The CREST syndrome often accompanies this form of systemic sclerosis.

68. Define the CREST syndrome.

C = **C**alcinosis
R = **R**aynaud's phenomenon
E = **E**sophageal dysmotility
S = **S**clerodactyly
T = **T**elangiectasia

69. What are the clinical manifestations of systemic sclerosis?

Most patients present initially with Raynaud's phenomenon and hand arthralgias or mild inflammatory hand arthritis. Months later skin thickening occurs. The skin looks shiny, taut, and smooth. Physical examination may reveal a speckled pattern on the skin and telangiectasias. Changes in the fingers may include swelling and ulcers on the tips. Progressive face and chest involvement includes limited movement, difficulty with swallowing, and difficulty with breathing. Renal failure, pericarditis, heart failure, pulmonary fibrosis, malnutrition, weight loss, and conduction defects may occur as the disease progresses.

70. How is systemic sclerosis diagnosed?

The diagnosis is based on the presenting skin lesions and appearance. A skin biopsy can confirm the diagnosis. Patients may also have ANA in their blood.

71. Describe the treatment for systemic sclerosis.

The goal of treatment is to treat the complications of the organ dysfunction. Progressive systemic disease is not treatable. Immunosuppressive medications, colchicines, and penicillamine may be tried but are usually not particularly effective.

NSAIDs can help with some of the pain and inflammation. Physical therapy can help prevent contractures. Vasodilators can help the spasms in the hands. Surgery is sometimes needed to debride ulcers or dilate the esophagus.

72. What should the nurse teach patients with systemic sclerosis?
Patients need to be taught to avoid cold exposure and to protect their fingers. They also need to be taught to exercise to prevent contractures and facial rigidity. A smoking cessation program is necessary to minimize the risk of vasoconstriction. The nurse can help patients set up a nutritional program with foods that are easy to swallow, have high calorie and nutrient content, and do not cause diarrhea. Patients should be instructed to practice proper dental hygiene to prevent ulcerations of the mucous membranes and inflammation in the mouth. The nurse should also inform them of the Scleroderma Foundation, which offers information and support for patients and families.

73. How can patients get more information about systemic sclerosis?
Patients can access the Scleroderma Foundation website at <www.scleroderma.org/>.

74. What is polymyositis?
Polymyositis is a diffuse, systemic, inflammatory disease of the symmetric proximal skeletal muscles.

75. How is polymyositis related to dermatomyositis?
Both diseases are subsets of idiopathic inflammatory myopathy, which refers to a group of seven inflammatory muscle diseases. Polymyositis and dermatomyositis are the two most common diseases in this group.

76. What causes polymyositis?
The cause is unknown, but the disease seems to have immunologic triggers. Other possible causes include bacteria, viruses, vaccines, stress, neoplasms, or parasitic agents.

77. Who develops polymyositis?
Adults aged 45–65 years, with a 2:1 ratio of females to males. There is also a juvenile form of the disease.

78. How is polymyositis diagnosed?
Five criteria are used to diagnose polymyositis: muscle weakness; increased creatinine kinase (CK); electromyographic (EMG) changes; muscle biopsy showing fibrosis, necrosis, and regeneration; and the typical skin rash. Patients may present with a history of increasing malaise and muscle weakness. They may have had a fall due to imbalance and may state that they have had skin and nail changes, difficulty with swallowing, palpitations, and a weak cough.

79. Describe the typical skin rash.
Violet or erythematous papules and small plaques at the proximal interphalangeal (PIP) joints; violet, erythematous symmetric rash around eyelids with edema; erythematous, smooth, scaly patches at the PIP joints; irregular, thickened cuticles with telangiectasias in nail beds, calcium nodules on the skin; and erythematous, scaling atrophic rash on the back.

80. What are the other symptoms of polymyositis?
Patients may have stiffness, pain, and redness of the joints. They also may have poor chest expansion and dyspnea as well as arrhythmias.

81. How is polymyositis treated?
High-dose oral corticosteroids are used initially. If they are not effective, intravenous corticosteroids, DMARDs (e.g., methotrexate), or immunosuppressants (e.g., azathioprine) may be used. Patients also need bed rest until the CK returns to normal. Physical therapy is encouraged to prevent contractures.

82. What do I need to teach patients about corticosteroids?
Patients need to be taught about the potential side effects of long-term corticosteroid use, such as increased risk of infection, increased appetite, weight gain, avascular necrosis, diabetes mellitus, bone necrosis, and facial swelling. They need to be taught to watch for sources of infection such as abrasions to the skin, mouth sores, low-grade fevers, and frequent urination. They need to be taught to take medication exactly as prescribed, never changing dose or discontinuing abruptly A medical professional should taper the dose slowly when the medication needs to be stopped. The nurse can also recommend that patients wear an identification tag stating that they are on corticosteroid therapy.

83. As an orthopedic nurse, what else do I need to teach patients with polymyositis?
Patients need to be taught fall prevention measures such as using assistive devices and following a passive and active range-of-motion physical therapy program. They also need to be taught aspiration prevention measures such as eating foods that are easy to swallow, eating in an upright position, and resting before meals.

84. What is Reiter's syndrome?
It is a chronic form of arthritis characterized by inflammation of the joints (arthritis), inflammation of the eyes (conjunctivitis), and inflammation of the genital or urinary system (urethritis or cervicitis) after an infectious disease.

85. What is another name for Reiter's syndrome?
Reiter's syndrome is also called reactive arthritis.

86. What does "reactive" arthritis mean?
This term refers to the theory that some people are genetically predisposed to react to certain bacteria in certain ways. In this case, it is thought that a bacterial infection of the genital, urinary, or gastrointestinal (GI) system triggers the immune system to react by causing subsequent arthritis and conjunctivitis.

87. How long after the infection do the other systemic symptoms appear?
Symptoms usually appear about 1 month after the initial infection.

88. Who is at risk for Reiter's syndrome?
Reiter's syndrome is found primarily in young men, but anyone who has had a recent genitourinary or GI infection and also has the HLA-B27 antigen may develop the disease. HLA-B27 is found in 80% of patients with Reiter's syndrome and is thought to correlate with the severity and chronicity of the syndrome. Males tend to be

affected 2 times more often than females after a genital infection. Males and females develop Reiter's syndrome equally after a GI infection. Children tend to get Reiter's syndrome after a GI infection.

89. Is Reiter's syndrome a severe disease?

Reiter's syndrome is a systemic rheumatic disease that can affect many organs in the body, including the heart, lungs, kidneys, skin, eyes, colon, and spine. It manifests in various levels of severity from mild self-resolving attacks to recurrent and progressively degenerating attacks. It can be progressively debilitating and cause functional disability in 20% of cases. Approximately one-half of patients with Reiter's syndrome eventually have a permanent disability.

90. How is Reiter's syndrome diagnosed?

On the basis of clinical signs and symptoms and history of infection. HLA-B27 is drawn to confirm the presence of the antigen. Urethral swabs can confirm the presence of a genital infection.

91. Do all patients with Reiter's syndrome have the triad of classic symptoms?

No. Less than 30% of patients have all three signs at time of diagnosis. Some patients also develop skin lesions on the genitals or feet.

92. Once the initial infection is treated, do the symptoms of Reiter's syndrome resolve?

Not necessarily. There is no cure for Reiter's syndrome. Treatment is symptomatic only; it has not been found to change the course of the disease. Patients can experience chronic, recurrent attacks. The bacterial infection is treated with antibiotics. The arthritis is treated with NSAIDs, physical therapy, and orthotic assistive devices. The conjunctivitis is treated with antibiotic eye drops. Prophylactic antibiotic treatment is controversial. Occasionally patients need knee surgery for persistent effusions and popliteal cysts that develop as a result of the disease.

93. As an orthopedic nurse, what do I need to teach patients with Reiter's syndrome?

Patients need to be taught to manage and understand the chronicity of the disease. They need to have a home exercise program that optimizes joint protection and energy conservation. The nurse should advise patients to practice safe sex and to avoid multiple partners as well as to follow a regular skin care program.

94. What is fibromyalgia?

It is a chronic, complex syndrome of fatigue and widespread nonarticular musculoskeletal pain that is noninflammatory, nonprogressive, and nondegenerative.

95. What causes fibromyalgia?

The cause is unknown. Research has investigated viruses and musculature abnormalities as potential causes, but at this point no definitive cause has been identified.

96. Can certain foods trigger exacerbations of fibromyalgia?

Yes. Foods such as dairy products, caffeine, wheat or corn cereals, citrus, and yeast are thought to trigger exacerbations.

97. What is the patient population?

About 80–90% of cases affect women, usually in their middle-aged years. Fibromyalgia has also been diagnosed in children.

98. Describe the clinical presentation of fibromyalgia.

Patients complain of pain, insomnia, fatigue, morning stiffness, and weakness. They have pain at 11 or more trigger points that are digitally palpated. They may also have localized erythema after point palpation and may have an anxious or flat affect.

99. What are the locations of the 18 specific trigger points?

Bilateral occiput	Bilateral low cervical
Bilateral trapezius	Bilateral second rib
Bilateral supraspinatus	Bilateral lateral epicondyle
Bilateral gluteal	Bilateral knee
Bilateral greater trochanter	

100. Describe the medical treatment for fibromyalgia.

Analgesics such as tramadol (Ultram), cyclobenzaprine (Flexeril), and capsaicin cream can be used for pain management. Local anesthteic or cortisone injections into trigger point areas can also relieve painful soft tissues and stop muscle spasms. NSAIDs have not been found to be particularly effective for fibromyalgia pain. Other medications may be used to help improve sleep, such as low-dose tricyclic antidepressants, low-dose selective serotonin reuptake inhibitors, and benzodiazepines. Amitriptyline (Elavil), fluoxetine (Prozac), and zolpidem (Ambien) are commonly used for sleep.

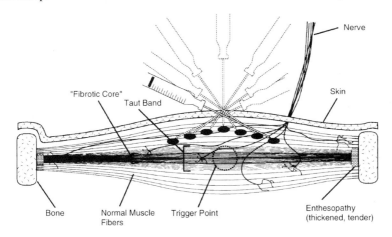

Under sterile conditions, using a 25- or 27-gauge needle, trigger points can be injected with 1-2 cc of a local anesthetic (e.g., lidocaine or a combination of lidocaine and bupivacaine). (From Lennard TA: Pain Procedures in Clinical Practice, 2nd ed. Philadelphia, Hanley & Belfus, 2000, with permission.)

101. What other interventions are used for treatment of fibromyalgia?

Other interventions that can be tried include low-impact aerobic exercise, physical therapy, relaxation techniques, transcutaneous electrical nerve stimulation (TENS), massage therapy, reflexology, acupuncture, heat therapy, herbal therapy (e.g., St.

John's wort), stress management, visualization, meditation, various health food nutrients, and a dietary supplement called S-adenosyl-methionine (SAM-e).

102. Is it true that fibromyalgia is not considered a true physical diagnosis and that it is more psychological in origin?

No. Fibromyalgia is recognized as a true physical condition, not just a psychological condition. Orthopedic nurses need to understand and emphasize this point because many patients with fibromyalgia feel that no one takes them or their multiple complaints seriously. They often feel helpless, frustrated, and depressed because of their symptoms. They need to be instructed about specific symptomatic treatment so that they can manage the disease and decrease feelings of helplessness and frustration. In addition, they also need emotional support so that they can shift negative feelings to self-efficacy and hope.

103. What else should the nurse teach patients with fibromyalgia?

Nurses should educate patients about the chronic effects of fibromyalgia. Nurses should discuss techniques that optimize an effective sleep program and instruct patients in an effective exercise program. They should discuss medications, methods of managing symptoms, and potential side effect. Nurses can review nutritional aspects of the disease, such as food triggers, food nutrients, and dietary supplements. They should offer emotional support and discuss the patient's support systems. Nurses can also teach patients about time management and activity prioritization to ensure meaningful work balanced with leisure activities.

104. Where can patients obtain additional information about fibromyalgia?

They can access the National Databank for Rheumatic Diseases website at <www.fibromyalgia.org>.

BIBLIOGRAPHY

1. Bullough PG: Orthopedic Pathology, 3rd ed. London, Mosby-Wolfe, 1997.
2. Crowther CL: The effects of corticosteroids on the musculoskeletal system. Orthop Nurs 20(6):33-37, 2001.
3. Maher AB, Salmond SW, Pellino TA: Orthopedic Nursing, 3rd ed. Philadelphia, W.B. Saunders, 2002.
4. Salter RB: Textbook of Disorders and Injuries of the Musculoskeletal System, 3rd ed. Baltimore, Williams & Wilkins, 1999.
5. Schoen DC: Core Curriculum for Orthopedic Nurses, 4th ed. Pittman, NJ, Anthony J. Jannetti, 2001.
6. Turkoski BB: Orthopedic patients and the risk for peptic ulcer disease. Orthop Nurs 21:70-74, 2002.

5. METABOLIC BONE DISEASE

Linda A. LaRocco, RN, MS, ANP-C

1. What are the basic steps of bone metabolism?

Bone formation (osteogenesis) involves three main steps: production of the extra-cellular organic matrix (osteoid); mineralization of the matrix to form bone; and bone remodeling, or metabolism, by two processes called resorption and formation. Two types of cells accomplish bone renewal: the osteoblasts, which are involved in bone formation, and the osteoclasts, which are involved in bone resorption. Osteoblasts aid in the synthesis of bone matrix, or collagen, and the osteoclasts absorb mineral matrix, or old bone.

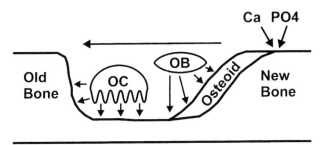

Process of bone formation. OC = osteoclast, OB = osteoblast, Ca = calcium, PO4 = phosphate. (From McDermott MT (ed): Endocrine Secrets, 3rd ed. Philadelphia, Hanley & Belfus, 2002, with permission.)

2. How does bone mass change as people age?

Bone remodeling is a lifelong process during which old bone is removed (resorption) and new bone is created (formation). As people progress through childhood and into adulthood, bones become larger, heavier, and denser. Bone mass increases until the age of 20–25 years, at which time it reaches the maximum bone density and strength, or peak bone mass. Bone mass remains unchanged for several years, during which there is equilibrium between bone formation and resorption. In postmenopausal women, bone mass starts to decrease.

3. What affects bone metabolism?

Bone formation and resorption are influenced by many factors. For example, parathyroid hormone (PTH) can affect calcium metabolism and increase the recruitment and structure of osteoblasts and osteoclasts. If the PTH level is too high, bone turnover accelerates. In people with a deficiency of vitamin D, the bone cycle is accelerated and results in bone loss. Vitamin D can increase the recruitment of osteoclasts and also aids in the mineralization of bone matrix. Too little vitamin D can impair mineralization, and an excess of vitamin D can cause bone loss. Other factors involved in bone remodeling include estrogens, calcitonin, glucocorticoids, progesterone, and androgens. Certain metabolic bone diseases may result from disturbances in the matrix, the process of remodeling, or endocrine, nutritional, or other factors that regulate skeletal and mineral equilibrium. Disorders can be hereditary or acquired and usually affect the complete skeleton. Acquired metabolic bone diseases are most common and include hyper- and hypoparathyroidism, Paget's disease of bone, osteoporosis, gout, osteomalacia, and rickets.

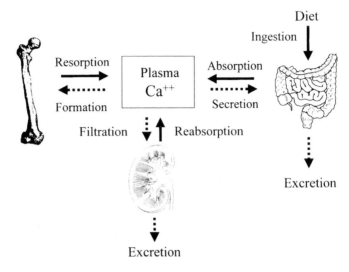

Calcium metabolism. (From McDermott MT (ed): Endocrine Secrets, 3rd ed. Philadelphia, Hanley & Belfus, 2002, with permission.)

4. What are the parathyroid glands?

The parathyroid glands are four small glands located in the neck on the posterior thyroid gland. These glands secrete PTH, which helps to maintain balance of the body's calcium and phosphorus.

5. What happens if the parathyroid glands secrete too much hormone?

The level of calcium in the blood rises (hypercalcemia). Increased calcium levels are a clue for health care providers to consider the cause. In addition, calcium increases in the blood may stimulate calcium loss from bones and excessive absorption of calcium from food. Urinary calcium may be increased and cause the formation of kidney stones.

6. What can cause hypercalcemia?

Possible causes of hypercalcemia include parathyroid adenoma (a benign tumor), enlarged parathyroid glands, and cancer of the parathyroids.

7. What causes hyperparathyroidism?

The causes of hyperparathyroidism include a benign adenoma. Many cases are idiopathic or unknown. Hyperparathyroidism can occur in patients with a family history of the disease.

8. How prevalent is hyperparathyroidism?

Approximately 100,000 people in the United States develop the disease annually. Women are affected more than men (2:1 female-to-male ratio). The risk of developing the disease increases with age.

9. Describe the symptoms of hyperparathyroidism.

Although symptoms do not always occur, they can range from mild (e.g., aches, pains, weakness, fatigue) to severe (e.g., nausea, vomiting, constipation, anorexia, confusion, polydipsia, polyuria). If bone thinning occurs, the person is at high risk for fractures. There is also an increased incidence of kidney stones due to the increase in calcium in the urine.

10. How is hyperparathyroidism diagnosed?

An increase in blood calcium (hypercalcemia) should lead the health care provider to check the blood level of PTH. Further testing should be done to determine whether the patient has suffered any complications of the disease, such as a bone density test to evaluate bone loss and testing for kidney damage and/or stones.

11. Describe the treatment for hyperparathyroidism.

The surgical treatment for hyperparathyroidism is excision of the enlarged gland(s). Excision is usually reserved for patients with symptomatic disease. If the disease is mild and asymptomatic, patients may require only periodic monitoring to avoid complications.

12. What nursing interventions are appropriate for patients with hyperparathyroidism?

For hospitalized patients with hyperparathyroidism, nursing interventions include administering medications as prescribed, monitoring intake and output, and monitoring vital signs. The nurse should encourage adequate hydration to promote calcium excretion and avoid fluid deficit. The nurse should also monitor for signs of volume overload and assess the lower extremities for pedal edema.

13. How should the nurse educate patients with hyperparathyroidism?

In light of the potential for multiple complications, patients with hyperparathyroidism need to be fully informed about their diagnosis. They should know the names, dosages, and possible side effects of medications and when to follow up with the health care provider. The patient and family also need to be aware of signs and symptoms of hypocalcemia. Fluid balance must be maintained and monitored. In the case of surgical excision of the glands, the nurse may be asked to teach postoperative wound care and may have to interpret test results for the patient and family as well as arrange for follow-up care.

14. What happens if the parathyroid glands secrete too little PTH?

If the parathyroid secretes too little PTH, a condition called hypoparathyroidism occurs. Hypoparathyroidism causes serum hypocalcemia, which may result in tetany. Tetany causes painful muscle spasms and tremors. In addition, hypoparathyroidism can lead to metabolic alkalosis, decreased bone resorption, altered mental state, and symptoms similar to Parkinson syndrome.

15. What causes hypoparathyroidism?

Causes include accidental surgical removal of the parathyroid gland in conjunction with thyroidectomy, irradiation of the parathyroid, genetic absence of the gland, or idiopathic causes. Cancer, trauma, or tuberculosis can also cause the disease. Disorders that affect vitamin D availability in the body can lead to hypoparathyroidism. Examples include pancreatitis, renal disease, liver disease, and surgery of the stomach or intestines. A history of alcohol abuse can predispose a person to hypoparathyroidism.

16. How prevalent is hypoparathyroidism?

The exact occurrence in the United States is unknown. Hypoparathyroidism is very rare, occurs equally in men and women, and may affect all ages. Children tend to develop forms of the disease that are correctable or reversible, whereas adults tend to develop forms of the disease that are irreversible.

17. Describe the symptoms of hypoparathyroidism.

In addition to tetany, other symptoms of hypoparathyroidism and subsequent hypocalcemia include weakness, muscle cramps, paresthesias of the hands, excessive nervousness, loss of memory, headaches, malformations of the teeth, and malformed fingernails. Patients may develop very brisk deep tendon reflexes and possibly a positive Chvostek's sign. Some hypoparathyroid patients may also develop pernicious anemia, dry and coarse skin, alopecia, vitiligo, and mental depression. Patients may have short stature and short metacarpal bones. A patient can develop cardiovascular symptoms, including congestive heart failure, tachycardia, and prolonged QT and/or ST interval.

18. How is hypoparathyroidism diagnosed?

Investigation of the presenting symptoms leads the health care provider to order serum PTH levels. Common lab findings include decreases in serum calcium, alkaline phosphatase, vitamin D, and urinary calcium. Potentially increased lab findings include serum phosphorus, magnesium, chloride, uric acid, and creatinine. An electrocardiogram (EKG) is also beneficial, because the condition can cause cardiac problems such as prolonged QT interval, decreased myocardial contraction, or first-degree heart block

19. Describe the treatment for hypoparathyroidism.

Treatment consists of the administration of calcium supplements and vitamin D to increase the absorption of calcium and help to maintain normal blood calcium levels. This treatment is lifelong.

20. What nursing interventions are appropriate for patients with hypoparathyroidism?

As a result of hypocalcemia, patients with hypoparathyroidism may experience integumentary changes, including dry skin. This condition requires appropriate skin care, such as turning patients on bed rest every 2 hours, using special devices to relieve pressure, and monitoring skin integrity (especially over bony prominences) for changes in skin condition.

Because patients with hypoparathyroidism are at risk for seizures, maintenance of seizure precautions is imperative. Suction equipment must be readily available, and the bed rails should be padded for patients with ongoing seizures. The nurse must administer antiseizure medications as ordered.

21. How should the nurse educate patients with hypoparathyroidism?

As with any other disease, the nurse must provide the patient and family with pertinent and current information about the condition, including instructions for medication administration, diet, and skin care. The patient and family also need to be aware of the importance of frequent follow-up appointments and monitoring of serum calcium and kidney function, EKG changes, and bone density changes.

22. What is Paget's disease?

Paget's disease, also called osteitis deformans, is a metabolic bone disease. It is a skeletal disorder affecting bone turnover and resulting in excessive resorption and destruction of bone followed by subsequent abnormal repair. It typically affects the cranium, pelvis, spine, and long bones and slowly worsens over time.

23. What causes Paget's disease?

Abnormal osteoclasts reproduce, causing disproportionate resorption of bone. The rapid pace of resorption prevents normal bone formation. Instead of normal new bone, fibrous tissue is formed, increasing the thickness of bones. With abnormal bone resorption and formation, the surface of the bone becomes irregular and coarse.

24. How prevalent is Paget's disease?

Paget's disease affects males and females equally. It usually occurs in people over age 40. In the United States it is estimated to affect approximately 1–2% of the population.

25. What are the symptoms of Paget's disease?

The mild form of Paget's disease is asymptomatic. Later in the disease, symptoms may include bone pain, headaches, tinnitus, vertigo, and hearing loss. In more advanced cases the pain can be severe. As the disease progresses, bones may bend, the skull may become larger, and the spinal column may arch. Arching of the spinal column can cause the thoracic spine to become kyphotic. Pressure on nerves caused by enlarged bones can result in muscle weakness. If the skull becomes excessively enlarged, the result can be deafness, vision disturbances, dizziness, and tinnitus.

26. Are multiple bones always affected by Paget's disease?

Not in all cases. If only one bone is affected, the structure may become disfigured and the bone weakens, resulting in mild pain and stiffness. In bones subjected to the most stress, such as the femur, pelvis, and lower spine, pathologic fractures may occur.

27. How is Paget's disease diagnosed?

The disease is diagnosed by x-ray and/or bone scan, both of which show bone deformities. Serum alkaline phosphatase is elevated. Urinary hydroxyproline is elevated, and elevated urinary calcium can aid in the diagnosis and estimation of resorption. These tests are not specific for Paget's disease and may be influenced by other factors. Bone densitometry is used to measure bone mass. Bone densitometry measurements can estimate the risk of fracture. Bone biopsy may be performed if cancer or osteomyelitis is suspected.

28. How is Paget's disease treated?

Treatment includes the administration of drugs called bisphosphonates, which inhibit osteoclast-mediated bone resorption. These drugs include etidronate sodium (Didronel), alendronate sodium (Fosamax), and risedronate sodium (Actonel). A drug that may be used by people who cannot tolerate the bisphosphonates is calcitonin (Miacalcin), which is a nasal spray. Patients should also take daily calcium supplements of at least 1000 mg and 400 units of vitamin D. They should also be sure to get adequate exercise, maintain appropriate weight, and avoid undue stress on affected bones.

29. What are the possible complications of Paget's disease?

Possible complications include pain, deformed bones, degenerative arthritis, and fractures. Surgical replacement may be necessary for joints that are severely affected. The patient with Paget's disease may also develop hypertension, congestive heart failure, and hypercalcemia. Renal calculi, increased urinary calcium, and gout or pseudogout may develop with Paget's disease.

30. What nursing interventions are appropriate for patients with Paget's disease?

The patient and family need to be instructed about the correct way to take medication, including route of administration (teaching injection technique when appropriate). If medications such as alendronate (Fosamax) are prescribed, education includes taking the medication with at least 6 ounces of water on an empty stomach and remaining upright for at least 30 minutes. Also instruct the patient and family about possible medication side effects and interactions.

The nurse must conduct routine pain assessment and instruct the patient and family in the use of pain medication as well as scheduling periods of rest and activity. Teaching also includes fall prevention, nutrition counseling, referral to support services when necessary, and compliance with appropriate follow-up medical and laboratory appointments.

31. What is osteoporosis?

Osteoporosis is a metabolic disorder of bone in which the resorption rate exceeds the formation rate. Bone composition does not change; there is simply not enough of it. The bone becomes increasingly thinned as the disease progresses. The spongy bone usually has a dense honeycomb appearance that thins and is increasingly prone to fractures of the microarchitecture and leads to an overall decreased bony strength. As a result, bones become brittle and are more prone to fracture.

32. What causes osteoporosis?

Osteoporosis can be caused by malignancies or an endocrine disorder, but usually it is the result of aging. Bone loss begins around the age of 25, increases after age 40 and again after menopause. Other factors that influence the progress of the disease include hormone levels, overall physical fitness, and nutritional status. Because estrogen suppresses bone resorption, its decrease after menopause affects bone health.

33. How prevalent is osteoporosis?

More than 10 million people in the United States have osteoporosis, 80% of whom are women. Another 18 million have osteopenia, or a decrease in bone density, which increases the risk for developing osteoporosis. Osteoporosis is the cause of approximately 1.5 million fractures annually in the United States.

34. What are the risk factors for osteoporosis?

The disease can occur at any age, although risk increases with age. Risk is essentially equal for all ethnicities with slightly higher occurrence in Asian and Caucasian females. Additional risks include thin females over 50 years old who smoke and have a family history of osteoporosis. A woman has a higher risk for osteoporosis if she has had early menopause (including surgically induced menopause), late onset of the menstrual cycle, or amenorrhea from excessive exercise or anorexia. Certain medications, such as steroids, anticonvulsants, thyroid hormone, and certain antacids, can predispose the patient to osteoporosis. Other factors that can lead to osteoporosis include dietary calcium or vitamin D deficiency, sedentary lifestyle, and excessive alcohol consumption.

35. Describe the symptoms of osteoporosis.

Osteoporosis is often referred to as a "silent" disease, because bone mass can be lost without the development of symptoms. The first symptom that the patient develops may be a fracture of the wrist or hip from a fall or a vertebral compression fracture.

36. How is osteoporosis diagnosed?

Frequently, the disease is diagnosed only after a fracture occurs. The fracture may involve the hip, wrist, or vertebral body. Compression fracture of the vertebral body can lead to back pain, decreased height, and kyphosis. Osteoporosis is diagnosed by obtaining a bone densitometry, usually with a dual-energy x-ray absorptiometry (DEXA) scan.

37. How is osteoporosis treated?

Treatment is similar to that of Paget's disease. Bisphosphonate drugs are administered as tolerated. Estrogen use is also considered. Research has shown that these drugs increase bone mass, stop bone loss, and produce healthy bones in women who have been diagnosed with postmenopausal osteoporosis.

38. Can osteoporosis be prevented?

Prevention tactics include eating a balanced diet, including adequate amounts of calcium and vitamin D (which enhances absorption of calcium); engaging in a regular exercise program, including strength training; and avoiding the use of tobacco, caffeine, and alcohol. It is very important for adolescents to include ample amounts of calcium in the diet in order to achieve peak bone mass. An increase in dietary calcium is also warranted in women over age 60. The source may be foods or calcium and vitamin D supplements. Calcium intake for children and adolescents 9–18 years old should be 1800 mg/day, whereas adults 19–50 years old should take 1000 mg/day. Adults older than 51 years of age should take 1200–1500 mg/day. For menopausal women, use of estrogen replacement may preserve bone mass, thus preventing future fractures. Good dairy sources of calcium include milk, ice cream, cottage cheese, cheddar cheese, and Swiss cheese. Canned salmon with bones, broccoli, turnip greens, collard greens, and fortified orange juice are also good sources of calcium.

39. What nursing interventions are appropriate for patients with osteoporosis?

Education is essential not only for patients already diagnosed with osteoporosis but also for all women, including adolescent girls. Patients should be instructed to include appropriate amounts of calcium- and vitamin D-containing foods or supplements in their daily regimens. These measures may prevent hip and/or vertebral fractures. Calcium intake alone does not prevent osteoporosis in many cases. Antismoking education is very important as well as avoidance of alcohol and caffeine and an appropriate exercise program.

Fall prevention must be emphasized for the patient diagnosed with osteoporosis. Proper precautions must be initiated in the home. Encouragement of adherence to medication and exercise regimens is also important.

The administration of analgesics, use of massage, and application of heat or cold usually relieve pain due to fractures.

40. What is gout?

Gout is caused by an alteration in purine metabolism. Gout is a form of arthritis in which uric acid crystals are deposited in the joints, resulting in inflammation and extreme pain. The metatarsophalangeal joint of the great toe is the most commonly affected joint.

41. What causes gout?

Gout is caused by an excess of uric acid in the body, which may result from increased production, reduced elimination of uric acid by the kidneys, or an increase in intake of foods containing substances called purines. Purines are metabolized to form uric acid. Foods high in purine include organ meats, sardines, anchovies, herring, mackerel, scallops, and most wild game. Alcoholic beverages may also contribute to an increase in uric acid levels and may cause gout attacks. Gout may also be secondary to other conditions, including hemolytic anemia, psoriasis, renal insufficiency, and sarcoidosis.

42. How prevalent is gout?

Gout affects approximately 275 per 100,000 people; middle-aged males are most likely to develop the condition. Women rarely suffer from gout before menopause.

43. Describe the symptoms of gout.

The symptom that most frequently leads people to seek treatment is severe pain in the affected joint, usually accompanied by swelling, erythema, tenderness, and occasionally fever. Gout can also be asymptomatic, manifested only by the presence of excessive uric acid in the urine (hyperuricemia). The initial attack may subside after several days, even without treatment. In chronic gout, persistent symptoms may occur, including joint deformity. Over time, increased levels of uric acid in the blood can cause deposits around joints. These deposits can become crystal-like in formation and can lead to acute gout attacks. When crystals form in the urinary tract, kidney stones can result. Chronic gout can also result in the formation of tophi, or sodium urate deposits in the affected joint or areas, such as the Achilles tendon or the pinnae of ears.

44. How is gout diagnosed?

A presumptive diagnosis of gout can be based on subjective and objective information; however, a definitive diagnosis may be made only by smear and culture of aspirated joint fluid. The culture rules out infection, and the smear confirms or refutes the presence of urate crystals. Serum uric acid levels are elevated, but this finding is not specific for diagnosis of gout because elevated levels also may be seen in people who take daily low-dose aspirin or diuretics and in some people with renal insufficiency. If blood work is done during an acute attack, the white blood cell count and sedimentation rate may be elevated.

45. Describe the treatment for gout.

Gout is treated with analgesics and hypouricemic agents. Nonsteroidal anti-inflammatory drugs (NSAIDs) are given to manage pain and are considered first-line drugs. They include indomethacin (Indocin) and naproxen (Naprosyn). Agents used to decrease uric acid include allopurinol and probenecid. In addition to pharmacological management, patients are encouraged to decrease weight-bearing on the affected joint and may need joint immobilization.

46. What education is appropriate for patients with gout?

Patients need to be counseled about the importance of adherence to the prescribed medication regimen and medical and laboratory follow-up as well as correct joint immobilization and/or reduced weight-bearing. They should also understand that they need to drink more than 3 liters of fluid per day. Patients at risk for formation of renal calculi may be prescribed medication that alkalizes the urine.

47. What are osteomalacia and rickets?

Osteomalacia is the abnormal softening of bones as a result of lack of calcium or phosphorous in the bone matrix (osteoid). In children, the disease is called rickets, and the osteoid is affected at the growth plates. This discussion uses only the term *osteomalacia*; unless otherwise noted, the information is similar for both conditions.

48. What causes osteomalacia?

Osteomalacia is caused by inadequate dietary intake of vitamin D, lack of exposure to sunlight, or malabsorption of vitamin D (a fat-soluble vitamin) in the intestine. Other possible causes include renal failure, long-term antacid use, side effects of some antiseizure medications, liver disease (i.e., biliary tract obstruction and primary biliary cirrhosis), chronic pancreatitis, intestinal diseases (i.e., ileitis and celiac sprue), and surgical procedures (i.e., gastrectomy or resection of portions of the small intestine). In many of these conditions, intestinal mineral absorption is blocked. In the case of renal disease, the acid level of bodily fluids is increased, and the acids may erode the calcium in the bones, softening them. Osteomalacia is occasionally seen in strict vegetarians. Some patients with hypophosphatemia due to hyperparathyroidism may develop osteomalacia.

49. Describe the symptoms of osteomalacia.

Symptoms include bone pain and malaise. If not treated, osteomalacia causes softening of bones, which can cause pain and physical deformities, ranging from shortened stature to bow legs. Bones are also more prone to fracture. In infants, symptoms of rickets may include nocturnal fever, restlessness, pale skin, diaphoresis, progressive weakness, delayed dentition, and decrease in muscle tone.

50. How is osteomalacia diagnosed?

Patients with a mild-to-moderate deficiency of vitamin D may have symptoms typical of osteoporosis. However, the serum calcium level is low or low normal, the serum alkaline phosphatase level is high, and the serum phosphorus level is low. Radiographic findings are typically nonspecific. Abnormalities of the vertebrae are similar to those seen in osteoporosis. Bone densitometry is not of particular value in the diagnosis of osteomalacia, because results may be normal or even high because of the accumulation of partially mineralized osteoid. A bone biopsy may be done to arrive at a definitive diagnosis.

51. How is osteomalacia treated?

The treatment of osteomalacia depends on its cause. For patients who are suffering from vitamin D deficiency, treatment includes dietary and supplemental intake of adequate amounts of vitamin D. If malabsorption is the cause, osteomalacia is treated with oral or parenteral administration of vitamin D and possibly surgery to correct any causative intestinal disease. If the cause is found to be hypophosphatemia, phosphate replacement is necessary. Because phosphate can cause diarrhea, measures must be taken to minimize this effect. In all cases of osteomalacia, patients must maintain adequate intakes of calcium (1000–1500 mg/day).

52. What education is appropriate for patients with osteomalacia or rickets?

As with other metabolic diseases, patients need to be aware of appropriate nutritional measures, such as including sources of calcium and vitamin D in the diet and supplementation when prescribed. Also important in vitamin D deficiency is the need for adequate exposure to sunlight, which triggers vitamin D synthesis in the skin.

Patients and families need instruction about medical follow-up and laboratory testing, including the need for lifelong monitoring for liver, kidney, or gastrointestinal diseases. Vegetarians need counseling about appropriate vitamin D supplementation. It is important to advise patients of the need for regular weight-bearing activities for at least 30 minutes 3 times per week. For parents of children with rickets, teaching should include safety measures in the home, avoidance of accidents and injuries, and awareness of signs and symptoms needing intervention.

BIBLIOGRAPHY

1. Barnett G: A Tour around Paget's Disease of Bone. Available at <http://www.inpharm.com/netfocus/tours/medicaltours/tour_104.html>.
2. Bone Remodeling, 2001. Available at <http://www.medes.fr/Eristo/Osteoporosis/BoneRemodeling.html>.
3. Burke S: Boning up on osteoporosis. Nursing 2001 31(10):36, 2001.
4. Marieb E: Human Anatomy and Physiology, 2nd ed. Redwood City, CA, Benjamin/Cummings Publishing Co, 1992.
5. Mellors RC: Metabolic Bone Diseases, 1999. Available at <http://edcenter.med.cornell.edu/CUMC_PathNotes/Skeletal/Bone_04.html>.
6. National Institutes of Health Osteoporosis and Related Bone Diseases-National Resource Center: Paget's Disease of Bone, 2002. Available at <http://www.osteo.org/paget.asp>.
7. Porth CM: Pathophysiology: Concepts of Altered Health States, 3rd ed. Philadelphia, J. B. Lippincott, 1990.
8. Raisz LG: Metabolic bone disease. In Beers MH, Berkow R (eds): The Merck Manual of Geriatrics. Whitehouse Station, NJ, Merck, 2002.
9. Schoen DC: NAON Core Curriculum for Orthopaedic Nursing, 4th ed. Pittman, NJ, Anthony J. Jannetti, 2001.
10. Taber's Cyclopedic Medical Dictionary. Philadelphia, F. A. Davis, 1997
11. Uphold C, Graham M: Clinical Guidelines in Adult Health, 2nd ed. Gainesville, FL, Barmarrae Books, 1999.

6. INFECTIOUS CONDITIONS

Michael E. Zychowicz, RN, MS, NP-C

1. What are the human body's major defense mechanisms against infection?

The mechanical and chemical barriers of the skin and mucous membranes are extremely important in protection against infection. In addition to skin and mucous membranes, the body's inflammatory and immune responses are essential to fight off infection.

2. In general, how is the immune response different from the inflammatory response?

The inflammatory response is nonspecific and is activated relatively fast. The immune response is targeted against a specific foreign antigen and may take days to develop.

3. What is the purpose of the immune and inflammatory responses?

- Destroy an organism
- Limit damage to a certain area
- Prevent reproduction of an organism
- Clear debris and lay the groundwork for healing

4. What occurs when the inflammatory response is activated?

After any cellular injury, including that from an invading microorganism, the inflammatory response is activated. The main activators/mediators of the inflammatory response are the degranulation of mast cells; activation of the complement, clotting, and kinin systems; and release of cellular components of injured cells. The vascular component of acute inflammation is characterized by initial vasoconstriction near the site of injury, followed by vasodilation of arterioles and capillaries. This response leads to increased blood flow to the area, increased hydrostatic pressure, and increased capillary permeability, which causes plasma to move out of the blood vessels. The results are characteristic erythema, edema, and warmth of infection and inflammation.

Neutrophils, monocytes, and macrophages (phagocytes) are attracted to the inflammatory site by chemotactic factors. Neutrophils arrive first at 6–24 hours; monocytes arrive approximately 24–48 hours after injury. Margination occurs when phagocytes adhere to the blood vessel walls. The next step is emigration, when phagocytes slip out of the blood vessels through endothelial junctions into the tissues. Phagocytosis occurs as the white blood cell recognizes and attaches to the organism or antigen. The organism is engulfed, and degranulation, with release of destructive lysosomes, leads to death of the invading microorganism.

5. Discuss the role of the clotting cascade and the kinin and complement systems in inflammation.

When the **clotting cascade** is activated, it forms a mesh of fibrin to trap organisms and foreign bodies. It also provides a framework for healing as well as creates a clot to stop any bleeding.

The **kinin system** adds to vasodilation and vascular permeability as well as causes pain fiber stimulation.

The **complement system** has many purposes in the inflammatory process. First, it causes coating of organisms (opsonization), making them attractive to neutrophils and macrophages. Next, it attracts white blood cells by chemotaxis to the site of inflammation. Mast cells are also stimulated to degranulate by the complement system. Lastly, complement can directly lyse foreign microorganisms, leading to their destruction.

6. Summarize the role of the mast cell.

The mast cell is one of the main stimulators of the inflammatory response. By degranulating and releasing histamine, it immediately causes vasodilation and capillary permeability, leading to exudate formation. The mast cell also attracts neutrophils and eosinophils by releasing chemotactic factor. With prolonged inflammation, mast cells synthesize prostaglandin E and leukotrienes. Prostaglandin E leads to vasodilation, capillary permeability, and pain fiber stimulation, whereas leukotrienes cause vasodilation and capillary permeability.

7. Explain the two mechanisms of immune response to a foreign antigen.

The immune system is divided into the humoral and cell-mediated responses. The primary white blood cell of the humoral immune system is the B-lymphocyte. The T-lymphocyte is the primary white blood cell for the cell-mediated immune response. As a nonself antigen is identified by the immune system, the body's response is to activate the cell-mediated and humoral immune systems.

8. How does the humoral immune system operate?

As a B-lymphocyte encounters a foreign antigen for the first time, it becomes activated, divides, and differentiates into plasma cells. Plasma cells are located in the lymph nodes, spleen, and blood and at sites of inflammation. Plasma cells produce antibodies with specificity to the foreign antigen initially encountered. Antibodies can be released into the circulation and mucosal surfaces of the body. In addition to plasma cells, activated B-lymphocytes produce memory cells that ensure a more rapid and stronger antibody response when the specific antigen appears again.

9. What exactly do antibodies do?

Antibodies are glycoproteins produced by B-lymphocyte plasma cells. Antibodies, or immunoglobulins, have several primary functions in their protection of the body:
- Antibodies opsonize specific bacteria as well as activate the complement cascade. Thus, the inflammatory response is activated and makes the bacteria more recognizable, enabling phagocytosis.
- Antibodies attach to specific viral antigens. This action blocks the ability of viral antigens to attach to and enter a host cell, leaving them either to agglutinate or to be destroyed by phagocytes.
- Antibodies attach to the antigens of bacterial toxins, forming antigen-antibody complexes. This process enables the removal of the toxins and blocks binding to tissues where toxic effects can take place.

10. Describe the cell-mediated immune response.

T-lymphocytes are activated and proliferated in essentially the same way as the B-lymphocytes. A T-cell encounters a foreign antigen, becomes sensitized, then divides and develops into activated T-cells and memory cells. In addition to the memory cells, the specific types of T-lymphocytes include cytotoxic T-cells, helper T-cells, suppressor T-cells, and lymphokine-producing T-cells. The cytotoxic T-cells directly attack cells with the specific foreign antigens that they have been sensitized to recognize. Helper T-cells assist, and suppressor T-cells impede both the cell-mediated and the humoral immune response. As the name implies, the lymphokine-producing T-cells produce lymphokines, which act as a chemical messenger to stimulate other cells in the immune/inflammatory response.

11. Define cellulitis.
Cellulitis is an infection of the skin and subcutaneous tissues.

12. What infectious organisms usually cause cellulitis?
Streptococcal or staphylococcal bacteria are the usual causes of cellulitis infections.

13. What does the nurse usually find on physical exam of patients with cellulitis?
The patient with cellulitis usually presents with erythema, induration, fluctuance, edema, and pain. The patient may also exhibit fever, chills, and lymphadenopathy.

14. How does cellulitis develop?
Impaired skin integrity is one of the more common causes of cellulitis. It can result from any disruption of the skin, including a burn, laceration, abrasion, ulceration, intravenous line site, or surgical incision site.

15. Describe the usual treatments for cellulitis.
Adult patients with uncomplicated cellulitis can be treated with oral antibiotics for 7–10 days. An initial dose of a parenteral antibiotic may be warranted for uncomplicated yet more extensive infections. If the patient has significant underlying medical problems (e.g., diabetes) and severe cellulitis in addition to systemic symptoms, treatment should include parenteral antibiotics followed by oral antibiotic therapy after the infection has been diminished. The treating health care provider determines whether to treat the patient on an inpatient or outpatient basis based on the severity of the cellulitis and the existence of underlying medical problems.

16. Summarize the education of patients with cellulitis.
Patients should be instructed to keep all wounds clean and dry. The nurse should educate the patient about wound care and dressing changes as well as any medications or treatments. Patients with underlying medical conditions, such as diabetes, should receive education specific to their disease. The patient should also notify the health care provider if the infection worsens or does not respond to antibiotic therapy.

17. Define necrotizing fasciitis.
Necrotizing fasciitis is an extremely serious infection of the fascia that extends into the muscle. It can develop at the site of any disruption in skin integrity. The usual infectious organism is *Streptococcus* species. Other organisms that can cause necrotizing soft tissue infection include several fungi, anaerobic bacteria, gram-negative rods, and gram-positive cocci.

18. Why is necrotizing fasciitis such a serious concern?

Necrotizing fasciitis can be quite painful and spread quickly. Even if identified early and treated aggressively, necrotizing soft tissue infections can cause the patient to become septic and may ultimately end in death.

19. Describe the typical presentation of necrotizing fasciitis.

Initially, the infection may be difficult to differentiate from cellulitis; the patient may simply develop pain, erythema, edema, and warmth. This syndrome progresses rapidly to necrosis of the fascia and surrounding muscle, with bullae formation on the skin and watery discharge. The skin develops a bronze or purplish color and eventually becomes necrotic and sloughs. The patient can also develop gas, produced by the bacteria, within the tissues. The gas may be palpated as crepitus. Other signs and symptoms include confusion, fever, chills, hypotension, tachycardia, tachypnea, and decreased urinary output. Eventually the patient may develop multisystem organ failure and die.

20. Which diagnostic tests are useful in identifying and treating necrotizing fasciitis?

Gram stain, culture, and possibly biopsy determine what organism(s) is (are) responsible for the infection. Magnetic resonance imaging (MRI) or computed tomography (CT) scan can demonstrate the extent of the tissue involvement. An x-ray can be useful in the identification of gas within the tissues. Blood work usually shows an elevated white blood cell count. The patient may also show metabolic acidosis, electrolyte disturbance, dehydration, hypoalbuminemia, and dehydration.

21. How is necrotizing fasciitis treated?

The cornerstone of treatment includes broad-spectrum antibiotic administration with surgical debridement of the wounds. Nutritional and physiologic support is essential. If available, hyperbaric oxygen therapy may prove to be a useful adjunct. Proper and adequate pain management by the nurse is extremely important. The nurse should educate the family and patient about all treatments and medications and about the importance of proper nutrition. Depending on the patient's capacity and physical condition, wound care and dressing changes can be taught to the patient and/or family to assist the nurse with wound care and to prepare for eventual home care.

22. Which patients are predisposed to developing necrotizing soft tissue infections?

The patients with the highest incidence of necrotizing fasciitis are morbidly obese or diabetic. Other conditions that increase the incidence of necrotizing fasciitis include burns, trauma, foreign bodies, immunocompromise, intravenous drug use, surgery, and vascular disease.

23. Define osteomyelitis.

Osteomyelitis is an infection of the bone, which can frequently involve the marrow and surrounding tissue. The infection can be either chronic or acute. An organism causing osteomyelitis can be introduced by a hematogenous route, which often originates from a simple dental abscess, otitis media, or sinusitis. Spread from a neighboring infection to the bone is possible when the patient has cellulitis or infected bursitis. Bacteria can be seeded into the bony tissue after trauma, including open fractures or animal bites. Osteomyelitis can develop after surgical procedures with poor aseptic technique, poor wound care postoperatively, or inadequate pin care for patients with percutaneous pins.

24. Describe the pathophysiologic development of osteomyelitis.

The pathophysiology of osteomyelitis is essentially the same for all routes of infection. After the bone becomes infected, an inflammatory reaction occurs within the bone. The edema and exudate from the inflammatory response lead to sluggishness and thrombosis of the blood supply as well as blockage of the canaliculi within the bone. Decreased blood supply to the infected area of bone leads to necrosis. As the inflammatory response continues and exudate accumulates within the marrow, pressure increases within the bone, further compromising blood supply. The infection and exudate extend into the subperiosteal space, causing an abscess. As a result of the abscess, the periosteum lifts from the bone, disrupting blood supply through that area and further contributing to necrosis. Lifting of the periosteum occurs more frequently in children because the adult periosteum is more strongly attached to the bone. Adults, however, have a greater incidence of pathologic fracture through the osteomyelitis because of weakening of the cortical bone. The area of dead infected bone is called a sequestrum. Osteoblasts are stimulated to develop an involucrum, which is new bone surrounding the area of the sequestrum. Exudate may develop channels to the skin, where it can drain via sinus tracts.

25. What infectious agents most commonly cause osteomyelitis?

Osteomyelitis may be due to fungus, virus, bacteria, or parasite. The most common causative agent in adults is *Staphylococcus aureus*. In young children, *Haemophilus influenzae* is the most common offending organism. *Salmonella* species typically cause osteomyelitis in patients with sickle cell disease, whereas in patients with implanted orthopedic devices *Staphylococcus epidermidis* tends to be the offending organism. Osteomyelitis from animal bites is usually due to *Pasteurella multocida*, whereas osteomyelitis from human bites is usually due to *S. aureus*.

26. Describe the findings in the history and physical exam of patients with osteomyelitis.

Patients may have a history of a surgical procedure, open fracture, recent systemic infection, skin trauma, or infection. The patient may also have a past history of osteomyelitis, which has been inadequately treated. In addition, the patient may have other factors that increase the risk of developing osteomyelitis.

Symptoms obviously vary, depending on the site and extent of infection. Patients with acute osteomyelitis may exhibit acute onset of pain at the infected site, fever, and chills. Patients, especially children, may not bear weight on the infected limb. Back pain may be present if the spine is the site of osteomyelitis.

If untreated or inadequately treated, the infection progresses from acute to chronic. Chronic osteomyelitis may present with recurrent exacerbations of discomfort, and the skin may show erythema and edema with draining sinuses or abscesses.

27. Describe the x-ray findings in patients with osteomyelitis.

The x-ray of a patient with a bone infection usually shows no overt changes for up to 4 weeks after the infection. The x-rays are not necessarily useful in the early diagnosis of acute osteomyelitis; however, they may prove useful in diagnosing a pathologic fracture at the site of infection. As the infection progresses, x-ray findings include periosteal elevation and lytic lesions of the bone showing cortical defects and areas of bony destruction; reactive periosteal bone formation is seen as thickening of the periosteum. The soft tissues show edema with displacement of the usual fat lines.

28. Is an MRI or CT scan useful in the diagnosis of osteomyelitis?

Yes. Both MRI and CT scan are useful in making the diagnosis of osteomyelitis as well as assessing the extent of the infection. These tests can help make a diagnosis early in the infectious process and aid in differentiating between soft tissue infection and osteomyelitis.

29. Discuss the benefit of obtaining a bone scan for patients with osteomyelitis.

The bone scan is useful in diagnosing early acute osteomyelitis. The bone scan may show an area of increased uptake at the infection site within 1–3 days after the onset of infection. Early identification allows early treatment of the infection. If the patient is already diagnosed with osteomyelitis, the bone scan provides no additional valuable information.

30. What changes in lab data are seen in patients with osteomyelitis?

Common changes include a high erythrocyte sedimentation rate (ESR), elevated levels of C-reactive protein, and an elevated white blood cell count. Anemia may also be present in patients with chronic osteomyelitis.

31. Describe the management of osteomyelitis.

- For acute osteomyelitis the patient is usually treated with antibiotic therapy. Soft tissue or bony abscess drainage can produce significant pain relief. A surgeon may choose to debride the wound.
- In patients with chronic osteomyelitis, antibiotic therapy and surgical debridement are the usual course of treatment. Any dead space that remains after surgical debridement can be filled with tissue transfer. Antibiotic beads can be placed within the infected bone.
- Hyperbaric oxygen therapy may be used as an adjunct in treating chronic or acute osteomyelitis.

32. Summarize the nursing considerations in treating patients with osteomyelitis.

- Assess and manage pain.
- Educate patients about the disease process, treatment, and medications.
- Teach and provide proper wound care, dressing changes, and infection control.
- Assess and ensure proper nutrition.
- Teach and assist with range-of-motion exercises, or obtain an order for physical therapy

33. Do adults and children typically develop hematogenous osteomyelitis at different sites?

Yes. Adult patients develop hematogenous osteomyelitis more frequently in the small bones, pelvis, and spine. Children develop hematogenous osteomyelitis more frequently in the tibia, humerus, and femur.

34. Define septic arthritis.

Septic arthritis is an infection of a joint leading to rather serious complications. Septic arthritis is more common in adults than children. The infecting organism is introduced most commonly through hematogenous spread; however, spread may also result from a neighboring infection, such as osteomyelitis or cellulitis. Infection can also be caused by direct introduction from a puncture wound, trauma, laceration, fracture, or surgical procedure.

35. What organisms are typically responsible for septic arthritis?
The most prevalent infecting organisms are *Staphylococcus aureus* and streptococci in adults. *Neisseria gonorrhoeae* is another possible infecting agent in sexually active patients. Children are usually infected by *Haemophilus influenzae*. For patients with prosthetic joints, Staphylococcus epidermidis, *S. aureus*, *Pseudomonas* species, streptococci, and *Escherichia coli* are common infecting organisms.

36. Describe the history and physical findings in patients with septic arthritis.
The patient with septic arthritis usually complains of swelling, erythema, and warmth at a joint. General malaise, pain at the infected joint, fever, and chills are typical symptoms. A patient may guard the infected and painful extremity. If a joint in the lower extremity is infected, the patient may not bear weight on the affected leg or may walk with a limp because of the pain. Infants and children may be anorexic and irritable. The patient may also have limited active and passive range of motion at the infected joint. The examiner can elicit pain on palpation of the joint and may palpate a joint effusion.

37. Which joints are most frequently infected?
The patient with nongonococcal septic arthritis typically complains of monoarticular pain, most frequently involving the knee, hip, and shoulder. The knees are the most frequently infected joints in adults and the hip and knee in children. Patients with gonococcal septic arthritis often have polyarthralgia of the feet, ankles, hands, and wrists.

38. How is septic arthritis diagnosed?
In conjunction with a good history and physical exam, arthrocentesis is performed to remove fluid from the potentially infected joint. Gram stain, culture, glucose and protein analysis, and cell counts are performed on the fluid. In addition, analysis for uric acid crystals in the joint aspirate is useful in differentiating between gouty arthritis and septic arthritis. If the joint is infected, the aspirate may have a puslike appearance. Aspirated fluid from the septic joint shows leukocytosis with elevated polymorphonuclear neutrophils (PMNs) and grows the infecting nongonococcal bacteria with cultures. The glucose in the joint aspirate is decreased, and the protein level is elevated.

Other blood work may include complete blood count (CBC), ESR, and levels of C-reactive protein, antistreptolysin O (ASO), antinuclear antibody (ANA), rheumatoid factor, Lyme titer, and uric acid to rule out other causes of joint pain and swelling, such as Lyme disease, gout, rheumatoid arthritis, and other autoimmune disorders. Blood cultures may be performed. White blood cell count, ESR, and levels of C-reactive protein will be high if the patient has an infection.

39. Discuss the role of radiographic imaging in diagnosing and treating septic arthritis.
Within the first 2 weeks of infection, an x-ray of the joint space usually provides no information other than distention of the joint space due to effusion. It does not provide evidence of infection. As the infection continues untreated, the x-ray shows subchondral bone destruction and joint space narrowing due to destruction of the articular cartilage. Septic arthritis can develop a contiguous osteomyelitis with the correspond-

ing radiographic changes. MRI, CT scan, or bone scan is useful in identifying soft tissue and bony infection or abscess at joints that may be difficult to assess.

40. Why are identification and treatment of septic arthritis so important?

The complications from septic arthritis warrant early identification and treatment. Complications of untreated septic arthritis include ankylosis of a joint as the body attempts to heal, complete destruction of the articular cartilage, diminished or lost joint function, and growth-plate destruction leading to limb length discrepancy. In infants, whose epiphysis is still predominantly cartilaginous, significant joint destruction may lead to an unstable pseudarthrosis. Septic arthritis can lead to osteomyelitis, chronic joint infection, or avascular necrosis.

41. Describe the medical treatment for a joint infection.

Treatment for septic arthritis includes antibiotic therapy, pain management, and arthrocentesis of an effusion with the usual lab work. A surgeon usually irrigates the joint in the operating room. Rest and immobilization of the joint are followed by early mobilization of the joint after the acute symptoms have diminished. Pediatric patients may require traction after septic arthritis of the hip is surgically addressed. A continuous passive machine (CPM) is often used to assist with early mobilization of the affected joint.

42. Summarize the nursing care of patients with septic arthritis.

- Assess and manage pain.
- Ensure that immobilization devices are used properly.
- Educate patients about the disease process, treatment, and medications.
- Teach and provide proper wound care, dressing changes, and infection control.
- Assess and ensure proper nutrition.
- Teach and assist with range-of-motion exercises after the acute phase.

43. What organisms most commonly cause infection of a prosthetic joint?

The organisms that usually cause infection at a prosthetic joint are the same as those that cause septic arthritis of a nonprosthetic joint: *Staphylococcus aureus*, *Staphylococcus epidermidis*, *Pseudomonas* species, streptococci, and *Escherichia coli*.

44. What percentage of joint replacements become infected?

A relatively small number: 1–3%.

45. What are the main causes of a prosthetic joint infection?

- Hematogenous spread from medical procedures (e.g., dental work) or infection
- Direct infection due to postoperative wound infection

46. How can a prosthetic joint infection be treated?

Antibiotic therapy is a cornerstone of treatment. The surgeon may choose to irrigate the joint in the operating room. The surgeon may also choose to remove the prosthesis and debride the necrotic tissue at a later point to place another prosthesis.

47. Discuss the complications of untreated prosthetic joint infections.

Two of the major complications of an untreated prosthetic joint infection are chronic osteomyelitis and altered or lost function of the infected joint. In addition, failure of the prosthesis may require its removal.

48. Describe the usual findings in the history and physical exam of patients with a prosthetic joint infection.

On physical examination, the nurse notes pain and decreased range of motion at the infected joint. The usual signs of infection may be present, including fever, chills, erythema, warmth, and edema. The patient may have drainage from the operative site.

49. Summarize the nursing care of patients with an infected prosthetic joint.

The nursing care for patients with an infected prosthetic joint is essentially the same as for patients with septic arthritis (see question 42).

50. Which tests can assist in diagnosing prosthetic joint infection?

A bone scan can be performed to assist in making the diagnosis. Although x-rays of the prosthetic joint are not very helpful in diagnosis, they may show any cyst formation in the area or indicate whether the prosthesis is loose. Blood work shows the usual changes associated with infection, including increased ESR, elevated C-reactive protein, and increased white blood cell count. Fluid can be removed from the suspected site of infection for cell count, glucose and protein analysis, Gram stain, culture, and sensitivity testing. A surgeon may choose to perform a biopsy to confirm the diagnosis of prosthetic joint infection.

51. Does an infectious organism cause acute bursitis?

Typically bursitis results from excessive pressure, repetitive minor trauma to the bursae, or reactive inflammation from overuse. Septic bursitis usually develops secondary to an overlying cellulitis or some type of puncture wound that directly infects the bursae.

52. Does the patient with septic bursitis present differently from the patient without infection?

Patients with infected and noninfected bursitis develop similar symptoms of swelling, warmth, and pain with palpation and motion. The examiner may feel crepitus when palpating over the bursae. The patient with noninfected bursitis usually has a history consistent with overuse (e.g., painting), trauma to the area (e.g., falling on a hip), or excessive pressure (e.g., prolonged kneeling).

Patients with septic bursitis may present with symptoms of fever, chills, and malaise. They may have a history of a trauma to the skin overlying the bursae with a break in the skin or already established cellulitis. The patient may also have additional physical exam findings of an obvious laceration or puncture, drainage from a wound, lymphadenopathy, and lymphangitis.

53. How are infected and noninfected bursitis differentiated?

Although history and exam are useful, aspirating the bursae and sending the fluid for lab analysis confirms the diagnosis. Gram stain, culture, and cell count confirm the diagnosis.

54. How is septic bursitis treated?

Uncomplicated septic bursitis is usually treated on an outpatient basis with oral antibiotics. The bursa is aspirated to obtain fluid for analysis, which also relieves much of the pain due to pressure within the bursae. The patient should keep all superficial wounds clean, dry, and dressed appropriately. Any pain can usually be treated with nonsteroidal anti-inflammatory drugs (NSAIDs) or acetaminophen. Application of warmth to the area and rest may also provide comfort and aid in recovery.

55. What is postpolio syndrome?

Postpolio syndrome (PPS) is a cluster of symptoms that can affect patients who have had prior poliomyelitis. The specific cause is unknown, but theories about the development of the symptoms include degradation of altered motor units with aging. PPS is estimated to affect nearly 75% of people who previously had paralytic polio. Some researchers believe that all patients who had previously experienced paralytic polio will eventually develop PPS.

56. List the symptoms associated with PPS.

- Pain
- Cold or heat intolerance
- Breathing difficulties
- Swallowing difficulties
- Difficulty with speech
- Weakness or fatigue

57. What tests can be done to confirm PPS?

No tests can be performed to confirm the diagnosis of PPS, which is essentially a diagnosis of exclusion. Diagnostic tests, along with a thorough history and physical exam, should be used to rule out other potential causes of the patient's symptoms.

58. What medical treatment can be offered to patients with PPS?

Patients with PPS benefit from physical therapy and/or home exercise treatment, primarily to assist in fighting fatigue and activity intolerance. Discomfort can be treated appropriately with NSAIDs, deep heat, and massage. Refer the patient to a swallowing clinic if needed. Respiratory dysfunction may be treated with intermittent positive-pressure ventilation.

59. Summarize the nursing interventions for patients with PPS.

- Educate patients about the disease process and assistive devices.
- Advise and assist with smoking cessation.
- Promote physical activity with or without assistive devices.
- Promote activity and rest periods for energy management.
- Assess and manage pain.
- Educate patients about dietary and eating modifications (small sips, small bites, chewing food well).
- Educate patients about weight management.
- Provide psychosocial support for grieving, anxiety, or fear.

60. What bacterium causes Lyme disease?

The bacterium that causes Lyme disease is a spirochete called *Borrelia burgdorferi*. In North America, it is carried by the deer tick; in Europe the bacterium is carried by the sheep tick.

61. Do all people who are bitten by a deer tick become infected with Lyme disease?

No. Only 1–3% of people bitten by the deer tick become infected with Lyme disease. Three factors affect this relatively low percentage of infection:

- The tick must feed on the patient for approximately 24–48 hours for the bacteria to be transmitted.
- Healthy patients may have adequate immunologic defenses to fight off early infection.
- Not all deer ticks are infected.

62. Do any regions in North America have a higher prevalence of Lyme infections?
A majority of infections have been reported in the Northeast United States.

63. Can Lyme disease be transmitted from person to person?
Transmission of Lyme disease from one person to another has not been reported. Lyme disease has rarely been shown to cross from mother to fetus by way of the placenta.

64. List the three stages of Lyme disease.
- Stage 1: localized disease
- Stage 2: early disseminated disease
- Stage 3: late or chronic disease

65. What are the usual signs and symptoms of early localized Lyme disease?
Symptoms usually begin 1–4 weeks after exposure. The patient may develop the classic erythema migrans rash at the site of the bite, but the rash is present in only 60–80% of infected patients. Erythema migrans is typically described as a circular rash with a bull's-eye appearance. Erythema migrans from Lyme infection can be differentiated from the erythematous lesion that results from the tick bite because the bull's-eye rash expands rapidly. Patients may also complain of headache, fever, neck stiffness, fatigue, and muscle and joint aches.

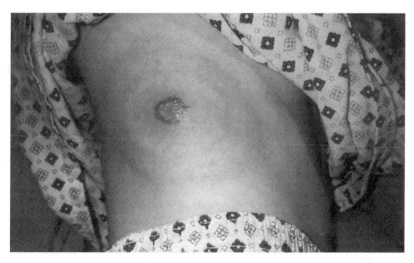

Erythema migrans. (From Eppes SO: Lyme disease. In Klein JD, Zaoutis TE (eds): Pediatric Infectious Disease Secrets. Philadelphia, Hanley & Belfus, 2003, pp 268–272, with permission.)

66. Describe the typical presentation of early disseminated Lyme disease.
Symptoms due to disseminated disease appear within weeks to months after exposure. Neurologic signs and symptoms may include encephalitis, meningitis, Bell's

palsy, radicular neuritis, photophobia, and memory loss. Cardiac signs and symptoms may include atrioventricular block or cardiomyopathy. Patients may also develop conjunctivitis, iritis, malaise, muscle and joint pain, or lymphadenopathy. Some patients develop hepatitis, hematuria, or proteinuria.

67. What are the common findings of late or chronic Lyme disease?

Late Lyme disease occurs within months to years after exposure. Signs and symptoms may include Lyme arthritis, fibromyalgia, and atrophic skin lesions. Neurologic disturbances range from mood or memory problems to neuropathies or encephalitis.

68. What tests are useful in diagnosing Lyme disease?

Diagnostic testing is used to rule in or rule out Lyme or other diseases that may cause similar symptoms, such as gonorrheal arthropathy, crystalline arthropathy, septic arthritis, and fibromyalgia. Blood work may consist of Lyme titer, rheumatoid factor, uric acid, CBC, ESR, ANA, ASO, and enzyme-linked immunosorbent assay (ELISA). Any joint aspirate should be tested for crystals, cell count, glucose, Gram stain, and culture.

69. Summarize the current treatment for Lyme disease.

- Initiate appropriate antibiotic therapy.
- Use NSAIDs for myalgia and arthralgias.
- Initiate appropriate treatment for any neurologic and cardiac complications.
- Patients with cardiac dysfunction may require a temporary pacemaker.
- Patients with painful chronic synovitis may benefit from surgical synovectomy.

70. What tick bite prevention techniques can the nurse teach?

Patients with the potential for tick exposure should consider the following prevention strategies:
- Wear long pants with the ends tucked into the socks.
- Use approved tick repellant on the clothing (e.g., Permanone).
- DEET insect repellent can be used on the skin.
- Wear light-colored clothing for easy identification of brown-colored ticks on the body.
- Check all pets, self, and others for attached ticks shortly after potential exposure.

71. Who should consider obtaining the Lyme vaccine?

Patients between the ages of 15 and 70 years old should consider the Lyme vaccine if they work or engage in frequent activities associated with a high-to-moderate risk of exposure.

72. How does musculoskeletal tuberculosis (TB) develop?

Patients who develop musculoskeletal TB initially become infected by way of the airborne *Mycobacterium tuberculosis*. After pulmonary TB develops, the infection may eventually spread by a hematogenous or lymphatic route to the bones and/or joints. A patient can also develop musculoskeletal TB due to hematogenous or lymphatic spread from another site of extrapulmonary TB.

73. Is musculoskeletal TB communicable from person to person?

Musculoskeletal TB is not spread casually from person to person. Patients with active pulmonary TB can certainly infect others; however, only 50% of patients have both active pulmonary TB and musculoskeletal TB. A patient with musculoskeletal TB can infect health care providers if the bacterium is aerosolized during surgery or debridement.

74. How common is the development of musculoskeletal TB?

Only 2–3% of all TB cases involve infection of the bone and/or joint.

75. What is the most common site for musculoskeletal TB infection?

The most common site for musculoskeletal TB is the spine (also known as Potts disease). When a patient has TB of the spine, the most common site for infection is the thoracic spine.

76. What may the health history reveal in patients with musculoskeletal TB?

The health history may reveal exposure to a person with active TB or a known history of TB. Patients also have some type of underlying immune compromise or history of drug or alcohol abuse.

77. Describe the common symptoms of musculoskeletal TB.

Signs and symptoms of bone and joint TB are usually rather insidious in development. Initial signs and symptoms are rather vague and nonspecific. Typical examples include night sweats, unexpected weight loss, loss of appetite, bone or joint pain, weakness, fever, and chills. Patients may notice redness or swelling of the joints or a change in the shape of the back, possibly due to gibbus deformity or compression fractures.

78. What are the typical physical findings in patients with spinal TB?

The physical examination of a patient with TB of the thoracic or lumbar spine may show decreased range of motion and discomfort or pain with movement and palpation over the spine. The patient with sacroiliac joint infection typically develops unilateral buttock discomfort. The examiner may palpate increased warmth over the infected area. A patient may eventually develop a gibbus deformity or kyphosis due to compression fractures of the infected vertebral bodies. Compression fractures or abscess formation at the infection site may place pressure on the spinal cord, possibly leading to paraplegia. A patient can develop peripheral neurologic symptoms, which may include altered sensation, extremity weakness, and pain along a nerve root distribution.

Cervical TB is less common than thoracic infection. In addition to the warmth, pain, and decreased range of motion mentioned above, the patient may develop cervical lymphadenopathy and torticollis. Dysphagia and hoarseness also may develop.

79. Describe the typical exam findings in patients with TB of the appendicular skeleton.

The typical exam findings include warmth, edema, erythema, and pain over the infection site. Patients may develop decreased motion at a joint, weakness, and muscle atrophy. TB osteomyelitis can develop abscess formation; sinus tracts from the abscess to the skin may eventually lead to drainage.

80. Discuss the pathophysiology of TB infection within the appendicular skeleton.

Bone can become infected with TB by way of hematogenous or lymphatic spread. Destruction of the bone results from the infection. Unlike other osteomyelitis infections, TB osteomyelitis does not result in reactive bone formation and typical sequestrum formation to wall off bacteria. Because there is no sequestrum formation, extension of the infection into the joint space is made easier. Because of inflammation and necrosis from the infection, exudate and necrotic material lead to increased pressure within the bone with eventual abscess formation. The abscess can eventually develop a sinus tract and drain through the skin.

Joints can also become infected by a hematogenous source as well as extension of TB osteomyelitis. An infected joint produces granulation tissue, which eventually covers the articular surface and causes erosion of articular cartilage. The joint eventually develops a fibrous ankylosis across the joint space. The synovial tissues of the joint thicken and produce increased synovial fluid because of the normal inflammatory process. The joints develop an effusion from a combination of excessive synovial fluid, exudate, and necrotic debris from the infection. As with bone infection, an abscess may form and eventually drain through the skin by way of a sinus tract.

81. Describe the pathophysiologic destruction associated with spinal TB.

Destruction at the spine usually begins in the anterior subchondral bone of the vertebral body. As the infection progresses, destruction of the bone eventually leads to a compression fracture and collapse of the vertebral body. The collapse of the vertebra results in an anterior wedge formation that causes a kyphotic or gibbus deformity of the spine. With the collapse of the vertebral body comes abscess formation as the accumulated necrotic material is squeezed into the paravertebral space. Patients may develop spinal cord compromise and paraplegia secondary to paravertebral abscess formation and the collapse of the vertebral body. Intervertebral disc destruction is also caused by spinal TB infections.

82. Define gibbus deformity. How is it different from a kyphotic deformity?

A gibbus deformity is essentially a variation of the kyphotic deformity and is characterized by a sharp kyphotic angulation of the spine at the site of vertebral body collapse. The typical kyphotic deformity is described as more of a sweeping curve of the spine due to incompletely collapsed wedge-shaped vertebral bodies. Multiple wedges stack upon each other, giving the accentuated sweeping curve of the kyphotic deformity.

83. How are TB bone infections different in adults and children?

- Children develop bone TB more frequently in the upper thoracic vertebrae, whereas in adults the lower thoracic and upper lumbar vertebrae are more frequently infected.
- Children usually have spontaneous healing of the TB lesions, which is rare in adults.
- Children develop abscess formations less frequently than adults.
- Children frequently have a growth deformity of the affected extremity due to the proximity and involvement of the growth plate with the infectious site.

84. What are the potential complications of untreated musculoskeletal TB?

- Chronic pain
- Deformity of the spine
- Deformity of the bones or joints
- Fractures
- Dysfunctional joints

85. What diagnostic tests prove useful in evaluating and confirming musculo-skeletal TB?
- Chest x-ray shows the presence of pulmonary TB.
- An x-ray of the suspected TB skeletal infection shows the characteristic bony destruction.
- MRI assists in giving a clearer understanding of the bony and soft tissue destruction.
- The purified protein derivative (PPD) skin test confirms exposure to TB.
- Synovial fluid shows increased protein, decreased glucose, poor mucin clot, and elevated white blood cells with elevated PMNs.
- Acid-fast stain, Gram stain, and culture of synovial fluid assess for *M. tuberculosis* or other bacteria.
- Blood work may show elevated ESR, leukocytosis, and hypochromic anemia.
- Biopsy of the bony lesion confirms the diagnosis.

86. Summarize the nursing management of patients with musculoskeletal TB.
- Educate the patient about the disease process.
- Educate the patient about medical, surgical, and pharmacologic interventions.
- Educate the patient about proper nutrition.
- Ensure that any required public health reporting is performed.
- Emphasize the necessity for compliance with the long-term pharmacologic regimen.
- Medication is occasionally managed through direct observation by a home health nurse or daily clinic visits because of frequent noncompliance with the pharmacologic regimen.
- Assess and manage pain.
- Address impaired physical mobility through active/passive range of motion, home exercises, or physical therapy.

87. How is musculoskeletal TB treated surgically?
Surgical intervention is indicated for spinal instability, neurologic symptoms, or a large paraspinal abscess. The goal is to provide stability to the spine by performing a spinal fusion to prevent or decrease neurologic compromise. Patients may also undergo a synovectomy at infected joints to remove large areas of infection, loose bodies, and synovial pannus. A joint fusion or eventually an arthroplasty may be performed when joint destruction and pain are severe.

88. What precautions should operating room personnel observe when a patient has bone or joint TB?
Musculoskeletal TB can infect health care providers if the bacterium is aerosolized during surgery or debridement. Therefore, all providers should wear the appropriate respirators because aerosolized TB is spread through an airborne route.

89. Discuss the current pharmacologic treatment of musculoskeletal TB.
Current pharmacologic treatment for the patient with musculoskeletal TB is a multidrug approach similar to that for pulmonary TB. The length of pharmacologic treatment is usually between 1 and 2 years. The medication regimen typically consists of isoniazid (INH), rifampin, and one or two of the following: pyrazinamide, ethambutol, streptomycin, or cycloserine.

BIBLIOGRAPHY

1. Apley AG, Solomon L: Concise System of Orthopedics and Fractures, 2nd ed. London, Reed Educational and Professional Publishing, 1996.
2. Huether S, McCance K: Understanding Pathophysiology, 2nd ed. St. Louis, Mosby, 2000.
3. Lewis SM, Heitkemper MM, Dirksen SR: Medical Surgical Nursing: Assessment and Management of Clinical Problems, 5th ed. St. Louis, Mosby, 2000.
4. Maher AB, Salmond SW, Pellino TA: Orthopaedic Nursing, 3rd ed. Philadelphia, W.B. Saunders, 2002.
5. Schoen DC: NAON Core Curriculum for Orthopaedic Nursing, 4th ed. Pittman, NJ, Anthony J. Jannetti, 2001.

7. ORTHOPEDIC TRAUMA

Michael E. Zychowicz, RN, MSN, NP-C, *Jill Brennan-Cook*, MS, RN, CEN, and *Barbara Krajewski*, RNC, MSN, FNP-C

1. Define trauma.

Trauma refers to any injury that a person sustains. Trauma ranges widely in the level of severity and can be as simple as a small contusion or benign grade I ankle sprain or as significant as open skull fractures, gunshot wounds, or traumatic amputations. When health care providers refer to trauma, they are usually speaking of severe injury. Trauma is the most common cause of death for people less than 40 years of age and is the fourth leading cause of death among people of all ages.

2. Define multiple trauma.

Multiple trauma is defined as injuries involving two or more body systems. Examples of injuries that can cause multiple trauma include crush, penetration, blast, and head injuries as well as gunshot wounds.

3. What guidelines are available for assessing patients with traumatic injury?

In caring for patients with traumatic injury, rapid, methodical assessment and treatment of life- and limb-threatening problems are essential. The initial assessment consists of the primary and secondary surveys, followed by definitive treatment of injuries.

The American College of Surgeons (ACS) has developed Advanced Trauma Life Support guidelines and a certification program for the assessment and treatment of trauma. Physicians, nurse practitioners, and physician assistants use these guidelines. The Emergency Nurses Association (ENA) has developed the Trauma Nurse Core Course (TNCC) and the Course in Advanced Trauma Nursing (CATN). Both ENA courses teach guidelines for nurses that complement the ACS guidelines for physicians.

4. List the elements of the primary survey.

The primary survey is done rapidly and addresses life-threatening conditions with standard resuscitation of the patient. In a basic sense, the primary survey has expanded on the ABCs of cardiopulmonary resuscitation to develop the ABCDEs:

A = **A**irway and cervical spine control
B = **B**reathing
C = **C**irculation and life-threatening bleeding
D = **D**isability (neurologic)
E = **E**xposure of all injuries

5. What are the main tasks and considerations for airway and cervical spine control?

Ensure that the patient's airway is open and clear. Open and maintain the airway as needed. Use the jaw thrust to open the airway unless cervical spine injury has been ruled out. Look for and remove any foreign material in the mouth. Maintain proper cervical spine precautions, keeping the neck immobilized in a neutral position. Assume

85

cervical spine injury exists if obvious deformity, neck pain, head injury, or decreased level of consciousness is present or if the mechanism of injury might lead to cervical spine injury (e.g., diving injury, fall from height greater than 8 feet).

6. What is involved in assessment of breathing?

Assess the patient for spontaneous breathing and adequacy of air movement. The normal respiratory rate is 12–20 breaths per minute. Patients with neurologic dysfunction may have a respiratory rate less than 12 breaths per minute. Patients with hypoxia, shock, or acidosis may have a respiratory rate greater than 30 breaths per minute.

7. Explain the assessment of circulation and life-threatening bleeding.

Circulatory assessment at this stage gives a gross estimate of cardiovascular status. Pulse is assessed for presence, quality, and regularity. Capillary refill normally occurs within 1–3 seconds. If refill requires more than 3 seconds, common causes may include shock, medications, or hypothermia. Skin color, skin temperature, and mucous membrane color are assessed. Direct pressure is placed on any bleeding site, typically large arterial vessels, that is potentially life-threatening.

8. How is the patient assessed for neurologic disability?

The examination for neurologic disability consists of general assessment of cerebral function and oxygenation. The level of consciousness should be assessed. The **AVPU** mnemonic can be used for labeling the patient's level of consciousness:

A = **A**lert
V = Responds to **V**erbal stimulus
P = Responds to **P**ainful stimulus
U = **U**nresponsive

The Glasgow Coma Score is more widely used in assessing the patient's level of consciousness. Patients with diminished level of consciousness may have decreased cerebral oxygenation due to hypoxia or hypoperfusion, central nervous system injury, drug or alcohol overdose, or metabolic derangement. The nurse should also remember that a belligerent, combative, or uncooperative patient may be hypoxic.

9. What is meant by exposure of all injuries?

Undress the patient completely. Cut off clothes if necessary. The trauma team cannot treat what they cannot see. However, modesty and hypothermia should be considered in exposing a patient. Avoid unnecessary exposure to minimize hypothermia, and take the patient's core temperature as soon as possible. Scenarios involving cold and/or water exposure before arrival at the hospital can also contribute significantly to hypothermia.

10. List the elements of the secondary survey.

The secondary survey is performed to identify any limb-threatening and other less significant injuries in addition to performing a head-to-toe examination of the patient. The secondary survey continues with the alphabetical sequence:

F = **F**ahrenheit (temperature)
G = **G**et vital signs
H = **H**istory and Head-to-toe assessment
I = **I**nspect the posterior surfaces of the patient

11. What should the nurse do if the patient develops a life-threatening problem during the secondary assessment?

Patient resuscitation is well under way during the secondary survey; life-threatening problems of the airway, breathing, and circulation already have been addressed. If the patient develops a life-threatening problem during the secondary assessment, the trauma team changes focus to address airway, breathing, and circulation again.

12. Summarize the special considerations in obtaining the vital signs of patients with trauma.

The goal during the secondary survey is to obtain a baseline set of vital signs. For critical trauma patients, vital signs generally are recorded at least every 5 minutes during the resuscitation period. In general, rectal temperatures should be taken for an accurate core temperature in all patients with trauma.

13. What are the guidelines for obtaining a brief but adequate patient history?

A mnemonic for obtaining a rather rapid patient history is **AMPLE**:

A = **A**llergies
M = **M**edications or drugs
P = **P**ast medical history
L = **L**ast meal
E = **E**vents preceding the injury

14. What is the Glasgow Coma Scale (GCS)?

The Glasgow Coma Scale is used to assess the trauma patient's level of consciousness and severity of brain injury. The score ranges from 3 to 15 and is calculated based on the patient's best eye-opening, motor, and verbal responses. As a patient's score decreases, the probability of concomitant morbidity and mortality increases. The GCS score also enables health care providers to quantitatively track a patient's progress after a brain injury. A score of less than 9 is indicative of severe head injury; a score of 9–12 indicates a moderate head injury; and a score of 13–15 indicates a mild injury.

Glasgow Coma Scale

Eyes		
Open	Spontaneously	4
	To verbal command	3
	To pain	2
No response		1
Best motor response		
To verbal command	Obeys	6
To painful stimulus	Localizes pain	5
	Flexion—withdraws	4
	Flexion—abnormal (decorticate rigidity)	3
	Extension (decerebrate rigidity)	2
	No response	1
Best verbal response		
Arouse patient with painful	Oriented and converses	5
stimulus if necessary	Disoriented and converses	4
	Inappropriate words	3
	Incomprehensible sounds	2
	No response	1
Total		3–15

15. What should the nurse evaluate during the basic trauma assessment?

The examiner should perform regional examinations consisting of look, listen, and feel.

- Look for ecchymosis, deformity, hemorrhage, swelling, and abnormal skin indentations.
- Listen for crepitus, air from a punctured chest wall, and breath sounds.
- Feel all bones and joints for abnormal movement, crepitus, pain, pulses, and skin temperature.

16. What should the nurse look for when the trauma exam is performed region by region?

- Inspect the head for contusions, abrasions, lacerations, bony asymmetry, hemorrhage, and abnormalities of eye, ears, nose, or mouth. Palpate for crepitus, deviation, or bony depression.
- Observe the neck for contusions, abrasions, lacerations, jugular vein distention, swelling, deformity, or tracheal deviation. Palpate for crepitus, tracheal deviation, and cervical spine tenderness.
- The chest is observed for paradoxical movements, contusions, abrasions, deformity, equal chest expansion, accessory muscle use, and bulging or retractions. Observe the patient for splinting or guarding of an injury. Listen to the lungs bilaterally.
- The abdomen and pelvis are inspected for abrasions, ecchymosis, distention, laceration, or other obvious injury. Palpate the abdomen and pelvis, including the iliac crest and symphysis pubis. Twenty-five percent of patients with a seatbelt sign (a band of ecchymosis across the abdomen) have intestinal injury or rupture. They also have a high incidence of lumbar fractures.
- At the extremities, palpate all bones and joints for crepitus, unusual movement, or pain. Look for obvious hematoma, deformity, bleeding, lacerations, abrasions, ecchymosis, or edema. Palpate for the presence of pulses in the extremities, and assess capillary refill and skin temperature.
- Inspect the posterior surfaces from head to toe by log-rolling the patient. Use more than one person, and stabilize the cervical spine. Inspect and palpate for any obvious wounds and potential weapons because trauma is frequently associated with violent crimes. Listen to the posterior lung fields while the patient is in this position.
- Perform a cursory neurologic exam, assessing sensory and motor function and noting any weakness, loss of sensation, or paralysis.

17. Does cervical immobilization need to be implemented for patients with no neck pain?

Spinal immobilization in a trauma patient is a high priority. The orthopedic nurse should be aware of the potential for cervical spine injury in all trauma patients. Patients must be treated as if a cervical fracture is present with either manual or rigid cervical collar immobilization until it is ruled out by diagnostic imaging. Advanced Trauma Life Support (ATLS) protocols recommend immobilizing the cervical spine until all aspects of the cervical spine have been adequately evaluated and injury is ruled out. The cervical spine should be positioned in a neutral position and not hyperextended or flexed. This protocol is especially important in patients who had a transient loss of consciousness or who require intubation.

18. How is a fracture diagnosed?

History, physical exam, and diagnostic testing help to diagnose a fracture. When the nurse obtains the history, patients usually describe some type of trauma of varying degrees. They may note that they heard a pop or snap during the injury along with pain and disability. On examination, the examiner can elicit point tenderness over the suspected fracture site. Obvious angulation or deformity, ecchymosis, edema, soft tissue trauma, or bone ends protruding through the skin may be seen on physical exam.

Radiographs are the most frequently used test to evaluate and diagnose a fracture. The x-ray may or may not show a fracture. Other tests that are useful in evaluating and diagnosing a fracture include magnetic resonance imaging (MRI), bone scan, computed tomography (CT) scan, plain tomography, fluoroscopy, and myelography.

19. What are the different types of fractures? How are they caused?

Fracture Type	Cause	Clinical Example(s)
Pathologic fracture	A weak portion of bone breaks with little or no force applied.	Bone metastasis, bone cyst, osteomyelitis or osteoporosis.
Stress fracture	Repetitive stress to the bone leads to damage of the microarchitecture causing cracks in the bone. Eventually the bone may collapse and fracture completely.	Dancers, athletes, and military recruits significantly stress the metatarsals, tibia and/or fibula from overtraining.
Compression fracture	A heavy axial load is applied to a bone, compressing the cancellous bone.	Vertebral body of osteoporotic patients.
Penetrating injury	A projectile penetrates a bone.	Gunshot wound or blast injury.
Rotational injury	A twisting stress to the bone may result in a spiral type fracture.	Twisting injury to the tibia from a fall while skiing.
Traction injury	A strong pull at the insertion of a tendon or ligament, causing an avulsion fragment.	Sprained ankle
Tapping injury	A forceful direct blow results in a fracture with mild-to-moderate soft tissue injury.	A soccer player accidentally kicking another player's leg.
Crush fracture	A crush injury injures soft tissues and causes a transverse or comminuted fracture.	A hand struck by a sledgehammer.
Angulation fracture	A force is applied laterally, causing an angulated fracture.	A patient hit in the lower leg by the bumper of a car.

20. What does mechanism of injury mean?

The mechanism of injury is essentially the method by which the force or trauma was applied to the human body in causing the injury. The mechanism of injury gives the health care provider information and insight into the extent and degree of potential underlying injuries.

21. Aside from bone injury, what bodily damage can accompany fractures?
- Edema, ecchymosis, and hemorrhage
- Joint dislocation

- Ruptured tendons and ligaments
- Nerve injury
- Damaged blood vessels
- Injured body organs
- Skin and muscle damage

22. How are fractures described?

Providers in the orthopedic community commonly use classic descriptors and names to describe a variety of specific fractures. The mechanism of injury, type of fracture line, and specific anatomic location of the fracture site are used to describe fractures. Anatomic alignment of the fracture fragments, degree of displacement, amount of angulation, and specific features of fracture appearance are additional descriptors. Finally, if the fracture causes a break in the skin, it is described as open; closed fractures do not cause a break in the skin.

23. Describe various fracture lines.

- **Avulsion** fractures are small pieces of bone pulled off by tendon/ligament injury or force.
- **Comminuted** fractures usually have more than two fragments of broken bone.
- In **oblique fractures** the fracture line extends in an oblique fashion.
- **Greenstick fractures** are characterized by splintered bone on one side and curvature on the other.
- In **impacted** fractures fracture segments are impacted into one another.
- In **longitudinal** fractures the fracture line extends the length of the bone.
- In **spiral** fractures the fracture line extends in a spiral fashion around the bone.
- **Transverse** fractures extend across the bone shaft at a right angle to the longitudinal axis.

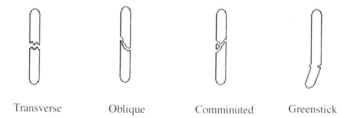

Transverse   Oblique   Comminuted   Greenstick

Types of fractures. (From Mehta AJ: Management of fractures. In O'Young BJ, Young MA, Stiens SA (eds): Physical Medicine and Rehabilitation Secrets, 2nd ed. Philadelphia, Hanley & Belfus, 2002, pp 305-311, with permission.)

24. What is an occult fracture? How is it evaluated?

A fracture is described as occult if the fracture line is not visualized on standard x-ray examination. Frequently occult fractures are visualized with a repeat x-ray examination within 2 weeks because the necrotic tissue around the fracture site is removed and the fracture line may become more visible. Some early reactive bone formation may also be seen on follow-up x-rays. Occult fractures can be further evaluated using other diagnostic testing, including bone scan and MRI. If the patient has an occult fracture, the bone scan shows increased uptake of the injected radionuclide at the fracture site; the MRI shows bony edema and possibly a fracture line.

25. What anatomic locations are used to describe fractures?

- **Articular**: the fracture involves the articular surface.
- **Intra-articular**: the fracture extends into joint surface.
- **Periarticular**: the fracture is located near a joint but does not extend into the joint.
- **Condylar**: the fracture extends into the condyle.
- **Diacondylar (transcondylar)**: the fracture extends across the condyle.
- **Supracondylar**: the fracture is located above the condyle.
- **Apophyseal**: the fracture involves an avulsion of a portion of the apophysis.
- **Diaphyseal**: the fracture extends through the shaft of the bone (diaphysis).
- **Epiphyseal**: the fracture extends through the growth plate (physis) and/or end of the bone (epiphysis).
- **Metaphyseal**: the fracture is located between the epiphysis and diaphysis.
- **Extracapsular**: the fracture is near but does not extend into the joint capsule.
- **Intracapsular**: the fracture extends into the joint capsule.
- **Cortical**: the fracture involves disruption or buckling of the bony cortex.
- **Subperiosteal**: the fracture does not disrupt the periosteum.

26. Describe the Salter-Harris classification of epiphyseal fractures in children.

Various classification systems exist for describing epiphyseal fractures; the Salter-Harris method is widely accepted in clinical practice. The Salter-Harris classification of fractures is used to describe epiphyseal fractures in children with open epiphyseal plates. Traditionally, five Salter-Harris classifications are used to describe fractures in clinical practice:

- **Type I**: disruption through the epiphyseal plate with or without movement of the epiphysis and metaphysis at the epiphyseal plate. No true fracture line through the bone can be visualized.
- **Type II**: disruption is present through the epiphyseal plate with a fracture line extending into the metaphysis.
- **Type III**: disruption is present through the epiphyseal plate with a fracture line extending through the epiphysis into the articular surface.
- **Type IV**: the fracture extends from the metaphysis through the epiphyseal plate and epiphysis into the articular surface.
- **Type V**: a crushing injury that involves the epiphyseal plate.

27. Why are epiphyseal fractures potentially problematic?

Although most children with epiphyseal fractures heal and recover without dysfunction or deformity, epiphyseal fractures are potentially problematic because the fracture traverses through the growth plate. Approximately 10% of children sustain growth disturbances of the injured limb. The patient can develop early closure of the epiphyseal plate, angular growth disturbance, or limb length discrepancy from growth cessation. Type IV and V Salter-Harris fractures have a relatively high incidence of subsequent growth disturbance.

28. What is the difference between stable and unstable fractures?

A **stable** fracture is well reduced and has a good probability of remaining reduced without movement of the bones at the fracture site during immobilization. In an **unstable** fracture, the fractured bone ends do not remain in adequate alignment despite attempts at closed reduction and immobilization.

29. Describe the five stages of fracture repair.

- **Stage I** occurs immediately after the fracture. Bleeding at the fracture site causes a hematoma, clot, and inflammation. Bony necrosis surrounding the fracture results from blood vessels that are injured and compressed by inflammation and hematoma.
- In **stage II** the clot serves as a fibrin network for cellular invasion, which occurs between day 3 and 14. Phagocytes begin the process of removing necrotic debris.
- In **stage III** fibroblastic cells, blood vessels, and osteoblasts invade the hematoma, forming granular tissue. Between 2 and 6 weeks after injury the body develops a callus at the fracture site, which is essentially fibrous tissue that adds stability to the fractured bone ends.
- **Stage IV** occurs between 3 weeks and 6 months after the fracture. The callus that bridges the fracture gap becomes ossified and is slowly replaced by trabecular bone. Phagocytic cells continue to remove callus and remaining necrotic bone and tissue.
- **Stage V** is characterized by remodeling, which occurs over the remaining year. Bone is reabsorbed and produced due to physical stresses and the needs of the body.

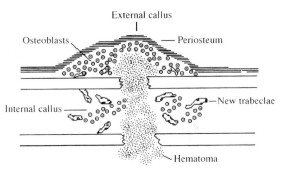

Fracture repair.

Summary of fracture repair. (From Mehta AJ: Management of fractures. In O'Young BJ, Young MA, Stiens SA (eds): Physical Medicine and Rehabilitation Secrets, 2nd ed. Philadelphia, Hanley & Belfus, 2002, pp 305-311, with permission.)

30. What factors enhance bone healing?

- Proper immobilization
- Appropriate weight bearing for long bones
- Bone fragment contact
- Sufficient blood supply
- Proper nutrition
- Adequate growth hormone, thyroid hormone, calcitonin, insulin, and vitamins A and D
- Energy field or ultrasound bone stimulators

31. What factors inhibit bone healing?

- Extensive local trauma and bone loss
- Inadequate immobilization

- Space between bone fragments
- Infection, avascular necrosis, or metabolic bone disease
- Irradiated bone and bony malignancy
- Intra-articular fracture
- Older age
- Corticosteroid use
- Loss of innervation

32. How long does it usually take for an uncomplicated fracture to heal in adults? In children?

On average, most adult fractures heal within 6–8 weeks; children's fractures heal somewhat faster.

33. What methods are used to realign displaced or angulated fractures?

Fractures are reduced by closed reduction, open reduction, or traction.

34. Why are open fractures more dangerous than closed fractures?

Because fractured bone penetrates through the skin, an open fracture involves the risk of serious infection. Bacteria or dirty materials may contaminate the wound.

35. Describe the classification of open fractures.

Type	Contamination	Size	Soft Tissue Injury	Usual Fracture
I	Clean	<1 cm	Minimal injury	Oblique or transverse
II	Moderate	>1 cm	Moderate injury	Moderately comminuted or crushed
III	Significant	>1 cm	Extensive possible amputation	Unstable or severely comminuted
III-A	Significant	>1 cm	Severe injury but good soft tissue coverage over the fracture	Severely comminuted or segmental
III-B	Significant	>1 cm	Bony exposure, periosteum stripped, severe injury with tissue loss	Severely comminuted
III-C	Significant	>1 cm	Any degree	Any fracture with arterial injury necessitating repair

36. How are open fractures initially treated?

Because of the risk for infection, broad-spectrum antibiotics are used prophylactically. Tetanus toxoid is provided if the patient's immunization is not up to date. The wound may then be irrigated, debrided, and cleansed in the operating room with reduction of the fracture. (See Chapter 13 for more information about open reduction and internal fixation [ORIF].)

37. What is the time frame for irrigation and debridement of an open fracture in the operating room?

It is safe to wait for 6 hours. After 6 hours the risk for infection and further tissue damage is significantly increased.

38. Explain closed reduction of a fracture.

Fractures can be manipulated and repositioned to their previous anatomic position by applying traction and countertraction. This technique is done by a trained professional and involves pulling and pushing the bones back into their original position and alignment. Because closed reduction can be quite painful, hematoma block and possible sedation should be used before the procedure is done. Once the fracture is reduced, repeat x-rays are taken to ensure proper fracture position, length, and alignment. A cast, splint, brace, or traction may then be applied to maintain the original position until the fracture heals.

39. What are the indications for closed reduction of a fracture?

If a fracture has greater-than-acceptable angulation or neurovascular compromise due to angulation, closed reduction should be attempted.

40. What are the potential consequences if a fracture is not reduced?
- Angulation, deformity, and malunion
- Delayed union or nonunion
- Posttraumatic arthritis
- Pseudarthrosis
- Neurovascular compromise

41. What are the major nursing considerations in assisting with fracture reduction?
- Educate the patient about the procedure.
- Provide adequate pain management.
- Assist with the reduction and application of splint or cast.
- Educate the patient about cast care and fracture care after the procedure.

42. What methods can be used to immobilize a fracture?

A fracture can be immobilized using a sling, splint, brace, cast, traction, and external or internal fixation. (For further information see Chapter 14.)

43. List potential adverse outcomes of almost any fracture.
- Delayed union, nonunion, malunion and pseudarthrosis
- Posttraumatic arthritis and joint stiffness
- Osteomyelitis
- Limb shortening
- Muscle damage, including loss of strength, scarring of tissues, and myositis ossificans
- Nerve damage, including severed nerves, nerve palsy, and reflex sympathetic dystrophy
- Compartment syndrome
- Fat emboli syndrome

44. What is the usual treatment for strains, sprains, and dislocations?
See Chapter 8.

45. Describe reflex sympathetic dystrophy.

Reflex sympathetic dystrophy (RSD), also know as causalgia or complex regional pain syndrome (CRPS), is a potential complication of any musculoskeletal trauma with an onset at approximately 1 month after trauma. The pathophysiologic cause is not well understood, but it is believed to be due to altered pain processing by the brain and abnormal sympathetic response. RSD frequently occurs after a relatively minor trauma, such as a sprained ankle or wrist fracture. The brain possibly perceives the minor trauma as more significant than it actually is, resulting in a significant autonomic response.

46. What are the signs and symptoms of RSD?

The classic signs and symptoms of RSD are pain out of proportion to the injury, edema, local skin moistness, joint stiffness, and vasomotor instability with cool/pale or warm/flushed skin. Patients usually complain of significant pain with light touch to the affected area or with movement. Severe cases may be associated with sparse hair distribution on the limb, trophic skin changes, and brittle nails.

47. Are any tests useful in the early diagnosis of RSD?

Usually the diagnosis of RSD is made clinically; however, a bone scan may be useful if the diagnosis is unclear. The bone scan may show increased activity in the affected limb. An x-ray is usually negative but may show diffuse patchy osteoporosis in severe or prolonged RSD.

48. How can RSD be treated?

Management of RSD should begin as early as possible. Treatment may consist of pain medication, physical therapy for desensitization treatment, nerve blockade, transcutaneous electric nerve stimulation, dorsal column stimulators, or sympathectomy. Frequently patients with RSD are referred to a pain management service. In addition, patients with RSD, like many patients with chronic pain, may develop emotional and behavioral disturbances that are best treated with a psychiatry referral.

49. Can someone other than an orthopedic surgeon safely realign a deformed, pulseless, fractured extremity?

Yes. It is generally believed that more benefit than damage results from gentle traction and realignment of a pulseless extremity. The traumatic force required to injure the extremity has already done the major damage. If the patient is in the hospital, the nurse should ask a physician, nurse practitioner, or physician assistant to perform the reduction. A paramedic, nurse, or emergency medical technician can reduce a pulseless angulated fracture in the prehospital setting to address this limb-threatening problem. If a pulseless extremity is left uncorrected for a prolonged period, vascular compromise leads to hypoxic and necrotic injury to the tissues. After reduction, the pulse is rechecked to ensure that it has been restored. The extremity should be splinted and elevated, and ice should be applied.

50. What should the nurse do if profuse bleeding is associated with a fracture?

The nurse should apply direct pressure and determine whether the bleeding is arterial or venous. If arterial bleeding is present, prolonged pressure is required. With predominantly venous or capillary bleeding, the extremity may be splinted and elevated after pressure is applied. If the bleeding is unresponsive, more aggressive treatment may be required, including cautery.

51. How are clavicle fractures usually treated?

Clavicle fractures with acceptable angulation and displacement are usually treated with a sling or figure-of-eight clavicle strap. Mobility of the upper extremity must be maintained to avoid stiffness.

52. How can humoral fractures be treated?

Humoral fractures are frequently treated with a sling or humoral fracture brace if angulation and displacement are acceptable. The patient should begin early mobilization of the humerus with gentle range-of-motion exercises to prevent stiffness and adhesive capsulitis. If the fracture is unstable or has significant displacement and angulation, it can be stabilized surgically.

53. Is a cast required for a supracondylar fracture of the elbow?

Supracondylar fractures are typically treated with a long arm cast or posterior elbow splint. Unstable fractures can be treated with ORIF.

54. Is closed treatment for combined radial/ulnar fractures the same as treatment for isolated fractures of the distal radius?

No. Closed treatment for isolated fractures of the distal radius consists simply of a short arm cast for approximately 6 weeks. The initial nonsurgical treatment for a combined forearm fracture is a long arm cast, which is converted first to a short arm cast and eventually to a removable brace for further protection. Combined forearm fractures may take up to 10 weeks to heal.

55. Are toe and finger fractures treated in the same manner?

Both toe and finger fractures can be treated with buddy taping or by taping the injured digit to the adjacent digit. A finger fracture often is treated with a splint for the first few weeks, followed by conversion to taping to avoid stiffness.

56. What is the most common cause of pelvic fractures?

The most frequent cause of a severe pelvic fracture is a motor vehicle crash.

57. What is the initial concern with a pelvic fracture?

Hemodynamic stability and assisting with resuscitation are the orthopedic nurse's initial goals in the emergency setting when the patient has a pelvic fracture.

58. What are the major potential complications of pelvic fractures?

Pelvic fractures may cause serious complications such as hemorrhage from lacerated veins and arteries, neurologic injury, colon laceration, and genitourinary damage.

59. How much blood can be lost with a pelvic fracture?

Severe pelvic fractures can result in the loss of up to 6 liters of blood. The bleeding may be severe enough to cause hypovolemic shock or death.

60. How are pelvic fractures diagnosed?

Physical exam, x-ray, CT scan, bone scan, and MRI can aid in diagnosing a pelvic fracture.

61. List the various types of pelvic fractures.
- Isolated fractures without disruption of the pelvic ring
- Pelvic ring fractures
- Acetabular fractures
- Sacrococcygeal fractures

62. How does an isolated fracture of the pelvis occur?
Isolated pelvic fractures are usually relatively benign, depending on the extent of soft tissue injury. An isolated pelvic fracture usually results from an avulsion fracture, stress fracture, or direct trauma. An avulsion fracture occurs at a musculotendinous attachment on the pelvis, usually in athletes. Patients with osteoporotic bone may sustain a stress fracture due to poor bone density. Patients who have direct injury to the pelvis can have isolated fractures.

63. How are pelvic ring fractures classified?
A generally accepted method for classifying pelvic ring fractures uses four categories based on the type of force that caused the injury:
- **Anteroposterior compression fractures** lead to the classic open-book injury to the pelvic ring. They are characterized by anterior disruption and widening at the symphysis pubis and posterior disruption at the ilium or sacroiliac joint. A possible mechanism of injury is a pedestrian struck anteriorly by a car.
- **Lateral compression fractures** generally result in pubic rami fractures and fractures at the ilium and sacroiliac joint. Frequently they occur when a pedestrian is struck laterally in the hip by a car.
- **Vertical shear fractures** are due to falls from a height. They are generally unstable and have a high incidence of neurovascular or visceral complications. Because of fractures at the pubic rami and sacroiliac joint, the affected hemipelvis is displaced vertically.
- **Complex pelvic ring fractures** are a combination of two or three of the above pelvic fractures.

64. What are the usual causes for acetabular and sacrococcygeal fractures?
Fractures of the acetabulum frequently result from a fall with direct impact to the side of the hip or from motor vehicle collision (MVC). The patient typically is not wearing a seat belt during the MVC and hits the knees into the dashboard on impact, causing the femur to displace posteriorly and disrupting the acetabulum in the process. Sacrococcygeal fractures frequently result from falls in which the patient lands directly on the sacrococcygeal area.

65. Describe the signs and symptoms of pelvic fractures.
Signs and symptoms vary in severity, depending on the amount and complexity of the injury. The patient may simply have mild point tenderness on palpation, discomfort or pain with ambulation and mild discomfort when the injured area is stressed. More complicated pelvic fractures may exhibit signs and symptoms of shock from bleeding into the pelvis. Patients may have neurovascular compromise of one or both of the lower extremities, blood in the urine, ecchymosis, pain and crepitus with palpation of the pelvis, and obvious deformity.

66. How can a pelvic ring fracture be stabilized?

In the emergency department the nurse may use military antishock trousers (MAST) or pneumatic antishock garments (PASG) to splint the pelvis. Another way to immobilize the pelvis is to wrap the patient with a sheet or towel and knot it at the front. The pelvis may also be secured to a long board or bed in a criss-cross fashion with tape. The trauma or orthopedic surgeon may choose to stabilize the pelvis with external or internal fixation.

67. What should the nurse do once the pelvis has been immobilized?

The nurse should reassess neurovascular status, mobility, and capillary refill of the lower extremities.

68. When is a Foley catheter contraindicated in patients with a suspected pelvic ring fracture?

A Foley catheter should not be placed in patients with blood at the meatus, inability to void, or gross hematuria. In these settings a catheter may cause further injury by tearing the urethra.

69. How are pelvic ring fractures treated?

Treatment of a pelvic ring fracture ranges from bed rest or pelvic sling traction to skeletal traction with external fixation. The type and extent of treatment depend on the severity and stability of the pelvic fracture. Treatment may take from a few days to several weeks, depending on the method. The overall goal is to restore pelvic ring anatomy and maintain comfort while preventing further complications.

70. How do hip fractures usually occur?

Hip fractures in the elderly most often result from a fall. Common factors leading to falls include tripping on a curb, animal, or throw rug. Decreased muscle strength may contribute to loss of postural stability.

71. Why are the elderly most likely to sustain a hip fracture?

The elderly are more prone to hip fractures because of the effects of aging and decreasing bone mass. Poor vision, effects of medications, and alterations in balance, proprioception, and coordination, combined with decreased bone mass, explain why the incidence of hip fractures increases with aging.

72. Describe the usual presentation of a hip fracture.

The affected extremity may be shortened and externally rotated. Severe pain, ecchymosis, and tissue swelling may be evident.

73. How are hip fractures treated?

Initial treatment includes immobilizing and stabilizing the extremity with a foam immobilizer. Later skin or skeletal traction may be necessary to maintain proper alignment before surgical treatment. ORIF, percutaneous pinning of the hip, or total hip arthroplasty may be necessary to stabilize the hip and prevent future complications. The goals of treatment are early mobilization and restoration of the hip to its original alignment. The hip must be reduced and realigned to provide stability and restore original structure length.

74. What does a femur fracture look like?

A femur fracture may or may not be clinically obvious. The patient may have a grossly deformed swollen thigh with a large amount of pain in the affected area. The affected leg may be rotated internally or externally and may be markedly shorter than the unaffected leg.

75. What complications are associated with femur fractures?

Femur fractures frequently result from major trauma. A large amount of blood may be lost because of the disruption of the blood supply. A patient may lose up to 3000 ml of blood from an isolated femur fracture. Femur fractures may also lead to neurovascular injury and fat emboli syndrome.

76. How are femur fractures treated initially?

Initially the patient must be hemodynamically stabilized and the leg must be re-aligned. After reduction and splinting or immobilizing with skin or skeletal traction, neurovascular status must be reassessed.

77. What is the difference in treatment of stable combined midshaft tibial and fibular fractures compared with stable ankle fractures?

Stable ankle fractures are treated with a short leg cast or an immobilization boot, whereas combined tibial/fibular fractures are treated with a long leg cast. Both should be addressed surgically if they are unstable or open.

78. Is a cast necessary for metatarsal fractures?

Stable metatarsal fractures can be treated conservatively with a short leg cast, hard-soled shoe, or an immobilization boot. If the fracture is unstable, surgical intervention may be required, including ORIF or percutaneous pinning.

79. What orthopedic problems can result from chest wall trauma?

Chest wall trauma can result in fractures to the ribs or sternum.

80. Which ribs are most frequently fractured in patients with chest wall trauma?

The third through ninth ribs are the most frequently fractured. The first and second rib are well protected by the muscles and bones of the shoulder girdle. If the first two ribs are fractured, the nurse must consider a forceful mechanism of injury and should be astute in looking for other underlying injury.

81. What considerations accompany rib fractures?

Rib fractures, in general, lead to the possibility of injury to underlying organs, including lungs, spleen, and liver. In addition to underlying injury, the nurse must address the patient's pain and potential for secretion retention and ineffective ventilation.

82. Describe a flail chest injury.

A flail chest injury occurs when multiple rib fractures are present. The patient may also have a sternal fracture. The flail segment is described as moving paradoxically when the patient breathes. In paradoxical respiration, the flail segment bulges out and the rib cage moves in when the patient exhales; the flail segment retracts and the rib cage expands when the patient inhales. The combination of the flail segment and pain leads to decreased air movement.

83. Summarize treatment of a flail chest.
- Administer oxygen and manage the airway.
- Manage pain.
- If spinal fracture is ruled out, position the patient with the injured side down.
- Surgical repair of the flail segment may be required.

84. What complications may arise from sternal fractures?

A sternal fracture is associated with high-force chest wall trauma. The underlying injuries are a major concern for the health care team. The patient can have significant underlying organ injuries, including cardiac contusion, pulmonary contusion, pneumothorax, hemothorax, and aortic tear.

85. What populations are at risk for spinal fracture and cord injury?

The majority of spinal fractures and cord injuries occur in young men as a result of motor vehicle crashes. Alcohol and drug use is also a contributing factor. Highly active sports, such as motocross racing, skydiving, football, and diving, are associated with spinal fracture and cord injuries. Violent crimes are also a significant contributor to spinal cord injuries. In older adults, spinal fracture and cord injuries are often caused by a fall.

86. What types of injuries can result in spinal fracture and potential spinal cord injury (SCI)?

Spinal fractures have several mechanisms of injury and can be traumatic or nontraumatic. Traumatic causes include motor vehicle accidents, diving injuries, blunt trauma, and falls. When bone density is decreased or weakened, as in patients with bone cancer or osteoporosis, a nontraumatic vertebral fracture can easily occur. Forces applied to the spine that can cause vertebral fractures include axial loading, rotation, hyperextension, and hyperflexion. In addition, penetrating injuries, as with a bullet or knife wound, can cause spinal fracture and SCI.

87. What types of vertebral fractures can occur?
- **Compression fractures** result from axial compression, as in patients who fall and land directly on the buttocks. Compression fractures can also result from hyperflexion injuries to the spine. Such fractures are generally stable if the vertebral ligaments remain intact.
- **Burst fractures** also result from axial loading of the spine. They are significantly more problematic than compression fractures because fragments of the vertebrae and intervertebral disc can cause compression and injury to the spinal cord and nerve roots.
- **Teardrop fractures** are caused by a combination of compression and flexion forces and characterized by fracture of the anterior portion of the vertebral body. A potential problematic complication is posterior migration of the vertebral body, which may cause injury to the spinal cord.
- **Simple fractures** at the spine are usually stable and typically affect the pedicle, facet, spinous process, or transverse process.
- **Vertebral dislocations** are caused by flexion injuries and involve sprained or ruptured ligaments of the vertebrae with dislocation of one or both facet joints. The vertebral dislocation is characterized by spondylolisthesis.

- As the name implies, a **fracture-dislocation** is a combination of a vertebral fracture with subsequent dislocation. These injuries are frequently unstable and associated with spinal cord compromise.

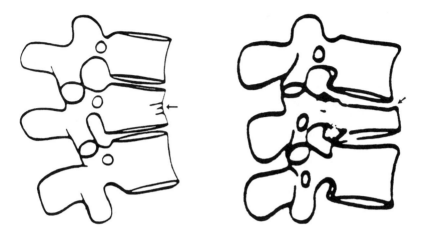

Left, Compression fracture (arrow). *Right,* Burst fracture (arrow). (From Callewart CC: Traumatic injuries of the lumbar spine. In Cole AJ, Herring SA (eds): The Low Back Pain Handbook. Philadelphia, Hanley & Belfus, 1997, pp 399-404, with permission.)

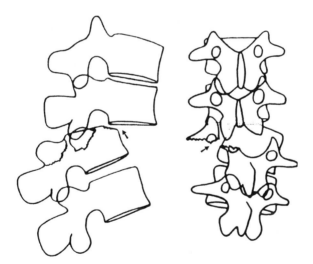

Fracture-dislocation (arrows). (From Callewart CC: Traumatic injuries of the lumbar spine. In Cole AJ, Herring SA (eds): The Low Back Pain Handbook. Philadelphia, Hanley & Belfus, 1997, pp 399-404, with permission.)

88. What is the most frequent level of spinal injury?

The cervical and lumbar areas are the most mobile and therefore the most frequently injured. The thoracic vertebrae are protected by the rib cage and are much less mobile.

89. What is special about high cervical fractures?

The high degree of movement between the skull, C1, and C2 makes this area vulnerable to potentially life-threatening SCI. Jefferson fractures are essentially burst fractures of C1. A fracture of high-energy force can cause dislocation between the skull and C1. Fractures of the odontoid process of C2 can result in displaced or nondisplaced fractures of the atlantoaxial joint. Hangman's fractures occur through the pedicles and/or lamina of C3 and can lead to potential instability at C2–C3.

90. Describe the physical exam of patients with potential spinal injury.

The nurse must perform a complete neuromuscular assessment, which includes assessment of deep tendon and superficial reflexes, motor function and strength, and sensory status (see Chapter 1). In addition to the neuromuscular assessment, the nurse should be cognizant of the mechanism of injury and potential associated injuries. The nurse must perform at least vascular, cardiothoracic, and abdominopelvic exams in addition to the neuromuscular exam. The initial trauma assessment is discussed in the beginning of this chapter.

91. How are stable vertebral fractures frequently managed?

Stable vertebral fractures are generally treated rather conservatively with various immobilization techniques, including a cervical collar or brace, thoracolumbosacral orthoses (TLSO), lumbosacral orthoses (LSO), or corset braces. Patients should be educated about avoiding stress and strain to the spine from activities such as stooping, lifting, pushing, or pulling. The associated soft tissue injuries can be treated as indicated.

92. What are the immobilization options for unstable vertebral fractures?

Immobilization options for unstable vertebral fractures include surgical stabilization with fusion, decompression, and/or instrumentation. Other nonoperative treatment includes the halo apparatus and skull tongs. Options for vertebral fractures are further discussed in Chapter 14.

93. Summarize the basic nursing interventions in caring for patients with a vertebral fracture.

- Maintain proper immobilization of the patient as ordered.
- Turn and position the patient using log-rolling or other turning devices as needed.
- Educate the patient about injuries, treatments, and possible complications.
- Assist the patient with ADLs as needed.
- Assess and manage pain.
- Discuss the patient's home and work concerns and possible modifications.
- Maintain proper nutrition and hydration.
- Monitor for changes in vital signs or neuromuscular status.
- Monitor for skin integrity problems or infection.
- Monitor for signs of altered bowel or urinary elimination.
- Monitor pulmonary function and oxygenation.

BIBLIOGRAPHY

1. Brown DE, Neumann RD: Orthopedic Secrets, 3rd ed. Philadelphia, Hanley & Belfus, 2003.
2. Greene WB: Essentials of Musculoskeletal Care, 2nd ed. Rosemont, IL, American Academy of Orthopedic Surgeons, 2001

3. Hanson TH, Swiontkowski MF: Orthopedic Trauma Protocols. New York, Raven Press, 1993.
4. Holleran RS: Pre-hospital Nursing: A Collaborative Approach. St. Louis, Mosby, 1994.
5. Jacobs BB: Trauma Nursing Core Curriculum, 5th ed. Chicago, Emergency Nurses Association, 2000.
6. Lewis SM, Heitkemper, MM, Dirksen SR: Medical Surgical Nursing: Assessment and Management of Clinical Problems, 5th ed. St. Louis, Mosby, 2000.
7. Maher AB, Salmond SW, Pellino TA: Orthopaedic Nursing, 3rd ed. Philadelphia, W.B. Saunders, 2002.
8. McQuillan KA, VonRueden KT, Hartsock RL, et al: Trauma Nursing: From Resuscitation through Rehabilitation, 3rd ed. Philadelphia, W.B. Saunders, 2002.
9. Morgan L: Advanced Trauma Life Support Course, 6th ed. Chicago, American College of Surgeons, 1997.
10. Schoen DC: NAON Core Curriculum for Orthopaedic Nursing, 4th ed. Pittman, NJ, Anthony J. Jannetti, 2001.
11. Staheli LT: Pediatric Orthopedic Secrets, 2nd ed. Philadelphia, Hanley & Belfus, 1997.

8. SPORTS MEDICINE

Amy L. Hite, MSN, FNP-C, ONC

1. What is sports medicine?

The role of sports has become increasingly important in the United States. The beginning of sports medicine dates back to the second century AD, when Galen served as the team physician for gladiators. Sports medicine is a general term that is difficult to define specifically. For the purpose of simplicity it includes the medicine behind sports injury. However, with increased research and emphasis on the prevention of injuries and rehabilitation after injuries, sports medicine involves a broad understanding and commitment to athletes and their specific injuries. The sports medicine team now consists of people from multiple disciplines.

2. Who benefits from sports medicine?

Sports medicine in the 21st century does not apply only to professional athletes. It includes self-directed exercise enthusiasts, weekend softball players, little league ball teams, weight-lifters, league bowlers, aerobic queens and kings, geriatric aquasizers, and people of all ages who participate in athletics. Despite reports that society in general is more sedentary and obese, with a direct relationship to the increase in diabetes and cardiovascular and pulmonary diseases, participation in recreational and intramural sports, health club memberships, purchase of home gym equipment, public exercise accessibility (walk/bike/skate parks, nature trails), and exercise classes have increased. The health care industry must be prepared to promote and maintain people involved in fitness or athletic participation by understanding the nature of stresses on the body that each activity can cause and the proper approaches to injury prevention, diagnosis, treatment, and rehabilitation.

3. Who makes up the sports medicine team?

Many people are involved in the sports medicine team, each with individual and overlapping roles. The physician is the team leader, making the final decision about eligibility for athletic participation. The team physician "oversees all aspects of the sports medicine program, including conditioning to prevent injury, an emergency care protocol for injuries, illnesses, as well as the treatment and rehabilitation of those conditions."[15] Team physicians vary from family physicians, orthopedic surgeons, pediatricians, chiropractors or other medical specialists. Allied health care professionals may include nurse practitioners, physician assistants, nurses, nutritionists, orthotists, pharmacists, physical and occupational therapists, psychologists, or emergency medical technicians and paramedics. The coach and athletic trainer are integral members of the team

Other members of the sports medicine team can include parents, families, or guardians; athletic administrators; team owners, general managers, or boards of trustees; superintendents, principals, and school boards; lawyers or sports managers; and equipment managers, conditioning coaches, or personal trainers.

4. What is the role of the athletic trainer?

The athletic trainer is "a qualified allied health care professional educated and experienced in the management of health care problems associated with sports participation."[15] The athletic trainer is an integral member of the team and has the most direct contact with the athletes. The roles of the athletic trainer include risk management, injury prevention, injury recognition, evaluation and immediate care, administration, and initiation of treatment and rehabilitation.

5. How does the coach fit on the sports medicine team?

The coach serves as an educator to the athlete by teaching techniques and strategies that prevent injuries. The coach must maintain communication among the physicians, athletic trainers, and athletes to optimize team performance and promote safety. The athlete should be willing to work with and learn from the sports medicine team to ensure safety and enhance participation.

6. What college sports have the highest reported injury rates?

The National Collegiate Athletic Association (NCAA) developed the Injury Surveillance System (ISS) in 1982 to analyze trends in intercollegiate sports injuries. According to the NCAA,[12] the following three sports have the highest reported injuries for the 1998–1999 seasons (in descending order):

- Injuries in practice: spring football, wrestling, women's soccer
- Game injuries: football, wrestling, men's soccer
- Percentage of all injuries in practices and games: women's gymnastics, women's volleyball, wrestling
- Practice injuries resulting in 7 or more lost days of participation: spring football, women's gymnastics, wrestling
- Game injuries resulting in 7 or more lost days of participation: football, wrestling, ice hockey
- Practice injuries resulting in surgeries: spring football, women's gymnastics, wrestling
- Game injuries resulting in surgeries: football, wrestling, women's soccer.

7. What are the most common acute injuries in sports?

Common sports injuries include fractures, strains, sprains, bruises/contusions, acute compartment syndrome and dislocations/subluxations.

- A **fracture** is a crack or breaks in a bone and can be open (the bone comes through the skin) or closed (the bone remains in the skin).
- A **strain** is a stretch, tear, or complete rupture of a muscle or tendon.
- A **sprain** is a stretch, tear, or complete rupture of a ligament.
- A **bruise** or **contusion** involves bleeding in the muscle as the result of a direct blow.
- **Acute compartment syndrome** develops as a sequela to the injury. Swelling and increased pressure in the compartment result from bleeding and cause compression of the involved nerves and blood vessels.
- **Dislocations** occur when the ball of a joint is forced out of the socket or when the articulating bones of a joint are separated.
- **Subluxations** occur when a partial dislocation or a brief dislocation immediately reduces (pops back into place).

8. Which acute injury requires immediate medical attention?

Acute compartment syndrome is a medical emergency that requires a fasciotomy to prevent irreversible tissue damage. Fractures and dislocations also require early medical evaluation.

9. What are overuse and chronic injuries?

An overuse injury results from continuous repetitive stress or loading of tissue, causing a wide variety of muscle, tendon, ligament, and bone abnormalities. Such injuries can cause tissue disruption and inflammation or tissue degeneration. Chronic injuries can last for months or even years and are characterized by persistent symptoms. The main differences between a chronic and acute injury are that chronic injuries show long-term inflammation, scar tissue accumulation, degenerative changes, and muscle atrophy.

10. Give examples of chronic injuries.

Tendinitis, bursitis, fasciitis, neuritis, chronic compartment syndrome, stress fractures, chondromalacia, and osteochondritis dissecans.

11. Differentiate among tendinitis, bursitis, fascitis, and neuritis.

Tendinitis is the inflammation in the tendon due to microtears. Tendinitis is most often seen in the Achilles, rotator cuff, biceps, and patellar tendons.

Bursitis is inflammation of a bursa sac due to repetitive forces that cause swelling from increased synovial fluid in the area. Bursitis is common in the shoulder, elbow, hip, and knee.

Fasciitis involves inflammation and microtears of the fascia, the overlying connective tissue. Plantar fasciitis of the foot and overuse compartment syndromes are the most common examples.

Neuritis is irritation or inflammation of nerves. Repetitive mechanical stretching, friction, or compression of the nerve by overlying tissues or bones causes neuritis.

12. Describe compartment syndrome and stress fractures.

Chronic compartment syndrome results in increased intracompartmental pressure due to muscle hypertrophy and increased muscle volume from exercise.[4] **Stress fractures** occur in the presence of microdamage to the bone from abnormal or repetitive stresses applied without the proper rest for the normal reparative process. The cause of a stress fracture usually includes repetitive over-exercising and new or increased training programs. Stress fractures can occur in any bone but usually are seen in weight-bearing bones.

13. What is the difference between chondromalacia and osteochondritis dissecans?

Chondromalacia is the softening of the articular cartilage due to abnormal stress or excessive pressure. The repetitive microtrauma can lead to degenerative changes and is common in the knee, hip, and shoulder.

Osteochondritis dissecans is due to injury to the subchondral bone, resulting in necrosis, fragmentation, and separation of the bone with loose bodies in the joint. This condition is caused by repetitive microtrauma in the joint. It is common in the ankles and knees of children and the femoral condyles of adult knees.

14. What is the most common treatment of all sports injuries?

The most important treatment of any sport-related injury is RICE: **r**est, **i**ce, **c**ompression, and **e**levation. This treatment should begin as soon as the injury occurs. Immediate use of RICE can reduce disability time and improve recovery time. The principle behind RICE is to minimize and control swelling and inflammation. Often nonsteroidal anti-inflammatory drugs (NSAIDs) are used along with RICE for the management of pain and inflammation.

15. What is the importance of the pre-participation physical exam?

The pre-participation physical exam is instrumental in preventing sports injuries. All athletes should have a pre-participation physical exam; it is required for most school-related, community, and organized sports. However, anyone beginning athletic or fitness participation should discuss this decision with a health care provider and have a thorough physical exam to detect potential problems, assess the chosen sport individually, and make safety recommendations.

16. Discuss the safety aspect of using the proper sports equipment.

The use of proper equipment is necessary for participation and safety. The most important factor is shoes. The right footwear (shoes and socks) can prevent injuries and optimize performance. Appropriate clothing for the sport and climate is essential. Men are encouraged to wear athletic support straps, and women should invest in a high-quality, supportive sports bra. Outdoor fitness after dark should always include several items that glow in the dark and a luminous vest.[10]

Specific equipment for each sport or fitness activity should be evaluated for safety and durability. Equipment that is broken or unfamiliar should not be used. Safety equipment for specific sports should always be properly fitted by a professional familiar with the equipment. Examples include helmets, eyewear, mouth guards, throat protectors, pads, chest protectors, facemask, and chinstraps.[1]

17. Why are warming up and cooling down important?

The key to preventing injuries is warming up and cooling down. Warm-up or sweat suits should be used in cold weather for insulation and warmth of the muscles, tendons, and ligaments. For safe and effective stretching a warm-up is essential. Exercises that are good for warm up include five minutes of walking, light jog, stationary bike, or marching in place. The warm-up increases intramuscular temperature, making the muscles more elastic and lubricated, creating less friction in joints, improved nerve impulse transmission to muscle fibers, and enhanced reflexes. Warm-up should be followed by 5–10 minutes of stretching, which should include performing slow stretches for each major muscle group and holding each stretch between 20 and 60 seconds. Flexibility decreases with age and injuries, both of which warrant more emphasis on stretching, especially in problem areas. Each stretch should be held to the point of tension, not pain. Bouncing is not recommended for stretching and can be more damaging.[10]

Participation should be followed by 5 minutes of cool-down and 5 minutes of stretching. This practice allows the heart rate to slow down, prevents muscle spasms and tightening, and maintains or improves flexibility.

18. What is a contusion?

A contusion, or bruise, results from a direct or indirect blow that applies blunt force to a muscle. Contusions involve the deep muscle fibers, whereas a strain involves the superficial muscle fibers. The injury to the muscle fibers causes bleeding, which results in ecchymosis. A severe contusion or continuous activity after the contusion can lead to a hematoma (pooling of the blood in the tissue under the skin). Any muscle can be involved in a contusion, but the most commonly affected muscles are the quadriceps and gastrocnemius.

19. Describe the treatment for a contusion.

The treatment for a contusion includes RICE, prevention of hematoma formation by early intervention, and early motion in associated joints (24-48 hours). Rehabilitation should start with stretching (independent stretching only-absolutely no assisted stretching), progression to isometric exercises, and then progressive resistance exercises. The athlete should practice and participate in noncontact sports before fully resuming his or her specific sport. The most common problems are overtreating and returning to activities too quickly, which can exacerbate symptoms and prolong recovery. With a mild-to-moderate contusion, recovery and return to full participation usually occur within 2 weeks. A moderate-to-severe contusion takes 3–5 weeks, and a severe contusion can take 5–8 weeks for recovery and return to sports.

20. What is a charley horse?

A charley horse is a quadriceps contusion due to blunt trauma to the anterior thigh. This injury is seen most often in contact sports and sports with a higher potential for falling (football, basketball, soccer, and hockey). Symptoms include localized pain, exquisite tenderness to palpation, swelling, ecchymosis, and limping. Severe contusions can cause an effusion in the ipsilateral knee.[1,4,5]

21. What is the recommended treatment for quadriceps contusions?

The treatment for quadriceps contusions can be divided into three phases.
- **Phase I**: during the first 24 hours, RICE and crutch walking. Immobilization should maintain the knee in full flexion to prevent muscle shortening.
- **Phase II**: restoring motion with ice treatments and passive and active knee flexion and extension. Crutches should be continued until the patient has 90° of knee flexion, good quadriceps control, and minimal limp.
- **Phase III**: knee flexion to 120° without pain and excellent quadriceps control, followed by progression to sports. Extra padding at the site of injury should be used for participants in contact sports for 3–6 months.[15]

22. What are the complications of quadriceps contusions?

The two serious complications of quadriceps contusions result from severe bleeding: compartment syndrome and myositis ossificans. Both should be considered even in mild contusions if the patient has a bleeding disorder.

23. What are the symptoms of compartment syndrome?

Acute anterior compartment syndrome is an emergency that requires surgical intervention by a fasciotomy. Symptoms of compartment syndrome after quadriceps contusion include abnormal pain; firm or tense swelling; decreased distal pulses; sensory deficits along the anterior knee and medial aspect of the lower leg and foot (femoral and saphenous nerve distributions); and increased pain with flexion of the knee or elevation of the affected leg.[5,8,15] Compartment pressure measurements can definitively diagnose compartment syndrome.

24. What is myositis ossificans?

Myositis ossificans is a result of trauma to the muscle and periosteum, caused by severe compression on underlying bone. Heterotopic bone begins to form adjacent to the injury. Myositis ossificans should be considered if a firm mass begins to develop at the contusion site after approximately 3–4 weeks. Radiographs demonstrate densities in the soft tissue mass and reactive bone changes. The use of heat and ultrasound for the treatment of contusions has been found to increase the risk of myositis ossificans.

Treatment depends on the severity of functional disability, and surgical excision is a last resort that should not be attempted before 6–12 months.[3,5,15]

25. What medication is often used to prevent myositis ossificans?

Indomethacin (Indocin) has been shown to decrease the risk of myositis ossificans because of its ability to deter bone formation. It is occasionally used immediately after severe contusions and after surgical excision to prevent recurrence. The use of other NSAIDs after severe contusions is controversial. Some studies have shown that they increase bleeding and potentiate myositis ossificans, whereas other studies have shown that they are beneficial in treating inflammation and pain. Without a doubt, the most important treatments are ice and keeping the knee immobilized in a flexed position.

26. What is involved in a strain?

A strain, also known as a pull or tear, is the most common injury to a muscle or tendon. It results from stretching at or near the musculotendinous junction. The injury can range from overstretching of a few muscle fibers to complete tears between the muscle and tendon. Minor strains are characterized by pain at the site of injury, swelling, ecchymosis, or a small palpable defect. More severe cases are associated with the minor symptoms plus limited function, muscle spasms, pain with range of motion (ROM), and a large palpable or visual deformity.

27. Describe the recommended treatment for strains.

The treatment depends on the severity of the injury. General treatment for acute injuries includes rest, NSAIDs, ice, and elevation. In severe cases the use of crutches may be warranted for lower extremity strains. If a strain is severe enough to require immobilization, the muscle should be immobilized at full length to prevent contractures and atrophy. Early use of gentle stretching reduces the formation of scar tissue and muscle shortening, but overstretching can be more harmful. The return to strengthening and practice or sport participation should be individualized and may take up to 4 weeks. Isometric strengthening should be used before weight or resistance strengthening, and practices should precede return to games. Prevention of muscle strains is crucial to limiting injuries. A period of vulnerability during which the risk of reinjury is believed to be greatest occurs with incomplete healing time and quick return to play without complete rehabilitation. The period of disability is much longer with continual reinjury and lack of full healing, which can lead to chronic problems.

28. How can strains be prevented?

Warm-up before stretching is the single best way to reduce muscle strains. The muscle that is properly warmed up before stretching has a more forceful contraction and recovers more quickly to produce increased strength and speed.[10]

29. What muscle is involved in groin strain?

The adductor longus muscle is involved. Its site of origin is the pubic rami near the symphysis pubis, and it inserts into the posterior femur. The action of the adductor longus includes adduction, flexion, and external rotation of the thigh. Strains to the muscle most often occur with a leg that is abducted and forced into external rotation or with forceful adduction of the leg. Groin strains are most often seen in soccer, hockey, and tennis.

30. Describe the symptoms of groin strains.

Groin strains cause immediate stabbing pain in the groin, weakness or inability to adduct the leg, swelling and ecchymosis in the groin, and tenderness to palpation. Pain from a groin strain can be elicited with passive abduction or resisted adduction of the affected leg.

31. How are groin strains treated?

The treatment for a groin strain includes RICE initially; ROM and NSAIDs after 24–48 hours; and crutches as needed. Rehabilitation depends on the severity of the injury but should include early pain-free stretching and slow progression to resistance exercises. The recurrence rates for groin strains are highest when healing time is incomplete before return to activities. Most people recover from groin strains within 2–8 weeks.

32. What muscles make up the hamstring?

Three muscles make up the hamstring: semimebranosus, semitendinosus, and biceps femoris. The primary actions are knee flexion and thigh extension. The muscles span the entire posterior thigh. The biceps femoris tendon is the most commonly injured of the group.

33. What is the significance of the hamstring?

The hamstring group is significant because all three muscles cross both hip and knee joints. They are attached proximally at the ischial tuberosity, and the insertion is below the knee. Because two joints and a large muscle mass are involved, the action of the hamstrings is highly synchronized and complex.

34. What causes hamstring strains or pulls?

Hamstring strains are one of the most common injuries in sports (and most sensitive to treat). Several factors are responsible for hamstring strains, including inadequate warm-up; failure to stretch properly; muscle imbalance between the hamstring and quadriceps; poor endurance, technique, or posture; overstretching; and leg length discrepancies.[5,10]

A hamstring strain is more likely to be seen in sports that require sudden start-stop running motions, explosive increases in speed while running, or excessive stretching demands. Examples include runners (especially sprinters), football players, gymnasts, and dancers.

35. How are hamstring injuries evaluated?

The complaint after hamstring strains is an immediate onset of posterior thigh pain with rapid activity. Sometimes a pop is heard. The hallmark signs are localized tenderness and reproduction of the pain with passive extension of the knee with the hip flexed at 90°. More severe injuries cause ecchymosis; rarely are defects in the muscle palpated. Muscle spasms are common in the hamstring and often are the major cause of the pain.

36. Discuss the recovery time and rehabilitation for hamstring strains.

The recovery time of hamstring injuries depends on the severity of the injury and can take between 3 days and 3 weeks. Early return to sports is the worst mistake because it leads to re-injury.

Initial treatment should begin immediately with RICE. Pain medication is usually not necessary, but NSAIDs are beneficial. For severe muscle spasms, a muscle relaxant may be necessary. Slow progression to stretching and strengthening should be started as tolerated. Return to sports should be considered only after complete resolution of pain with activities and attainment of hamstring stretching and strengthening.

37. How can I remember the difference between a sprain and strain?

The key is proper identification. A strain involves a tendon or muscle, and a sprain involves a ligament. Remember that there is a "t" in strain and a "t" in tendon and that tendons are attached to muscles.

38. What is a sprain? How are sprains classified?

A sprain is a traumatic joint injury resulting in stretching, tearing, or rupture of the ligament between two bones. Sprains are classified as grades I to III.

- **Grade I**: mild sprain with stretching of only a few ligament fibers; characterized by mild tenderness, slight swelling, no limitation of motion or instability in the affected joint, and minimal discomfort in weight-bearing joints.
- **Grade II**: moderate sprain with stretching or tearing of up to half the ligament fibers; characterized by swelling, ecchymosis, localized pain, slight limitation of motion and instability in the affected joint, and some discomfort with weight-bearing.
- **Grade III**: severe sprain with complete tearing and separation through the ligament or avulsion at the insertion site to the bone. Symptoms include severe swelling, ecchymosis and pain, inability to bear weight, and marked limitation of motion with joint instability.[10,14]

39. What is the most common type of sprain?

In the lower extremity, the ankle is the most common site. In the upper extremity, the wrist is the most common site.

40. Describe the usual mechanism of injury in ankle sprains.

The most common mechanism is an inversion injury (the foot rolls inward), which causes a lateral ankle sprain. Lateral ankle sprains account for more than 80% of ankle sprains. They are often seen with stepping on uneven surfaces and sports such as tennis, basketball, football, volleyball, and skating. Medial ankle sprains are significantly less common but can be more troublesome to treat.

41. Describe the recovery time and rehabilitation of ankle sprains.

The severity of the sprain determines the length of recovery. In general, grade I ankle sprains recover in 1–4 weeks, grade II sprains in 2–6 weeks, and grade III sprains in 6–8 weeks. Early initiation of treatment lessens symptoms and promotes earlier return to activity. Initial treatment for grade I and II ankle sprains should include RICE, NSAIDs, short period of immobilization, protective weight-bearing as tolerated, and early motion exercises. The motion exercises should emphasize dorsiflexion and plantarflexion. Grade III ankle sprains should include the basic care of grades I and II, but prolonged immobilization and protective weight-bearing are necessary. Grade III sprains or chronic instability due to recurrent ankle sprains may require surgical fixation.

42. How can an ankle sprain be differentiated from an ankle fracture?

The only reliable way to determine a fracture is by radiographic studies. Indications for determining the need for x-rays include exquisite bone tenderness (medial malleolus or lateral malleolus) or inability to bear weight on the affected ankle joint. Follow up x-rays are also indicated if there is delay in the expected recovery time.

43. What joints and bones make up the knee?

The knee consists of two joints and three bones. The joints are the tibiofemoral joint (with medial and lateral compartments) and the patellofemoral joint. The bones are the femur, patella, and tibia. The knee is a complex joint that is vulnerable to injury in almost all sports.

44. What are the key questions to ask a patient who complains of a knee injury?

- Where is the area of the most pain?
- Is the knee buckling (giving out)?
- Is the knee catching or locking (*not* popping)?
- Is the knee swelling?

45. What is the hallmark sign of a knee injury?

An effusion (swelling) of the knee joint is always a sign of some form of internal derangement in the knee. The amount of swelling often indicates the severity of injury or the lack of treatment. If the knee continues to swell with rehabilitation, consider three possibilities: premature return to activity, overuse, or incorrect original diagnosis. If the knee joint is aspirated, the color and content of the fluid can also reveal a great deal about the injury. If the fluid is straw-colored, think of meniscal injury; if the fluid is bloody, think of ligament injury; and if fat globules (most easily seen in a steel pan) are present, think of chondral injury or fracture.

46. Can knee injuries be prevented?

The majority of nontraumatic knee injuries in sports can be prevented or risk factors can be modified. Risk factors include muscle imbalances between the hamstring and quadriceps, past history of knee injuries, female gender, failure to participate in preseason conditioning, anatomic predisposition, improper shoewear, artificial playing surfaces (Astro Turf), and ligament laxity (loose-jointed). All attempts should be made through conditioning, exercise, coaching, and equipment to minimize the risk of knee injuries in sports.

47. What is the usual direction of patella dislocations?

Almost all patella dislocations are lateral. A medial patella dislocation is so rare that most orthopedists never see one in their career. However, because the medial femoral condyle is uncovered and prominent, people often think that the knee is displaced medially. If the patella does not immediately reduce, it can easily be palpated laterally. Patients with a dislocated patella hold the knee in flexion.[4]

48. Who is at risk for patella dislocations?

Most people with patella dislocations have an underlying or anatomic predisposition. It is important to assess the opposite uninjured knee to determine any predisposition. Several studies have shown that two-thirds of all patients with patella dislocations have a predisposition. Predisposing factors include patella alta (high-riding patella); shallow trochlea; ligament laxity; severe genu valgum (knock-knees); femoral anteversion (intoeing); and increased patella mobility.[5] Patella dislocations are most common in sports that involve cutting, pivoting, or contact.

49. What is the mechanism of injury in patella dislocations?

A patella dislocation usually occurs with one of the following mechanisms: a twisting injury with strong contraction of the quadriceps muscle; a direct blow to the medial side of the patella that pushes it laterally; or a direct blow to the lateral side of the leg that forces the knee into valgus.[5,15] Rarely does a direct fall onto the patella result in patella dislocation.

50. How are patella dislocations managed?

The majority of acute patella dislocations reduce immediately if the person fully extends the knee. Often in sports injuries the athlete feels two pops in the knee, first the dislocation and then the reduction. Usual symptoms include immediate swelling and pain over the medial side of the knee.

Once the patella is reduced, immobilization for 4–6 weeks with the knee in full extension allows healing of the disrupted medial structures. A commercial knee immobilizer is usually used, but sometimes a cylinder cast is used for guaranteed patient compliance. During immobilization, quadriceps strengthening can be achieved with straight leg raises and quadriceps sets. Return to activity is not allowed until complete recovery and rehabilitation are attained. With return to activity a knee sleeve or wrap with a patella cutout or lateral compression pad is often used to help maintain normal patella tracking. Surgical treatment is not usually necessary with acute, isolated dislocations. Surgery may be indicated for chronic, recurrent patella dislocations or for correction of an anatomic predisposition.

51. What are the possible complications of a dislocated patella?

A patella dislocation may result in an osteochondral fracture of the femoral trochlea or patella or an avulsion fracture of the medial aspect of the patella. Osteochondral fractures may result in loose bodies within the knee joint. Radiographs should be used for this diagnosis, and surgical intervention may be necessary to stabilize the patella.

52. Describe the role of the meniscus.

The meniscus is a C-shaped structure that acts as cushion cartilage to absorb loads put on the knee joint and protects the articular surfaces of the knee joint. The knee has both a medial and a lateral meniscus, corresponding to the inside and outside of the knee. The menisci also aid in joint stability of the knee.

53. What is the usual mechanism of injury in acute meniscal tears?

Meniscal injuries are uncommon isolated injuries in athletes under 20 years of age, and an anterior cruciate ligament injury should be carefully considered. Wrestlers and weightlifters have increased risk of injury to the menisci because of the increased time spent kneeling and hyperextending the knees,[15] but overall meniscal injuries have the highest incidence in football, basketball, and wrestling.[5]

Meniscal injuries usually result from a twisting or shearing force in the knee of a young person. In people over the age of 35, degenerative tears are more common. Medial meniscal injuries are more common than lateral meniscal injuries. The main types of meniscal injuries are shown below.

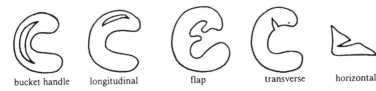

bucket handle   longitudinal   flap   transverse   horizontal

The five main types of meniscal tears. (From Brown DE, Neumann RD (eds): Orthopedic Secrets, 2nd ed. Philadelphia, Hanley & Belfus, 1999, with permission.)

54. What are the common symptoms of meniscal injuries?

Meniscal injuries usually present with pain in the knee (specifically pain over the joint line of the affected side), catching or locking, and buckling. Symptoms may include swelling and limitation of motion, especially lack of full extension. Pain is elicited at the joint line with squatting. This test is especially sensitive with posterior lateral meniscal tears, which are associated with exquisite posterior lateral joint-line pain with squatting because the lateral meniscus is compressed.

The most sensitive tests for meniscal injuries are the McMurray and Apley grind tests or any other test that manipulates the knee into a position that can displace or compress the meniscus. Pain with these tests and a palpable or audible click as the meniscus displaces or reduces are highly indicative of meniscal tears. Plain radiographs of the knee are not useful in diagnosing a meniscal injury because the meniscus is soft tissue. However, they should be obtained for all knee pain to rule out fractures or bony lesions. Weight-bearing radiographs are used to estimate the amount of joint space. Magnetic resonance imaging (MRI) scans are the mainstream approach to meniscal injuries and, according to most research data, are between 90% and 96% accurate.

55. What is the usual treatment of meniscal injuries?

There are several answers to this question. First of all, the symptoms and desired return to activities must be analyzed. The meniscus does not have a good healing potential, especially with isolated injuries. Vascular supply to the meniscus is limited, and the synovial fluid provides many of the nutrients. However, many meniscal tears are asymptomatic after recovery from the acute injury, and the person is able to return to activities without complications.

Options in treatments for meniscal injuries include conservative treatment and arthroscopic repair or removal. A number of variables must be considered before determining the appropriate treatment plan. There is some concern that untreated symptomatic meniscal injuries increase the risk for early arthritis in the knee. The option of arthroscopic repair or resection of the torn meniscus depends on the age of the patient, the stability of the knee, the location of the tear, and the integrity of the meniscus.[5]

56. Describe the main ligaments of the knee and their function.

Four main ligaments provide stability to the knee:
- Anterior cruciate ligament (ACL)
- Posterior cruciate ligament (PCL)
- Medial collateral ligament (MCL)
- Lateral collateral ligament (LCL)

The ACL provides stability against anterior forces applied to the tibia, and the PCL provides stability against posterior forces applied against the tibia. The MCL provides medial stability against valgus stress, and the LCL provides stability against varus stress. Although these ligaments are responsible for the majority of stability in the knee, they are assisted by several contributing structures.

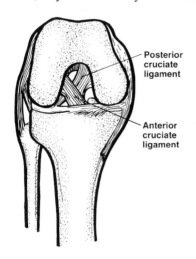

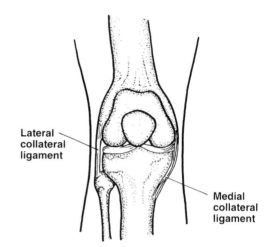

Anterior and posterior cruciate ligament structures. (From Frontera WR, Silver JK (eds): Essentials of Physical Medicine and Rehabilitation. Philadelphia, Hanley & Belfus, 2002, with permission.)

Medial and lateral collateral ligaments. (From Frontera WR, Silver JK (eds): Essentials of Physical Medicine and Rehabilitation. Philadelphia, Hanley & Belfus, 2002, with permission.)

57. What tests are used to assess ligament injuries?

The ACL can be assessed for integrity with the Lachman, anterior drawer, or pivot shift test. The PCL can be assessed with the posterior drawer test. The LCL should be assessed with varus stress testing and the MCL with valgus stress testing. All tests assess the integrity and the potential for laxity or looseness while a load is applied to the specific ligament. If the stress or load results in no firm endpoint of stability, the amount of laxity often determines the degree or grade of injury. The injured knee should always be compared with the opposite knee.

58. Where do most ligament injuries occur in sports?

Ligament injuries occur when the leg is planted and a force is applied or a sudden change in direction takes place. The majority of ligament injuries in the knee occur with twisting, cutting, and pivoting sports, such as basketball, football, tennis, soccer, snow skiing, rugby, volleyball, and gymnastics. Frequently injuries to the knee result in combined ligament damage or ligament and meniscal involvement.

59. Describe the mechanism of MCL injuries.

MCL injuries occur when the knee is forced inward (valgus force) by a twist or direct blow on the lateral side of the leg. There is pain along the MCL, and valgus stressing causes pain and laxity. Associated cruciate ligament injuries can occur and should be assessed. Meniscal injuries are uncommon. Soft tissue swelling may occur, but there should be no joint effusion if the injury is isolated. MCL disruption is common with PCL injuries.

60. How are MCL injuries treated?

Treatment depends on the severity of the injury and is usually nonsurgical. RICE should be initiated, but immobilization is usually not necessary except in severe cases or for comfort. Early ROM should be initiated. Weight-bearing and strengthening exercises are started when the patient has full, pain-free ROM and no swelling. Lateral or bilateral hinged braces can be used to protect the ligament during healing and for return to sports.

61. Describe the mechanism of LCL injuries.

The majority of lateral knee stability is not derived from the LCL but from several structures that make up the lateral complex. Lateral complex injuries are uncommon, except in wrestlers, because they require a medial blow or twisting of the knee resulting in varus stress. Lateral complex injuries result in lateral knee pain and laxity with varus stressing. The peroneal nerve should always be assessed by resisted dorsiflexion of the ankle and great toe because of associated traction injuries.

62. How are lateral complex injuries treated?

The treatment of lateral complex injuries depends on their severity. Associated injuries are often present and may require surgical intervention.

63. Describe the usual mechanism of PCL injuries.

Although PCL injuries are less common and disabling, they are often missed or misdiagnosed. PCL injuries result from a direct blow to the anterior tibia by another player or from a fall onto the ground, twisting injuries, or hyperflexion. PCL injuries are often asymptomatic, and swelling, if present, ranges from trace to mild. The patient feels little-to-no pain, and many times no interruption in sports participation is necessary. Occasionally patients may complain of knee pain with running or difficulty in slowing down or stopping.

64. How are PCL injuries treated?

The majority of PCL injuries heal without intervention; bracing or detailed rehabilitation is rarely required.

65. What is the significance of ACL injuries?

Many ACL injuries are season- or career-ending injuries for athletes. The majority of ACL injuries are complete tears that require consideration of surgical intervention and prolonged rehabilitation. ACL injuries usually occur in team competitive sports with a noncontact twisting, jumping, deceleration, or pivoting maneuver in response to an opponent. The foot is planted, and there is a violent twist, hyperextension, or rapid start–stop activity. Often a pop is felt or heard, along with a tearing sensation in the knee. Players are unable to continue participation and often need assistance with ambulation.

66. Describe the physical exam findings in patients with ACL injuries.

The knee exam after an ACL injury shows a large, tense effusion (aspiraton reveals a hemarthrosis); significant pain and laxity without firm endpoints with anterior stresses to the tibia; loss of full extension (due to blocking of joint motion by the torn ligament); and difficulty or inability to bear weight on the knee for ambulation.

67. How are ACL injuries treated?

Initial treatment includes RICE, immobilization, and crutches. Early ROM to the knee and quadriceps strengthening are important, whether the definitive treatment is surgery or conservative treatment. Plain radiographs are used to rule out a fracture (especially avulsion of the tibial spine). MRI studies are accurate in assessing ACL integrity. The decision to reconstruct or repair an injured ACL must be individualized. There must be clear understanding of the desired goals, activities, or lifestyle and the required rehabilitation.

68. What is the usual recovery time after ACL injuries?

An ACL injury that is treated conservatively with rehabilitation (and often bracing) takes approximately 3 months for return to competitive cutting and pivoting sports. In athletes with ACL-deficient knees who chose to avoid reconstruction and continue with high-risk sports, instability in the knee often leads to secondary injuries (usually meniscal tears).

The time required for recovery from ACL reconstruction and/or repair is 9–12 months. The goals of rehabilitation are full ROM, and equal strength and stability compared with the uninvolved knee. Various grafts are used for reconstruction of the ACL: patellar tendon, hamstring, iliotibial tract, cadaver grafts, or synthetic material. The timing of surgery varies from soon after the diagnosis to 3–4 weeks after the injury to allow restoration of maximum ROM, decreased swelling, and maximum quadriceps strength. Intense rehabilitation programs are started soon after surgery, and bracing is usually needed for 3–6 months after surgery. Competitive athletes often are braced for sports for 1–3 years after reconstruction.

69. Why are ACL injuries treated differently in younger athletes?

The skeletally immature patient (presence of open physes) presents special considerations when ACL disruption is suspected. Radiographs should be obtained to rule out avulsion fractures at the tibial or femoral ACL insertion and physeal fractures. The major problem lies in the risk of physeal disruption with surgical reconstruction techniques. Avulsion fractures can usually be treated with arthroscopically guided reduction and fixation, with good results for ACL integrity. Standard ACL reconstruction requires drilling of tunnels through the distal femur and proximal tibia that result in growth plate disruption and may lead to leg length discrepancy or deformity in limb alignment. The majority of skeletally immature patients must wait until maturity (approximately age 14 in girls and 15 in boys) to undergo reconstructive surgery. Conservative measures are used in the interim, such as knee braces, muscle strengthening, and prevention of further knee injuries due to ACL deficiency.[5,17]

70. Why are female athletes at increased risk for ACL injuries?

There are several intrinsic and extrinsic answers to this question. None can be offered with complete certainty; probably a combination of factors is involved. Many studies have shown that women tear the ACL between 4 and 10 times more than men in both recreational activities and competitive sports. Contributing factors may include poor conditioning, insufficient coaching, skeletal structure, lower extremity alignment, muscular development, ligament laxity, and hormonal changes.[2] Extrinsic factors may include different training principles, shoe-surface interface, and overall skill level.

During the menstrual cycle, estrogen and progesterone influence the integrity and structure of the ACL. The greatest risk of injury is during the ovulation phase, which causes increased ligament laxity. The risk is lower in women taking oral contraceptives.[7,13] Additional intrinsic risk factors for female athletes include greater quadriceps-to-hamstring imbalance, smaller intercondylar notch, greater ligament laxity, smaller overall ligament size, decreased muscle strength in proportion to body size, and limb alignment.[2,9,16,18,19]

Although such information is not meant to deter female athletes from participating in high-risk sports, additional steps need to be taken to decrease or eliminate the modifiable risks. Proper coaching, preseason conditioning, and shoewear help in this effort. Established conditioning programs have successfully lowered ACL injuries in female athletes.

71. What is considered the most serious sports injury to the knee?

Knee dislocation, which is a medical emergency because of the potential for neurovascular disruption and associated morbidity. This rare injury is most often seen in football, especially in tackles that involve several players (making visualization and early recognition difficult). The dislocation can occur in any direction and is based on the position of the displaced tibia. Posterior dislocations are most common; in any direction, however, the ACL and PCL are almost always involved.

72. How are knee dislocations treated?

The knee is often reduced by the time the player is reached, but sometimes the deformity is grossly obvious. Pedal pulses should be assessed immediately. Popliteal artery injuries are common and cannot be excluded by the presence of a pulse. Studies to ensure vascular integrity are mandatory (arteriograms or Doppler ultrasound). Nerve function should be assessed and documented, especially the tibial and peroneal portions of the sciatic nerve.

The athlete should be transported quickly to the closest medical facility with the leg splinted. Vascular studies and repair take precedence over knee structure injuries. If arterial disruption is prolonged for 6 hours or more, the risk of amputation is much higher.

Opinions about the time frame for surgical interventions vary from directly after the vascular repair is completed to weeks later. A high risk of amputation and compartment syndrome is associated with this injury, but early recognition and prompt evaluation and/or treatment can greatly reduce the morbidity.

Although knee dislocation is considered a rare injury, this author has been involved with two cases on the same football team in the same season. One injury occurred at practice and the other at a postseason playoff game. Although neither resulted in amputation, both required vascular repair. Treatment of the knee injuries was approached differently, and the results varied from minimal functional disability to permanent limitations. Neither player participated further in collegiate football.

73. Why is the shoulder a complex joint with high susceptibility to injury?

The shoulder consists of a complex coordination of systems that allows use of the entire arm. The shoulder consists of four articulations, three bones, more than 26 muscles, and innervation from the brachial plexus. Because of the shallow nature of the glenoid, the shoulder is not dependent on bony stability. The major stabilizing elements of the shoulder come from the muscles and, to a much lesser extent, the ligaments. All sports that involve use of any portion of the arm can result in either acute or overuse injuries to the shoulder. The most common sports to report general shoulder injuries include baseball (especially pitching), swimming, golf, tennis, and gymnastics. Shoulder dislocations and subluxations are common with any collision or contact sport.

74. Describe the anatomy of the acromioclavicular joint.

The acromioclavicular joint is composed of the distal clavicle and the medial surface of the acromium. The stabilizing structures are the acromioclavicular and coracoclavicular ligaments. The deltoid and trapezius muscles are dynamic stabilizers.

75. What is a shoulder separation?

A shoulder separation injury refers to sprains or tears of the ligaments and capsule of the acromioclavicular joint. A severe sprain or tear of the ligaments results in separation of the joint with superior displacement of the distal clavicle in relation to the acromion. The usual mechanism of injury is a direct fall on the lateral aspect of the shoulder, a fall on an outstretched arm, or a blow to the back.

76. Describe the symptoms of a shoulder separation.

The injury causes tenderness over the acromioclavicular joint and obvious deformity with prominence of the distal clavicle in severe cases. Pain is reproduced in the acromioclavicular joint with compression of the joint, as demonstrated with adduction of the arm across the body.

77. How are shoulder separations graded?

These injuries are rated in severity from grade I to grade III and usually require assessment by plain radiographs. Grade I involves stretching of the ligaments and capsule. Grade II results in tearing of the acromioclavicular ligament and slight upward migration of the distal clavicle. The coracoclavicular ligament remains intact but may be stretched. Grade III results in disruption of both the acromioclavicular and coracoclavicular ligaments and dislocation of the joint with upward displacement of the distal clavicle. Some classifications include grade IV–VI separations, which usually are caused by motor vehicle accidents rather than athletic injuries. The distal clavicle is displaced posteriorly, inferiorly, or superiorly.

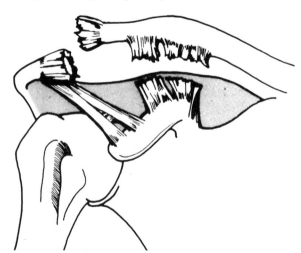

Grade III acromioclaviuclar joint injury. (From Mellion MB: Office Sports Medicine, 2nd ed. Philadelphia, Hanley & Belfus, 1996, with permission.)

78. How are acromioclavicular separations usually treated?

Grade I and II separations usually require minimal treatment. Once the diagnosis is confirmed, ice, NSAIDs, and a sling can be used symptomatically until pain subsides, followed by early ROM. Return to activities is indicated when the patient has pain-free motion and normal strength (usually by 1–2 weeks). Protective padding can be used to guard against repeat injuries with resumption of sports participation.

Grade III separations should be placed in a shoulder immobilizer or sling. The approach to treatment varies. Patients may need surgical intervention or longer rest from sports, early ROM, and gradual progression of rehabilitation. Return to sports varies from 3 to 8 weeks.

79. What makes up the glenohumeral joint?

The shoulder joint is made up of the articulation between the humerus and glenoid. There is significant mobility of the shoulder joint, but little stability is derived from the bones. The glenoid labrum and the glenohumeral ligaments support the glenohumeral joint.

80. How are injuries to the glenohumeral joint classified?

Injuries are usually classified by instability or labral pathology. Almost any sport that requires throwing can cause injuries, and there is also a high incidence of glenohumeral insults in contact/collision sports, swimming, and racquet sports.

81. What causes glenohumeral instability?

Sprains result from stretching or tearing of the ligaments and joint capsule. Subluxations are caused by joint laxity, which allows the humeral head to partially translate over the glenoid. Dislocations occur when the joint is unstable and the humeral head loses contact with the glenoid. Anterior/inferior instability and dislocations are most common, but posterior dislocations and multidirectional instability also occur.

All shoulder subluxations and dislocations require careful assessment of the neurovascular system. The axillary nerve can be stretched, torn, or contused with anterior dislocations or subluxations. The neurovascular assessment should be repeated after reduction.

82. What injuries are associated with shoulder dislocations?

Anterior shoulder dislocations may cause two typical lesions. The **Bankart lesion** is a tear of the anterior, inferior glenoid labrum. The **Hill-Sachs lesion** is an indention or fracture of the humeral head, caused by the force of the humeral head against the glenoid rim. These injuries can predispose the joint to recurrent instability.

83. What causes glenoid labrum tears?

Glenoid labrum tears most often occur in throwing athletes and athletes with chronic shoulder instability. Although labral tears can be acute injuries due to falls on an outstretched arm or direct force to the shoulder, most are due to repetitive insults that cause microtears.

84. Describe the symptoms of glenoid labrum tears. How are they treated?

Patients complain of snapping or clicking in the joint and pain that intensifies during the acceleration, release, and follow-through phases. Isolated labral pathology usually responds to rehabilitation strengthening exercises and motion limitation, but if symptoms persist, arthroscopic debridement of the labrum is indicated.

85. What is a SLAP lesion?

An injury that involves the biceps tendon and the anterior glenoid labrum is referred to as a SLAP lesion (superior labral, anterior to posterior). The SLAP lesion is classified according to the severity of labral tearing and biceps detachment.

86. What makes up the sternoclavicular joint?

The sternoclavicular joint is made up of the sternum and the medial aspect of the clavicle. It is one of the least commonly injured joints in the body, and most studies include a limited number of cases. The joint is relatively flat, and the majority of its stability is derived from the ligaments. Injuries are rare and usually result from motor vehicle accidents, but occasionally they occur in sports. Injuries are graded according to the degree of sprain to the ligaments and capsule and the degree of subluxation or dislocation of the joint.

87. Describe the symptoms and treatment of sternoclavicular sprains.

A sprain of the sternoclavicular joint causes pain and inflammation at the site of injury. A mild injury should be treated with ice for 12–24 hours, then with heat and NSAIDs. Moderate-to-severe sprains should be treated like a mild injury, with the additional placement of a figure eight (clavicle) splint and sling for stability and pain.

88. What is the most common type of sternoclavicular dislocation?

Most sternoclavicular dislocations are anterior and are easily recognizable on exam because of the prominence of the affected clavicle. Treatment depends on the severity of the dislocation and is usually conservative with figure eight splints and slings. Occasionally closed reduction is necessary, but usually it does not result in a more stable joint initially and requires splinting and sling.

89. What is important to remember in sternoclavicular dislocations?

The immediate anatomic position of the great vessels posterior to the sternoclavicular joint is important, especially in the rare case of dislocation of the clavicle posterior to the sternum. Injuries to the great vessels, lungs, esophagus, and trachea are indications of a life-threatening emergency and should be ruled out initially.[1]

Sternoclavicular dislocations are rare in athletes younger than age 25 and usually represent an epiphyseal fracture. They do not usually cause growth deformity, and treatment is conservative in most cases. Although radiographs are difficult to obtain, it is important to identify this injury correctly.

90. What muscles make up the rotator cuff?

The rotator cuff muscles are the supraspinatus, infraspinatus, teres minor, and subscapularis. They originate from the scapula and insert in the proximal humerus. The rotator cuff is responsible for shoulder stabilization, internal and external rotation of the arm, and abduction and elevation of the arm. Injuries include tendinitis, partial or complete tears, and impingement syndrome.[14]

91. What causes rotator cuff injuries?

Repetitive use of the arm above the level of the shoulder is the usual cause of rotator cuff injuries. They are common in throwing and racquet sports (baseball, softball, volleyball, weightlifting, javelin, tennis, and swimming) and usually result from overuse, fatigue, or decreased flexibility.

92. What is shoulder impingement?

Impingement is most commonly seen in athletes over 35 years of age and results from narrowing under the acromion, which causes inflammation of the subacromial bursa (bursitis) and the underlying rotator cuff. Most patients complain of pain with overhead activities, night pain, and weakness with elevation and external rotation.

In athletes younger than 35, internal impingement is more common. Internal impingement results from anterior instability, glenoid labrum tear, partial tear of the posterior rotator cuff, and capsular laxity. The athlete complains of decreased strength and pain with throwing (especially in the cocking phase); instability is either subtle or not noticed.

93. What is calcific tendinitis?

Calcific tendinitis results from repetitive injuries to the rotator cuff at the insertion of the supraspinatus in the greater tuberosity of the humerus. Repetitive microtrauma results in tendon changes and deposits of calcium in the tendon. The usual symptoms are severe shoulder pain at rest, with ROM, and during sleep. Radiographs confirm the diagnosis. Treatment includes rest, ice, NSAIDs, sling, and modified resumption of activities.[4]

94. What causes rotator cuff tears?

Complete rotator cuff tears are unusual in athletes under 40 years of age. Most rotator cuff tears are chronic and result from degenerative tears in mature athletes. Patients usually complain of gradual loss of shoulder motion, and weakness and pain with overhead activities or at night. Occasionally the mature athlete has a single injury that causes a rotator cuff tear.

Younger athletes may recall a single episode of contact injury with rupture of the rotator cuff. The complaints include shoulder pain, rotator cuff weakness, and limitation of motion. Another entity in this population is acute hemorrhagic subacromial bursitis, in which the rotator cuff remains intact but suffers a contusion and moderate-to-severe subacromial bursitis.

95. How are rotator cuff injuries treated?

Rotator cuff injuries can be treated initially with conservative measures and attempts to return to activities. Early ROM is important to prevent adhesive capsulitis; passive ROM does not cause further injury. Complete tears in active people usually require surgical repair.

96. What are the most common causes of elbow injuries?

Elbow injuries are usually seen in repetitive throwing or racquet sports. Most elbow injuries result from overuse and indirect trauma. The elbow joint relies primarily on bony stability; ligaments provide secondary support. The location of the pain and precipitating factors are usually early diagnostic signs suggestive of the cause. Fractures in the elbow are common with skeletally immature patients and should always be ruled out with radiographs.

97. What is the most common cause of dislocated elbows?

Elbow dislocations are uncommon in athletes and the general population. They usually result from a fall on an outstretched arm that causes an abduction and hyperextension force. Most elbow dislocations are posterior and affect the nondominant upper extremity. Elbow dislocations are seen in football, skate boarding, and roller or ice-skating,

98. Describe the common symptoms of elbow dislocations.

The presentation of the elbow is often diagnostic, but radiographs should always be obtained for diagnosis and assessment of associated injuries. Symptoms include deformity, marked limitation of motion, swelling, and crepitus of the affected elbow. Careful assessment of neurovascular status is important and should be documented as soon as the dislocation is suspected.

99. How are elbow dislocations treated?

Treatment usually consists of closed reduction and splint immobilization. The earlier the reduction is attempted after injury, the easier it is. Comparison of neurovascular status after reduction is crucial, and patients should have serial exams.

The rehabilitation of elbow dislocations depends on the severity of the injury. Most often immobilization is for less than 2 weeks; then gentle ROM or hinged lockout braces are used. Gentle controlled strengthening is usually started around the third week and progressed slowly. A common sequela of elbow dislocations is loss of full extension, which can be prevented with early motion. Recurrent instability in the elbow is uncommon.

100. What are tennis elbow and golfer's elbow?

The two major overuse injuries to the elbow are related to irritation of the tendons that attach to the epicondyles of the distal humerus at the elbow joint. **Tennis elbow**, or lateral epicondylitis, is often the cause of pain on the lateral aspect of the elbow. The pain results from inflammation due to microtrauma in the extensor carpi radialis brevis (primarily) and in the extensor carpi radialis longus, extensor communis, and extensor carpi ulnaris as they cross the radial head and insert into the lateral epicondyle.

Golfer's elbow, or medial epicondylitis, is often the cause of pain on the medial aspect of the elbow. It involves repetitive use of the flexor and pronator muscles in the wrist and forearm. The inflammation occurs at the medial epicondyle insertion of the pronator teres, flexor carpi ulnaris, flexor digitorum sublimis, and flexor carpi radialis tendons. Golfer's elbow is much less common than tennis elbow.

101. Is tennis elbow seen in other sports?

Although a large number of tennis players develop tennis elbow, it is a common overuse injury in any upper extremity sport. Tennis elbow is frequently seen in baseball, swimming, softball, karate, bowling, gymnastics, racquetball, fencing, golf, and javelin or hammer throwing. Tennis elbow can result from improperly fitted equipment or poor technique. In children it is known as little leaguer's elbow and is very common in adolescent baseball players because of instability or chronic overuse.

102. What are the common complaints of patients with tennis elbow?

Patients with tennis elbow often participate in activities that require a significant amount of repetitive extension of the wrist or supination of the forearm. They complaint of pain in the outside of the elbow, weakness in the hand or wrist, and difficulty or pain when picking up a full glass, especially coffee cups ("coffee cup test").

103. Describe the physical exam findings in patients with tennis elbow.

Physical exam may demonstrate a slight limitation of flexion or extension of the elbow and pronation or supination of the forearm. Other findings include exquisite tenderness over the lateral epicondyle and a positive coffee cup test. Occasional findings include weakness in the grip strength of the ipsilateral hand. The hallmark sign is pain over the lateral epicondyle with resisted extension of the wrist and fingers while the elbow is fully extended and the forearm is pronated.

104. What treatment is recommended for tennis elbow?

Initial treatment includes rest from the repetitive activity with ice, compression Ace wrap, and NSAIDs. The key to ice therapy is deep massage, which can be obtained by freezing water in a small paper bathroom cup and using the cup for ice massage. As the symptoms decrease, stretching of the wrist and forearm, especially flexion of the wrist with the elbow in complete extension and the forearm pronated. A strengthening program for the forearm extensors and the hand is instituted once motion has returned to normal and pain is resolving.

The counterforce brace is often used for the treatment of tennis elbow. This 5 - to 6-cm band goes around the forearm just below the elbow. The brace should be used with the activities that cause the symptoms and otherwise removed. Other treatments include ultrasound, cortisone injections (no more than 3 in 1 year), adjusting equipment and form, and surgery.

105. What other sports may result in golfer's elbow?

People who participate in overhead throwing or hitting often develop golfer's elbow. Although it is seen in golfers, most patients with golfer's elbow participate in tennis, baseball, squash, racquetball, or softball. Medial elbow pain in young throwing athletes is common, but, as with any elbow pathology, it is important to differentiate other causes.

106. What are the hallmark signs of golfer's elbow?

The chief complaint is medial elbow pain and pain in the flexor muscle of the forearm. Weakness in the grip strength is more pronounced than with tennis elbow. The patient reports exquisite tenderness over the medial epicondyle to palpation and with resisted wrist flexion and supination.

107. How is golfer's elbow treated?

Treatment should be similar to that for tennis elbow, including the initial use of rest, ice, and NSAIDs. A medial counterforce brace is available, but it has not been found to be as beneficial as with tennis elbow. Stretching and strengthening should be directed at the wrist flexors. Injections at this site are less common, and special attention must be paid to the ulnar nerve because of its close proximity.

108. Why has appreciation of the female athlete increased?

The dramatic increase in literature and research related to the female athlete parallels the significant rise in female participation in sports. Male involvement in sports has remained the same or decreased. Since the passing of Title IX in 1972, female athletes must be given equal athletic opportunities as males. There is also a direct recognition that sport participation results in different stresses and injuries in females. Athletic participation during pregnancy must be carefully assessed, and safety issues must be reviewed and guided by the health care provider.

109. What differences are seen in female athletes?

Most female athletes enter sports at an older age and quit at a higher rate than their male counterparts. Female athletes usually are coached and supervised by males, and less emphasis is placed on pre-participation conditioning. Female athletes have a higher rate of ACL injuries, patella femoral pain, carpal tunnel syndrome, tennis elbow, posterior tibial tendinitis, ankle impingement, foot disorders, spondylolysis, stress fractures, eating disorders, and iron-deficiency anemia. Anatomically females have a wider pelvis, smaller heart, shorter legs, smaller lungs, narrower shoulders, and lower centers of gravity. Physiologically female athletes have increased body fat percentage, lower basal metabolic rates, increased cardiovascular resistance to fatigue, increased thermoregulation to cold, and less muscle mass per body weight. These generalized differences should not be used to categorize female athletes but as a guide to maximize potential and prevent injuries.

110. What is the female athlete triad?

The female athlete triad consists of disordered eating, amenorrhea, and osteoporosis. This complex syndrome occurs in physically active females. At the core of the problem is a psychosocial pressure to achieve or maintain a desired weight. The results of the triad can actually hinder athletic performance and lead to morbidity and even mortality.

- **Disordered eating**: a variety of harmful and ineffective behaviors in attempt to lose weight or achieve a thin appearance. Examples range from restricting food to bingeing or purging. Behaviors may include fasting, diet pills, enemas, laxatives, excessive exercise, or diuretics.
- **Amenorrhea**: the absence or delayed onset of monthly menstruation. Between 10% and 45% of athletic females experience amenorrhea. Physical activity results in suppression of the hormones responsible for menstruation.
- **Osteoporosis**: low bone mass and deterioration of bone tissue leading to increased risk of fracture.

Potentially all physically active females are at risk for developing one or more components of the triad. Females who display one component of the triad should be screened for the others. The long-term effects of the triad may be irreversible, if the components are not identified and treated. Early intervention is crucial and should involve a multidisciplinary approach that includes coaches, health care providers, and family.

BIBLIOGRAPHY

1. Andrews J, Clancy W, Whiteside J: On-Field Evaluation and Treatment of Common Athletic Injuries. St. Louis, Mosby, 1997.
2. Beim G: Sports injuries in women. Women's Health Orthop Ed 2:27-34, 1999.
3. Berg E: Deep muscle contusion complicated by myositis ossificans (a.k.a. heterotopic bone). Orthop Nurs 19(1):66–67, 2000.
4. Birrer R: Sports Medicine for the Primary Care Physician. Boca Raton, FL, CRC Press, 1994.
5. DeLee J, Drez D: Orthopaedic and Sports Medicine Principles and Practice. Philadelphia, W.B. Saunders, 1994.
6. Halloran L: Bilateral epicondylitis in a karate instructor. Orthop Nurs 17(5):28–30, 1998.
7. Hannafin J: More research in musculoskeletal medicine is essential. Orthop Today 18(2):72-74, 1998.
8. Harvey C: Compartment syndrome: When it is least expected. Orthop Nurs 20(3):15–23, 2001.
9. McGee P: Female college basketball players at greater risk of ACL injuries. Orthop Today 18(7):13–17, 1998.
10. Micheli L, Jenkins M: The Sports Medicine Bible. New York, Harper-Collins 1995.
11. O'Connor B, Budgett R, Wells C, Lewis J: Sports Injuries and Illnesses. Wiltshire, UK, Crowood Press, 1998.

12. Potts K, Dick R: Sports Medicine Handbook, 13th ed. Indianapolis, IN, National Collegiate Athletic Association, 2000.

13. Reuters Medical News: Risk of knee ligament injury tied to ovulation. In Reuter's Health, 2001. Available at <http://orthopdics.medscape.com/reuters/prof/2001/08.23/20010822clin005.html>.

14. Salmond S, Mooney N, Verdisco L: Core Curriculum for Orthopaedic Nursing. Pitman, NJ, Anthony J. Janetti, 1996.

15. Schenck R: Athletic Training and Sports Medicine, 3rd ed. Rosemont, IL, American Academy of Orthopaedic Surgeons, 2000.

16. Schnirring L: What's new in treating active women. Physician Sports Med 25(7), 1997. Available at <http://www.physsportsmed.com/issues/1997/07jul/shcnirr.htm>.

17. Stanitski C: Anterior cruciate ligament injury in the skeletally immature patient: Diagnosis and treatment. J Am Acad Orthop Surg 3(3):146–158, 1995.

18. Teitz C: The Female Athlete. Rosemont, IL, American Academy of Orthopaedic Surgeons, 1997.

19. Teitz C, Hu S, Arendt E: The female athlete: Evaluation and treatment of sports-related problems. J Am Acad Orthop Surg 5(2):87–96, 1997.

9. SPINE DISORDERS

Pamela Bilyeu, RN, BSN, CNOR, CURN, ONC,
and Michael E. Zychowicz, RN, MS, NP-C

1. When is back pain not just back pain?

When a patient exhibits "red flags" in addition to back pain, the examiner must consider certain relatively major, urgent, or emergent problems, including cauda equina syndrome, cancer, spinal tumor, spinal tuberculosis, or dissecting abdominal aortic aneurysm. Red flags include loss of bowel or bladder control, unexpected weight loss, fever and night sweats, pain that awakens the patient from sleeping, progressive upper or lower extremity weakness, abdominal pain or discomfort, and saddle anesthesia.

2. What is a low back strain?

A low back strain is an injury to the musculotendinous structures of the lumbar spine. Back strain is typically accompanied by an episode of low back pain that significantly impairs function from a few days to as long as 4 weeks. The patient may also complain of uncomfortable or painful muscle spasm. Paresthesias are occasionally felt into the buttocks or thigh.

3. What causes low back strain?

A low back strain can be caused by any injury that results in overexertion or overuse of the muscles of the low back. Low back strain may be caused by jobs that require heavy and repetitive lifting. People who are overweight are more likely to report back strain than people below or at normal weight.

4. What is the treatment for a minor low back strain?

Initial treatment for acute back strain is determined by the amount of disability that the patient experiences. If the patient has a minor back strain, treatment can consist simply of decreased activities (e.g., lifting, pushing, pulling), over-the-counter nonsteroidal anti-inflammatory drugs (NSAIDs), and gentle stretching. Initially, the patient can apply ice to the area, followed by heat (just as with any other strain). Many people with a minor back strain do not even seek treatment and recover without difficulty within a few weeks. Further work-up is indicated in patients with recurrent, unresolved, or worsening pain. In addition, they may benefit from physical therapy, massage therapy, or chiropractics.

5. Describe the treatment for patients with a more severe acute low back strain.

Patients with a more severe acute back strain usually seek treatment early. They typically experience significant back pain, possibly spasm of the paraspinal muscles, and occasionally discomfort into the upper thigh similar to sciatic discomfort. Treatment typically consists of a thorough exam, a lumbar spine x-ray, prescription of anti-inflammatory drugs, muscle relaxants, and possibly a narcotic medication if the pain is severe. Patients also benefit from early entry into physical therapy. For the initial injury ice can be applied for the first day, followed by heat thereafter. Bed rest should be limited to 1–2 days to avoid deconditioning.

6. What are the major parts of the intervertebral discs?

The intervertebral discs are made of two major components. The outer portion of the disc, or anulus fibrosus, is made of layers of fibrous tissue, whereas the nucleus pulposus makes up the inner portion of the disc material. The nucleus pulposus has the consistency of crabmeat with high water content.

7. What is the function of the intervertebral discs?

The intervertebral discs act as a type of shock absorber for the back. They aid with movement of the vertebrae as well as cushioning of loads.

8. What is degenerative disc disease?

Degenerative disc disease (DDD) is progressive degeneration of the intervertebral discs associated with decreased hydration of the disc, which may or may not be a pain generator. Plain radiographs may reveal decreased disc height. In addition, magnetic resonance imaging (MRI) may show decreased hydration of the disc as well as other potential complications, including spinal stenosis. DDD can affect both young and older adults and presents with predominantly low back pain. Onset is usually gradual onset, but DDD can be exacerbated by trauma.

9. How can a patient get relief from pain due to DDD?

Conservative treatment is the usual first-line approach to pain due to DDD: physical therapy, heat or ice, mobility exercises, anti-inflammatory medications, and modification of activities that cause pain.

10. Can surgery address or "fix" DDD?

Spinal fusion is an option for the pain due to DDD. Patients may also find pain relief from intradiscal electrothermoplasty (IDET)

11. How does IDET address pain due to DDD?

IDET is performed when a trained physician inserts a needle into the disc(s) that are pain generators as confirmed by discography. IDET is performed under fluoroscopy to confirm placement. A catheter that heats up is threaded into the disc. The purpose of heating the disc with the coil is to cause the disc to thicken and contract. The goal is to eliminate pain at the pain-generating level.

12. What is a disc herniation?

A disc herniation is a pathologic condition in which the nucleus pulposus of an intervertebral disc has protruded through the surrounding fibrocartilage or anulus fibrosus. Symptoms may result from pressure on the spinal nerves or the spinal cord.

13. Why do people have disc herniations?

Herniations occur for various reasons. A disc can herniate because of repetitive stress to the disc, which can cause dysfunction, weakness, and defects of the anulus fibrosus. The nucleus can herniate through these defects in the anulus. Nuclear material can also herniate through similar defects in the anulus due to DDD. Lastly, discs can herniate from trauma due to falls, car accidents, parachute accidents, or other causes.

14. What is the most common level of disc herniation?

The levels that are most frequently herniated in the cervical vertebrae are C5–C6 and C6–C7. In the lumbar spine, the most frequent levels for disc herniation are at the L4–L5 and L5–S1 level.

15. Who has a greater incidence of disc herniation, men or women?

Men typically have a higher incidence of disc herniation.

16. What are the various types of disc herniation?

- **Bulging**. As the name implies, the anulus of the disc bulges outward. There is not a true herniation of the nucleus. Many people with disc bulges have no pain or disability whatsoever.
- **Protrusion** occurs when the material from the nucleus herniates through the outer anulus without herniating through the posterior longitudinal ligament (PLL).
- **Extrusion** is the same as a protrusion with herniation of the nuclear material through the PLL.
- **Sequestration**. As with an extrusion, a portion of the nuclear material has extruded through the PLL; however, a fragment of the herniatied material has detached.

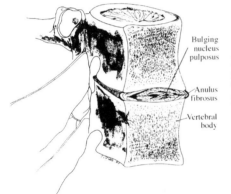

Disc space narrowing and circumferential bulging of the L4–L5 disc. (From Cole AJ, Herring SA: The Low Back Pain Handbook. Philadelphia, Hanley & Belfus, 1997, with permission.)

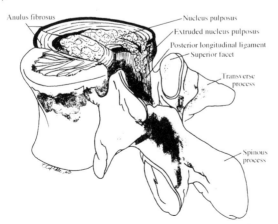

Extruded disc at L5–S1. (From Cole AJ, Herring SA: The Low Back Pain Handbook. Philadelphia, Hanley & Belfus, 1997, with permission.)

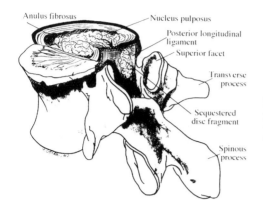

Anulus fibrosus
Nucleus pulposus
Posterior longitudinal ligament
Superior facet
Transverse process
Sequestered disc fragment
Spinous process

Sequestered disc herniation at the L5–S1 level. (From Cole AJ, Herring SA: The Low Back Pain Handbook. Philadelphia, Hanley & Belfus, 1997, with permission.)

17. What are the symptoms of lumbar disc herniation?
Pain usually begins in the low back and radiates to the sacroiliac region and buttocks. Radicular pain usually extends below the knee and follows the dermatome of the involved nerve root. The pain is generally worse in the leg than in the back. The patient may even have only leg pain and no back pain whatsoever. Pain may be intermittent and usually increases with activities, especially sitting in a car for a long time. Pain may be relieved by standing or bed rest. The hallmark is exacerbation of leg pain with straining, sneezing, or coughing. Weakness may be a complaint and is usually localized to the neurologic level of involvement. Paresthesias are common and follow the nerve root distribution for the sensory areas.

18. What is sciatica?
Lumbar radiculopathy (commonly called sciatica) is a condition with some degree of referred neurogenic dysfunction in the leg. Sciatica usually results when a herniated disc causes irritation of a lumbar nerve root. The pain results from direct mechanical compression of the nerve root and in part from chemical irritation by substances in the nucleus pulposus.

19. What is the cauda equina?
Translated from Latin, cauda equina means horse's tail. This name refers to the appearance of the nerves in the spinal canal after the spinal cord ends at the L1–L2 level.

20. What is cauda equina syndrome?
Cauda equina syndrome is caused by a large midline disc herniation that may compress several nerve roots of the cauda equina. The most common level is the L4–L5 disc. The onset of symptoms may be rapid or progress slowly. Perianal pain and back pain predominate, and disc symptoms are minimal. Difficulty with urination, increased frequency, or overflow incontinence may be present. Recent impotence may be elicited in men. Leg pain that progresses to severe numbness of the feet and difficulty with walking can also be present.

21. What is the usual treatment for cauda equina syndrome?
Urgent surgical intervention is the treatment of choice.

22. Aside from range of motion of the lumbar spine, what physical tests can be performed to diagnose a herniated lumbar disc?

- **Lumbar list**. With the patient standing, the examiner position him- or herself behind the patient and looks for a shift of the trunk to the right or left. A disc herniation can cause a list that is similar to a scoliotic curve. Record the direction of the list.
- **Heel walking**. Ask the patient to walk across the room on the heels. Patients with tight heel cords have difficulty with this test. Indicate whether the test result is positive due to heel cord tightness, exaggerated responses, lack of coordination, or weakness of the anterior tibial muscles. Heel walking tests the L4-innervated muscles.
- **Extensor hallucis longus (EHL) weakness**. With the patient seated, ask the patient to dorsiflex the great toe and compare strength on both sides. Indicate whether the test result is positive due to exaggerated responses or weakness of the muscle. EHL assessment tests the L5-innervated muscles.
- **Toe walking**. Ask the patient to walk across the room on tiptoes. Indicate whether the test result is positive due to exaggerated responses, lack of coordination, or weakness of the gastrocnemius soleus muscle group. Toe walking tests the S1-innervated muscles. The patient who has decreased strength and difficulty in performing the test or is completely unable to toe-stand may have a herniation compressing the S1 nerve root.
- **Straight leg raise**. With the patient supine, ask the patient to relax the leg as you cradle the foot in the palm of your hand. Elevate the leg until either the knee starts to bend or the patient indicates severe pain in the buttock or back. At that point, dorsiflex the ankle to see if this motion increases pain. Dorsiflexion increases sciatic tension and sciatic pain. Plantarflexion relieves sciatic tension, and increased pain in the back with this test is probably nonorganic. Record the degree of elevation at which pain occurs for each maneuver.

23. What are the physical findings in patients with unilateral disc herniation at the L3–L4 level?

Unilateral herniation at the L3–L4 disc generally involves compression of the L4 nerve root, with possible sensory deficits in the posterolateral thigh, anterior knee, and medial leg. Motor weakness is variable in the quadriceps and hip adductors. Changes also are apparent in the patellar reflex.

24. What are the physical findings in patients with unilateral disc herniation at the L4–L5 level?

The L5 nerve root is compressed with disc herniation at L4–L5. Sensory deficit occurs in the anterolateral leg, dorsum of the foot, and great toe. Motor weakness includes the extensor hallucis longus, gluteus medius, and extensor digitorum longus and brevis. Usually no reflex changes are present.

25. What are the physical findings in patients with unilateral disc herniation at the L5–S1 level?

Disc herniation at L5–S1 signifies compression of the S1 nerve root. Sensory deficits occur in the lateral malleolus, lateral foot, heel, and web of the fourth and fifth toes. Motor weakness involves the peroneus longus and brevis, gastrocnemius-soleus complex, and gluteus maximus. The Achilles reflex is usually diminished.

26. Describe the treatment for herniated nucleus pulposus (HNP).

The treatment of HNP depends on the severity of the patient's symptoms and how aggressively or invasively the patient wants to be treated. Initially, some patients are easily treated with an oral anti-inflammatory and/or narcotic medication; muscle relaxants are used for muscle spasm as needed. The use of short-term oral steroids may address chemical neuritis. An epidural steroid injection (ESI) series also addresses chemical neuritis. Many patients recover without surgery, which offers a final alternative.

27. What are the indications for surgery for HNP?

Indications for surgery include progressive neurologic deficit, intractable pain with the failure of conservative treatment, and bowel or bladder dysfunction.

28. What surgical procedure is used for the treatment of lumbar disc disease?

The traditional surgery is laminectomy and lumbar disc excision by means of a midline incision. The paraspinous muscles are stripped from the lamina of the vertebra on each side of the lesion. The lamina is identified, and the ligamentum flavum is excised. Portions of the superior and inferior lamina may be removed. After the nerve root is retracted, the disc herniation is identified and then removed, and the disc is dissected free of loose fragments. The closure is routine.

29. What is a microlumbar disc excision?

Microlumbar discectomy requires an operating microscope. The procedure is performed much like an open disc excision and laminectomy, except the laminae are not removed. Microlumbar discectomy requires less dissection and has the potential for less reactive scar tissue.

30. What are the complications of lumbar disc surgery?

- Cauda equina syndrome
- Thrombophlebitis
- Pulmonary embolism
- Wound infection
- Postoperative discitis
- Dural tears
- Nerve root injury
- Cerebrospinal fluid fistula
- Laceration of abdominal vessels
- Injury to abdominal viscera

31. What nursing interventions are essential for patients having spinal surgery?

The nurse caring for a patient who has had spine surgery should take adequate time to perform necessary preoperative teaching, explaining to the patient what to expect postoperatively with nursing and medical management. Postoperatively, the nurse should monitor for infection, constipation, urinary output, and hypovolemia. Adequate analgesia is essential for all patients. Vital signs and neurovascular assessments should be performed according to institutional policy and physician orders.

32. What is lumbar spinal stenosis?

Stenosis is a congenital or acquired narrowing of the spinal canal, usually worsening with age. It usually presents with an insidious onset of neurogenic (referred) leg pain. The age-related narrowing and inward buckling of the intervertebral disc, coupled with forward buckling of the interlaminar ligament and enlargement of arthritic facets, is the common cause.

33. What is found on examination of patients with spinal stenosis?

The examiner may find diminished patella and/or ankle reflexes. When the patient stands with the spine extended, pain reproduction indicates spinal stenosis. Weakness may be present with toe or heel walking as well as with great toe dorsiflexion. Sensation from pinprick and warm or cold temperatures are often abnormal, whereas light touch sensitivity is frequently normal.

34. What are the common clinical symptoms of spinal stenosis?

People with spinal stenosis complain of leg and/or low back pain that typically is exacerbated with walking. The clinician must differentiate stenosis from vascular insufficiency. Some patients may also experience bowel or bladder symptoms.

35. What is the most common position for relief of pain in patients with spinal stenosis?

Patients report that sitting or leaning forward typically relieves the leg or back pain. They may lean forward when shopping and essentially hang over the shopping cart to relieve pain while walking at the grocery store.

36. What radiographic examinations are used to diagnose spinal stenosis?

Computed tomography (CT) and MRI provide excellent delineations of the stenotic areas. True stenosis is considered absolute with a sagittal diameter of 10–12 mm.

37. Describe the treatment for spinal stenosis.

A vigorous physical therapy program is the nonoperative treatment for spinal stenosis. Biofeedback can be helpful. Transcutaneous electrical nerve stimulation (TENS) sometimes has been helpful. Patients should avoid extension activities that may aggravate the symptoms. The patient can also use oral anti-inflammatory medications, or an epidural steroid injection series may be performed.

38. What leads to the need for surgery in patients with spinal stenosis?

Surgical treatment for spinal stenosis is always the last resort. Indications for surgery include intractable pain with the failure of conservative treatment including epidural injections, physical therapy, anti-inflammatory medications, and bracing.

39. How is surgical treatment of spinal stenosis performed?

Removal of the lamina, ligamentum flavum, spinous process medial facets, and arthritic spurs in the lateral recesses. It is thought that portions of the facet joints should be left intact.

40. What are the potential complications of surgical treatment of spinal stenosis?

The most common complications after decompression are instability, arachnoiditis, nerve root injury, dural tears, infection, and epidural scarring.

41. Define spondylolysis.

Spondylolysis is a defect in the pars interarticularis, usually in the lumbar spine.

42. Define spondylolisthesis.

Spondylolisthesis is the slipping forward of an upper vertebra on a lower one.

43. What is found on examination of a patient with spondylolisthesis?
The neurologic exam may reveal a deficit. The patient usually presents with back pain and possibly leg pain. Physical appearance varies, depending on the degree of spondylolithesis. The buttocks may have increased prominence, the patient may show increased protuberance of the abdomen, or lumbar lordosis may be exaggerated. The examiner also may find a palpable step-off when palpating the spinous processes. The lateral spine x-ray shows slippage of one vertebra onto another, usually with the superior vertebra displaced forward onto the one below.

44. What are the five common types of spondylolisthesis?
Dysplastic, isthmic, degenerative, traumatic, and pathologic.

45. What is dysplastic spondylolisthesis?
Dysplastic spondylolisthesis is a deficiency in the inferior facets of L5 and/or the superior facets of S1, along with the elongation of the pars interarticularis.

46. What is isthmic spondylolisthesis?
Repetitive motion is the inciting factor in the development of isthmic spondylolisthesis. The repetitive hyperextension causes shear of the posterior elements of the spine. The incidence of this kind of spondylolisthesis is increased in gymnasts, football lineman, new Army recruits, and weightlifters.

47. How are slip percentage and slip angle determined?
Slip percentage represents the distance between the posterior border of the body of L5 and the posterior border of the body of S1 as a percentage of the anteroposterior diameter of S1. The slip angle is measured by drawing a perpendicular line to a line drawn along the posterior border of the sacrum and another line parallel to the inferior endplate of L5. The angle subtended by the intersection of these two lines is the slip angle.

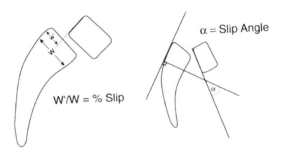

Slip percentage and slip angle. (From Brown DE, Neumann RD (eds): Orthopedic Secrets, 2nd ed. Philadelphia, Hanley & Belfus, 1999, with permission.)

48. How is spondylolisthesis classified?
Meyerding's system is the most commonly accepted classification for spondylolisthesis. No anterior slip of the upper vertebral body on the lower is classified as grade 0; 1–25% slippage is grade I; 26–50% slippage is grade II; 51–75% is grade III; and 76–100% is grade IV. Grade V, or spondyloptosis, is complete anterior dislocation of the upper on the lower vertebral body.

49. Which spinal segments are most commonly affected by spondylolysis and spondylolisthesis?

L5–S1 is the most common, followed by L4–L5 and then L3–L4.

50. What is the treatment of choice for spondylolysis and grade I spondylolisthesis?

Patients with a history of recent injury or short duration of symptoms are treated with minimal restrictions to avoid aggravating activities. In addition, they are prescribed a regimen of muscle strengthening for the back and abdomen. As treatment progresses, back pain and hamstring tightness decrease.

51. What is the treatment of choice for spondylolysis and grade II spondylolisthesis?

Asymptomatic patients should be followed with x-rays every 4–6 months. Patients with continuing symptoms should have an in situ posterior fusion without instrumentation.

52. What is the treatment of choice for spondylolysis and grade III spondylolisthesis?

In situ posterior fusion, including L4 in the arthrodesis, is the treatment of choice for spondylolysis and grade III spondylolisthesis. Anterior spine fusion may be used as part of this treatment modality.

53. What is the treatment of choice for spondylolysis and grade IV spondylolisthesis?

Posterior transpedicular reduction and fusion with instrumentation is the treatment of choice for spondylolysis and grade IV spondylolisthesis. During the postoperative period brace or casting may be used.

54. What two deviations of the spine must be present to classify a spinal curve as scoliosis?

A lateral curvature greater than 10° and rotation must be present for a patient to be diagnosed with scoliosis.

55. What are the signs of scoliosis on physical exam?

• One shoulder higher than the other
• One shoulder blade sticking out farther than the other
• Uneven waistline
• Hems hanging unevenly on girls and women
• Unilateral rib hump with forward bending
• Obvious curvature on inspection

56. List the various types of scoliosis.

The various types of scoliosis are idiopathic, congenital, paralytic, neurofibromatosis, traumatic, sciatic, and hysterical.

57. Of the various types of scoliosis, which is the most common form?

Idiopathic scoliosis is the most common form.

58. What causes idiopathic scoliosis?

Idiopathic scoliosis has no known cause.

59. What other physical findings may be seen in patients with scoliosis and neurofibromatosis?

The patient with neurofibromatosis and scoliosis may also have café-au-lait spots on the skin as well as vertebral scalloping on x-ray.

60. Can patients with a herniated vertebral disc present with scoliosis?

Yes. Patients who have a herniated disc or even a tumor that irritates the nerve root may present with scoliosis. This mechanism is an attempt to decrease pressure and irritation on the nerve root.

61. What are the major problems associated with significant scoliosis?

The patient with significant scoliosis has the possibility of developing overwhelming and/or chronic back pain. In addition, patients with a large thoracic scoliosis may develop cardiopulmonary disability.

62. Are patients with scoliosis more likely to have a curve to the right (dextroscoliosis) or left (levoscoliosis)?

If a patient's scoliosis is at the lumbar spine, it is more likely to curve to the left. A thoracic scoliosis is more likely to curve to the right.

63. How is a paralytic scoliosis different from the other types?

A paralytic scoliosis usually has a more elongated, less acute curve compared with the other types. In addition, paralytic scoliosis develops as a result of cerebral palsy, polio, spina bifida, or one of the many myopathies.

64. In infantile idiopathic scoliosis what is the most common curve pattern?

The most common curve pattern is a convex, left thoracic curve.

65. How is the curve pattern different in adolescents with idiopathic scoliosis?

With adolescent idiopathic scoliosis, a left thoracic curve is rare and often is associated with intraspinal pathology.

66. What causes congenital scoliosis?

An abnormal formation of the vertebral structures during early embryonic development is the cause of spinal curvature with congenital scoliosis. Patients with congenital scoliosis should have a spinal fusion that includes a mobile segment above and below the deformity as soon as the diagnosis is made.

67. What is currently the most widely used system for spinal radiograph measurement? How are radiographs measured with this system?

The Cobb method of radiographic measurement is currently the most widely used measurement system. A posteroanterior 3-foot standing radiograph is taken of the entire spine, including the iliac crest. The superior and inferior vertebrae of each curve are located. They are the vertebrae at the top and the bottom of the curve with the greatest tilt into the curve. Using a straight edge (i.e., goniometer) and wax pencil, a line is drawn parallel to the superior endplate of both the superior and inferior vertebrae of the curve being measured. Perpendicular lines are then drawn from the lines drawn in the previous step. The angle created by their intersection is measured using a goniometer. This angle corresponds to the number of degrees of the scoliosis curve.

68. What are the risk factors for progression of the curvature in adolescent idiopathic scoliosis?

The risk factors for progression of idiopathic scoliosis are curve magnitude (the larger the curve, the greater the risk), growth potential of the patient (the more growth remaining, the greater the risk), and the curve type (double curves have a greater risk of progression).

69. Describe the nonsurgical treatment of adolescent idiopathic scoliosis.

The use of a spinal orthotic (brace) is the only nonsurgical treatment of adolescent idiopathic scoliosis. The most common types of spinal orthotics are the Milwaukee brace (apex T8 and above), thoracolumbosacral orthotic (TLSO) or Boston brace (apex below T8), and the Charleston bending brace (nighttime use only).

70. What is one of the biggest challenges in treating adolescents with scoliosis?

Compliance is a major problem in adolescents.

71. What nursing considerations are important when a patient is braced?

Skin care is extremely important and should be aimed at avoiding skin breakdown. The patient can wear a cotton shirt or cotton liner under the brace to avoid direct irritation of the skin. The nurse should educate the patient to change the cotton undershirt daily as well as avoid body powder or lotions that may cause irritation of the skin.

72. What are the indications for operative treatment of adolescent idiopathic scoliosis?

Operative treatment of adolescent idiopathic scoliosis is recommended for curves greater than 40°–45° in skeletally immature patients, curves that progress despite bracing, or curves greater than 50°–60° in mature adolescents.

73. What is the operative treatment for adolescent idiopathic scoliosis?

The operative treatment for adolescent idiopathic scoliosis includes instrumentation of the surgeon's choice and spinal fusion for curves of more than 50°.

74. Define spina bifida.

Spina bifida refers to a defect of the lamina or vertebral arch. Myelomeningocele or meningocele may also be present.

75. Define kyphosis.

Kyphosis is a spinal deformity characterized by an increase in the posterior convex angulation in the sagittal plane. The normal posterior convex angulation of the thoracic spine is 20°–40°, as measured by the Cobb method.

76. What causes kyphosis?

The various causes of kyphosis include Scheuermann's disease, poor posture, laminectomy, trauma, paralysis, and congenital causes.

77. What is seen on radiographic examination of patients with Scheuermann's kyphosis?

- Three adjacent vertebrae with 5° or more of anterior wedging and a total thoracic kyphosis of greater than 45° measured from T5 to T12.
- Schmorl's nodes, which are punched-out areas in the endplate of a vertebral body that is surrounded by compact bone. Schmorl's nodes are due to intraosseous prolapse of the nucleus pulposus into the vertebral body. On lateral

radiographs, a Schmorl's node is seen as a radiolucency or hemispherical bone defect in the upper or lower margin of the body of the affected vertebra.
- Irregularity of the cartilaginous endplates.

78. Describe the treatment of Scheuermann's kyphosis.

Initial treatment for Scheuermann's kyphosis is nonsurgical and consists primarily of thoracic extension, abdominal strengthening exercises, and avoidance of heavy lifting. When the curve exceeds 70°, bracing is usually recommended. Surgical treatment is recommended when the curve exceeds 75° and the patient is symptomatic or neurologic signs appear. Curves of 100° may lead to restrictive lung disease.

79. What is the surgical treatment for Scheuermann's kyphosis?

Surgical treatment consists of an anterior release and fusion (preferably with anterior column support), followed by a posterior arthrodesis with instrumentation of the entire kyphotic segment.

80. How do metabolic disorders lead to kyphosis?

Osteoporosis and osteomalacia are two metabolic disorders that can predispose patients to developing compression fractures of the vertebrae. The compression fractures are due primarily to weakening of the vertebrae as a result of demineralization. When the vertebrae develop compression fractures, they can form into a wedge shape. This wedge shape can cause a kyphotic deformity of the spine, especially if the patient has multiple compression fractures.

81. What is the usual treatment for compression fractures due to osteoporosis?

Patients with compression fractures are usually treated with bracing for up to 3 months. If the kyphosis is progressive, surgical stabilization is a possibility. Kyphoplasty is also an option for patients with painful compression fractures. Bone cement is inserted into a cavity in the body of the vertebrae after a balloon is used to restore the shape of the collapsed vertebrae.

82. Define lordosis.

Lordosis is an anterior angulation of the spine in the sagittal plane. Excessive backward bending (apex anterior angulation) of the spine is seen, creating a swayback deformity.

83. Define lordoscoliosis.

Lordoscoliosis is a lateral curvature of the spine associated with either an increased anterior curvature or decreased normal posterior angulation in the sagittal plane. Increased lordosis can increase kyphosis, leading to pain and the possibility of surgical correction.

84. What is the most common thoracic spine disease?

The most common thoracic spine disease is thoracic disc herniation. Pain occurs near the midline, unilaterally or bilaterally, and may have characteristic radicular distribution along a dermatome. Numbness is the second most common symptom.

85. What level is most commonly affected by thoracic disc herniation?

A herniated thoracic disc generally develops below T8, with the highest incidence at the T11–T12 level. A central protrusion of the disc is generally found.

86. What is the most common symptom of cervical spine disease?

Radiculopathy with ipsilateral arm pain, weakness, and sensory changes are the most common symptoms of cervical spine disease. Radicular symptoms are the same, whether due to compression by an acute disc herniation or mechanical irritation by a chronic foraminal spondylotic spur.

87. What are the most common levels for cervical disc disease?

The most frequent levels for cervical disc disease are C5–C6 and C6–C7. C4–C5 and C7–T1 are less common, and C3–C4 is rare.

88. What other symptoms are associated with cervical disc disease?

Patients may have limited range of neck motion and complain of neck pain with movement.

89. What are the common indications for operative treatment of the cervical spine?

- Persistent and intolerable pain that has not been decreased by several months of comprehensive treatment
- Functional limitations of activities of daily living
- Severe or progressive muscle weakness

90. After cervical spinal surgery, what specific aspects of care should the nurse consider?

When caring for the patient who has undergone cervical surgery, the nurse should assess respiratory status and have a tracheotomy tray readily available. Cervical immobility and support should be used as ordered by the surgeon. The nurse should perform the usual pain assessment and neurovascular assessment in the upper and lower extremities.

91. What are the common surgical procedures for cervical radiculopathy?

Adequate decompression of the nerve roots is the goal of surgical procedures for cervical radiculopathy. The anterior approach is recommended for medial or central disc herniation or when fusion is contemplated. A posterior approach is necessitated by a posterolateral disc or osteophytes that are otherwise inaccessible.

92. What are the most common cervical spine procedures?

The most common cervical spine procedures include the anterior cervical discectomy (ACD), ACD with fusion (ACDF), ACDF with internal fixation, posterior foraminotomy, and posterior fusion.

93. How do ACD, ACDF, and ACDF with fusion differ?

ACD is indicated for patients with minimal neck pain, normal cervical lordosis, and single-level pathology to avoid the potential complications of fusion. ACDF is indicated for patients with symptoms of instability or more than one operative level. The risk of developing kyphosis from disc space collapse is also reduced. ACDF with internal fixation involves the addition of anterior plating. This procedure is recommended for multilevel fusions with documented instability or history of prior fusion failure. Internal fixation also allows early mobilization without bracing.

94. What is the purpose of a posterior foraminotomy?

A posterior foraminotomy involves removing one or more hemilaminae to remove osteophytes or lateral disc fragments. When it is used for soft disc herniation, the need for fusion is obviated.

95. When is posterior spinal fusion indicated?

Posterior spinal fusion is indicated for patients with posterior spinal instability. Instrumentation (plates and screws and/or wire) and fusion allow early mobilization if no paralysis is present.

96. Define failed back syndrome.

Failed back syndrome is essentially low back pain that has not responded to both conservative and surgical intervention.

97. Can anything be done to decrease pain due to failed back syndrome?

The patient with failed back syndrome can continue to receive relief with conservative treatment, including TENS, bracing, exercise, and acupuncture. The patient should be evaluated and treated as indicated by a pain management clinic. Surgical intervention is indicated only if a surgical problem arises. Nurses can provide interventions such as guiding the patient to participate in self-care to the greatest degree possible.

98. What complications of failed back syndrome should the nurse consider?

Depression is a common complication in patients with chronic back pain. The patient may develop narcotic dependency. In addition, the patient may have significant disruption of interpersonal relationships.

BIBLIOGRAPHY

1. Brown DE, Neumann RD: Orthopaedic Secrets, 2nd Ed. Philadelphia, Hanley & Belfus, 1999.
2. Brown KL: Cauda equina syndrome: Implications for the orthopedic nurse in a clinical setting. Orthop Nurs 14(5):35–36, 1998.
3. Dirschl DR, LeCroy CM, Obremskey WT: On Call Orthopaedics. Philadelphia, W.B. Saunders, 1998.
4. Maher AB, Salmond SW, Pellino TA: Orthopaedic Nursing, 3rd ed. Philadelphia, W.B. Saunders, 2002.
5. Mourad LA: Orthopedic Disorders. St. Louis, Mosby, 1991.
6. Rolak LA: Neurology Secrets, 3rd ed. Philadelphia, Hanley & Belfus, 1999.
7. Rothman S: The Spine, 3rd Ed. Philadelphia, W.B. Saunders, 1992.
8. Schoen DC: NAON Core Curriculum for Orthopaedic Nursing, 4th ed. Pittman, NJ, Anthony J. Jannetti, 2001.
9. Snider RK: Essentials of Musculoskeletal Care. Chicago, American Academy of Orthopaedic Surgeons, 1997.

10. NEUROMUSCULAR DISORDERS

Michael E. Zychowicz, RN, MS, NP-C,
and Valerie Armstrong, RN, MA, NP-C, CCRN, MSCN

1. What is cerebral palsy?

Cerebral palsy (CP) has been used as an umbrella term for varying disorders. Loosely translated, CP means brain paralysis. Generally, it refers to motor and postural abnormalities that are noted during early development. Despite advances in neonatal care, CP remains a significant clinical problem.

2. What causes CP?

CP is thought to be associated with maternal, prenatal, perinatal, or postnatal events of varying etiologies that cause an insult to the brain, leaving a static, nonprogressive encephalopathy. Events that may cause CP include:

- Intrauterine growth retardation
- Hyperbilirubinemia
- Hypoxic encephalopathy
- Intracranial hemorrhage
- Premature placental separation
- Preterm labor or premature birth
- Traumatic delivery
- Precipitous or prolonged labor

3. Discuss the learning needs of parents of children with CP.

Many children with the diagnosis of CP have normal or above-average intelligence. Expression of intellectual capacity may be limited by impairment in communication due to oromotor, fine motor, and gross motor difficulties. Without appropriate compensation, these difficulties have the potential to impair academic and social integration. A greater understanding of CP and the realization that children with CP have significant potential that simply needs to be unmasked allow parents and health care professionals to approach CP in a multidisciplinary manner and maximize rehabilitative efforts.

4. What complications may be associated with CP?

- Cognitive difficulties
- Frequent urinary tract infections
- Gastrointestinal dysfunction and malnutrition
- Dental caries
- Osteopenia from inactivity and associated fractures
- Sensory deficits
- Respiratory difficulty
- Seizure disorder

5. What signs and symptoms of CP may be found on examination?

The clinical expression of CP is subject to change as children and their developing nervous systems mature. Before the formal physical examination is done, observation may reveal abnormal neck or truncal tone; asymmetric posture, strength, or gait; or abnormal coordination. Spasticity may be evident in a tendency to keep the elbow flexed, the hips flexed and adducted, the knees flexed, and the ankles in equinus position, resulting in toe walking. Patients with dyskinetic or extrapyramidal CP may have decreased head and truncal tone with defects in postural control and motor dysfunction such as athetosis, chorea, and dystonia. Patients with CP may show the underdevelopment or absence of postural or protective reflexes and the persistence of primitive reflexes, including the Moro reflex or asymmetric tonic neck reflexes.

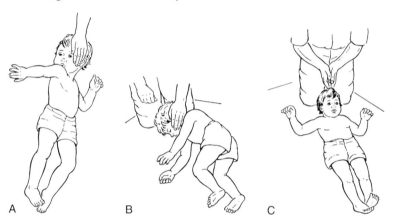

A   B   C

Signs of cerebral palsy in children. *A*, Asymmetric tonic neck reflex. Sharply turn the head to one side. The child responds with flexion of the limbs on the skull side and extension on the face side (abnormal after 12 months). *B*, Neck-righting reflex. Turn the head. The trunk and lower limbs follow the head as if rolling a log (abnormal after 12 months). *C*, Moro reflex. A clap of the hands, loud noise, or jarring the table elicits abduction of the upper limbs (abnormal after 12 months). (From Black EE: Cerebral palsy. In Staheli LT (ed): Pediatric Orthopedic Secrets. Philadelphia, Hanley & Belfus, 1998, pp 348-357, with permission.)

6. Define athetosis, chorea, choreoathetosis, and dystonia.

Athetosis is characterized as slow, writhing, involuntary movements, particularly in the distal extremities. **Chorea** is characterized as abrupt, irregular, and jerky movements. **Choreoathetosis** is a combination of athetosis and chorea. **Dystonia** is described as slow, rhythmic movements with muscle tone abnormalities and abnormal postures.

7. How is CP classified?

Many classifications of CP have been proposed based on body distribution, functionality, or severity of involvement. A modification of the system proposed by Crothers and Paine in 1959 divides CP into spastic (pyramidal), dyskinetic (extrapyramidal), and mixed types. Functional classification systems generally divide CP into mild, moderate, and severe types, depending on functional limitations. Alternatively, patients may be categorized more comprehensively by their abilities and limitations. Classic presentations of CP include spastic hemiplegia, spastic diplegia, dyskinesis, and spastic quadriplegia.

8. List the characteristics of spastic hemiplegic CP.

- One-sided upper motor neuron deficit that is more common in the arm than in the leg

- Early hand preference or relative weakness on one side
- Oromotor dysfunction
- Specific learning disabilities
- Possible unilateral sensory deficits
- Visual field deficits including homonymous hemianopsia and strabismus
- Seizures

9. **List the characteristics of spastic diplegic CP.**
   - Upper motor neuron findings that are more common in the legs than in the arms
   - Scissoring gait pattern (hips flexed and adducted, knees flexed with valgus)
   - Ankles in equinus position, resulting in toe-walking
   - Learning disabilities
   - Seizures (less common than in spastic hemiplegia)

10. **List the characteristics of dyskinetic (extrapyramidal) CP.**
    - Early hypotonia with movement disorder emerging between ages 1 and 3 years
    - More frequent involvement of the arms than the legs
    - Deep tendon reflexes that are usually normal or slightly increased
    - Some spasticity may be present
    - Oromotor dysfunction
    - Gait difficulties
    - Truncal instability
    - Risk of deafness in patients affected by kernicterus

11. **List the characteristics of spastic quadriplegic CP.**
    - Involvement of all limbs
    - Either truncal hypotonia with appendicular hypertonia or full-body hypertonia
    - Oromotor dysfunction
    - Increased risk of cognitive difficulties
    - Multiple medical complications
    - Seizures
    - The legs generally are affected equally or more frequently than the arms
    - Categorized as double hemiplegia if the arms are more involved than the legs

12. **What medications are useful in CP?**

Numerous medications can relieve the movement difficulties associated with CP. These drugs target dystonia, myoclonus, chorea, athetosis, and spasticity. Antiparkinsonian drugs (e.g., anticholinergic and dopaminergic agents) and antispasticity agents (e.g., baclofen) primarily have been used in the management of dystonia. Anticonvulsants, antidopaminergic drugs, and antidepressants also have been tried. Anticonvulsants, including benzodiazepines (e.g., diazepam), valproic acid, and barbiturates, have been useful in the management of myoclonus. Chorea and athetosis are often difficult to manage, although benzodiazepines, neuroleptics, and antiparkinsonian drugs (e.g., levodopa) have been tried. Benzodiazepines and baclofen are commonly used to manage spasticity.

13. **Is physical or occupational therapy beneficial for patients with CP?**

Regular physical and occupational therapy are crucial. The goals should be to maximize the functional use of the limbs, maximize ambulation, and reduce the risk of contractures.

14. What about nutritional therapy for severe CP?

Oromotor dysfunction may require limitations in the texture of food and liquid. Primary or supplemental feedings via gastrostomy or jejunostomy tube may be necessary to increase caloric intake and prevent aspiration.

15. What are neural tube defects?

Neural tube defects are dysfunctions and abnormalities in the formation of the spinal cord. Neural tube defects include spina bifida occulta, spina bifida cystica (meningocele and myelomeningocele), encephalocele, and anencephaly.

16. Describe spina bifida occulta.

As the name implies, it is an occult deformity often found incidentally when a spinal x-ray is taken. Spina bifida occulta is characterized by incomplete or nonexistent fusion of the posterior vertebral arch. Occasionally, the patient has a tuft of hair, dimpling of the skin, or skin pigmentation over the area.

17. What is the difference between encephalocele and anencephaly?

In patients born with anencephaly, some, if not all, of the brain is congenitally absent. Part of the top of the skull may also be congenitally absent. Such patients are typically born dead or die within a few days. In patients with encephalocele, a congenital defect in the skull allows herniation of the brain and meninges through the defect.

18. Compare meningocele and myelomeningocele.

Both meningocele and myelomeningocele are types of spina bifida cystica, which is a defect of the spine in which fusion of the posterior vertebral arch is absent. This disorder typically occurs in the lumbar spine. Meningocele is a herniation of the meninges through the incompletely closed vertebral arch; the herniation forms a cyst. The spinal cord is not involved, and this defect is rarely associated with neurologic compromise. Myelomeningocele is the same type of herniation, but it involves a portion of the spinal cord and nerves. An obvious cystic sac of varying size is usually present on inspection of the newborn's back.

19. What complications and dysfunction are associated with myelomeningocele?

Patients frequently develop hydrocephalus and Arnold-Chiari malformation of the brain. Motor and sensory deficits depend on the level of the spinal lesion. Common neuromuscular dysfunction includes partial or complete paralysis, contractures, sensory deficit, gait disorders, kyphosis, scoliosis, and clubfoot deformity. Frequently bowel and bladder dysfunction is present. Examples include bowel impaction, loss of anal sphincter tone, hydronephrosis, urinary tract infections, and lack of bowel or bladder control. Pressure ulcers, Charcot arthropathy, and latex allergies are additional complications associated with myelomeningocele.

20. What is Arnold-Chiari malformation?

Arnold-Chiari malformation is characterized by herniation of the cerebellum and brainstem through the foramen magnum at the base of the skull. The fourth ventricle is also herniated and obstructs the normal flow of cerebral spinal fluid (CSF), which leads to the characteristic hydrocephalus.

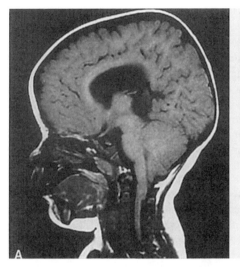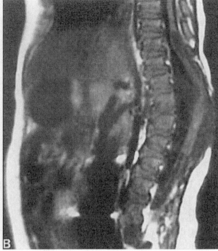

A, Unenhanced midsagittal T1-weighted MRI in a 6-month-old boy with Arnold-Chiari malformation. Note herniation or downward displacement of cerebellum and associated hydrocephalus. *B*, Unenhanced midsagittal T1-weighted MRI of lumbosacral spine in same patient. Note extensive thoracolumbar myelomeningocele associated with Arnold-Chiari malformation. (From Rolak LA (ed): Neurology Secrets, 3rd ed. Philadelphia, Hanley & Belfus, 2001, with permission.)

21. List the signs and symptoms of Arnold-Chiari malformation.
- Intermittent apnea
- Nystagmus
- Staring spells
- Stridor
- Vocal cord paralysis
- Abnormal or absent gag reflex

22. Why are ventriculoperitoneal (VP) shunts placed in patients with myelomeningocele?

Hydrocephalus with myelomeningocele is related to the Arnold-Chiari malformation. CSF flow is blocked, causing a subsequent hydrocephalus in approximately 80% of patients with myelomeningocele. A VP shunt is surgically placed to drain obstructed CSF into the peritoneal cavity to address the hydrocephalus. VP shunt dysfunction can lead to symptoms of hydrocephalus and development of hydromyelia, syringomyelia, or hydrosyringomyelia.

23. Describe hydromyelia, syringomyelia, and hydrosyringomyelia.

These three complications can result from a dysfunctional VP shunt, which causes increased pressure within spinal canal. Hydromyelia is a dilation of the central spinal canal within the spinal cord. Syringomyelia is a cavitation of the spinal cord parenchyma. Hydrosyringomyelia is a combination of the two disorders.

24. What anomalies may accompany myelomeningocele?

Myelomeningocele often occurs with multisystem congenital anomalies. Commonly associated anomalies are facial clefts, heart malformations, and genitourinary tract anomalies. Urinary tract anomalies, such as solitary kidney or malformed ureters, may contribute to increased morbidity in the presence of neurogenic bladder dysfunction.

25. What is the prognosis for ambulation in patients with myelomeningocele?

The level of the lesion and the strength of the lower extremity muscles are the most important factors influencing the achievement of ambulation in children with myelomeningocele. Approximately 50% of patients use wheelchairs as their primary form of mobility; 20% of these patients ambulate with orthotics and assistive devices as a form of therapeutic exercise. The remaining 50% of patients ambulate distances great enough to move around their home or local community. Up to 20% of ambulatory patients use some type of orthotic or assistive device.

26. How are the orthopedic dysfunctions of myelomeningocele addressed?

The actual cystic lesion is corrected surgically. Surgical intervention can correct or stabilize any joint or spinal deformity. Soft tissue contractures can also be surgically released if necessary. Various orthotic devices and braces for the limbs and trunk are available to provide support during ambulation. Standing frames or tables and parapodiums can be used to assist the patient in maintaining an upright position while ambulating. Range-of-motion exercises and/ or physical therapy may help to prevent contractures and enhance mobility. Wheelchairs are often required.

27. Summarize important aspects of nursing education for patients with myelomeningocele.

Preschool and school-aged children with myelomeningocele should be taught the use of adaptive equipment and alternative methods for self-care and performance of activities of daily living (ADLs). To become independent by school age, young children with myelomeningocele need to become active participants in skin care, bowel and bladder management, donning and doffing of orthotics, and traditional ADL tasks such as feeding and dressing. Acquisition of ADL skills is often influenced by attitudes and expectations. The multidisciplinary team members need to emphasize carryover of ADL skills in the home and school environments by providing anticipatory guidance to parents and caregivers.

28. What is Duchenne muscular dystrophy?

Muscular dystrophy is a myopathy that progresses with worsening weakness and muscle deterioration. The most common and severe type of muscular dystrophy is Duchenne dystrophy, an inherited X-chromosome disorder that only rarely is expressed in girls with Turner's syndrome. Duchenne dystrophy usually has a clinical onset of symptoms at 1–3 years of age and progresses rapidly; mental retardation frequently accompanies the disease. Duchenne dystrophy is characterized by pseudohypertrophy, a form of muscular degeneration and destruction in which lost muscular bulk is replaced by adipose and connective tissue. Less common and less severe types of muscular dystrophy include Becker's dystrophy, limb-girdle dystrophy, congenital dystrophy, fascioscapulohumeral dystrophy, and distal dystrophy.

29. Describe the pathophysiology and progression of Duchenne dystrophy.

Patients with Duchenne dystrophy have a defect of the short arm of the X chromosome with a mutation of the dystrophin gene. The dystrophin protein is normally present in both brain and muscle cells, but because of genetic mutation the dystrophin protein is altered, insufficient, or completely absent. Dystrophin is part of the cytoskeleton of muscle cells and helps maintain the structural integrity of the cell surface membrane. Muscle cells die because of cell wall structural dysfunction and the alterations that accompany cell injury. Cell wall injury causes fluid and electrolyte imbalance, including swelling and increased calcium uptake into the cell. Increased calcium in the cell causes dysfunction of the mitochondria with decreased or absent production of adenosine triphosphate (ATP). Without adequate ATP production, the cell is unable to drive aspects of cellular metabolism, including operation of the electrolyte pumps remaining in the cell wall and production of cellular components to repair the cell wall. The necrotic cells are eventually removed by phagocytes and replaced with adipose and connective tissue, resulting in the characteristic pseudohypertrophy.

30. Describe the usual history and physical findings of muscular dystrophy.

A patient may have a family history of muscular dystrophy or a personal history of progressive weakness with difficulty in performing or achieving developmental tasks such as sitting, standing, or walking. Patients may use a wide-based stance to maintain balance during standing. The child also appears clumsy and frequently falls because of difficulty with walking, running, climbing stairs, or hopping in place. During ambulation the patient exhibits a waddling gait caused by weakness of the gluteal and quadriceps muscles. Deep tendon reflexes may be absent or depressed, and lumbar lordosis is accentuated. Flexion contractures develop frequently, involving the hips, knees, and feet (with resultant equinovarus). The examiner sees the typical Gower's sign.

31. What is Gower's sign?

Gower sign is a typical finding and describes the method used by patients with muscular dystrophy to rise from the floor to a standing position. Patients are described as climbing up their legs to push the torso upward and achieve an upright position. This method is used to compensate for quadriceps and gluteal muscle weakness.

32. How is muscular dystrophy diagnosed?

In addition to history and physical exam, accuracy of diagnosis has been refined with recognition of the dystrophin gene defects and dystrophin staining of muscle biopsy specimens. Other typical diagnostic tests reveal elevated enzymes released from damaged muscles, including creatine phosphokinase (CPK), aspartate aminostransferase (AST), and aldolase. Electromyography and nerve conduction studies can assist the examiner in differentiating myopathy and neuropathy. If the patient has pulmonary or cardiac complications, pulmonary function testing, chest x-ray, and electrocardiogram may assist further assessment of these complications.

33. What supportive treatment can be given to patients with muscular dystrophy?
- Physical therapy
- Wheelchair, splinting, and orthotics as indicated
- Spinal fusion with instrumentation to address severe scoliosis
- Surgical tendon release to address muscle contractures

34. What complications often accompany Duchenne muscular dystrophy?

In addition to the muscular weakness and deterioration that defines muscular dystrophy, patients develop smooth muscle dysfunction, pulmonary dysfunction, cardiac involvement, and decreased IQ. Patients develop muscle contractures, typically involving the hip flexor muscles. Smooth muscle dysfunction, although rare, involves malabsorption, cramping pain, megacolon, and volvulus. Pulmonary dysfunction can be a consequence of kyphoscoliosis and wheelchair confinement, leading to respiratory insufficiency and pulmonary infection. Cardiac dysfunction occurs in up to 95% of patients with Duchenne dystrophy with a level of dysfunction ranging from tachycardia and ventricular hypertrophy to heart failure. Approximately 30% of patients with Duchenne dystrophy have some degree of mental retardation with an average IQ of 80.

35. What is the usual lifespan of patients with Duchenne dystrophy?
Approximately 75% die before they reach 21 years of age.

36. How can muscular dystrophy be detected in utero?
Both chorionic villus sampling and amniocentesis can provide a prenatal diagnosis of muscular dystrophy. Chorionic villus sampling can be performed earlier in the course of pregnancy than amniocentesis.

37. Define Friedreich's ataxia.
Friedreich's ataxia is an inherited degenerative disorder affecting boys and girls equally with a usual age of onset between 7 and 15 years. Degeneration occurs in the posterolateral columns of the spinal cord and parts of the cerebellum.

38. What testing is used to confirm the diagnosis of Friedreich's ataxia?
No testing is necessary. The diagnosis of Friedreich's ataxia is typically based on history and physical exam alone.

39. List the typical findings of the physical exam in patients with Friedreich's ataxia.
• Cavovarus deformity of the feet
• Muscle wasting and spasm
• Absent lower extremity reflexes
• Scoliosis
• Ataxia
• Speech and swallowing difficulties
• Proprioceptive and vibratory sense impairment
• Optic nerve dysfunction
• Cardiomyopathy

40. How can the complications of Friedreich's ataxia be addressed?
Patients with Friedreich's ataxia frequently develop muscle spasm. Appropriate nonsurgical treatment includes range-of-motion exercises, application of heat, massage, and muscle relaxants. Surgical intervention is considered if the patient is unable to sit because of muscle spasm. The complication of scoliosis can be addressed in the usual manner of observation, bracing, or surgical correction. Operative correction and joint fusion are options for patients with pes cavovarus deformity. Conservative treatment with orthotics is usually attempted before surgery is considered.

41. List appropriate nursing goals for patients with Friedreich's ataxia.
• The patient remains free of infection.
• Skin integrity is not impaired.

- The patient remains mobile within realistic limitations.
- Appropriate physical changes are made in the home environment
- Eating and drinking can be done safely, without aspiration.
- The patient sustains no injury.

42. What are neuromuscular junction disorders?

Neuromuscular junction dysfunction can result from medications, nutritional deficiency, or disease. Normally, the neurotransmitter is synthesized, packaged, and released by the presynaptic terminal at the neuromuscular junction. The neurotransmitter then travels across the synaptic cleft and binds to postsynaptic receptors on the muscle cell membrane. Neuromuscular junction disorders can interfere with neurotransmitter development, packaging, or release or cause interference at the binding site.

43. Define myasthenia gravis.

Myasthenia gravis is an autoimmune disorder that causes dysfunction at the neuromuscular junction. For an unknown reason, the acetylcholine receptor sites at the neuromuscular junction are perceived as nonself antigens. IgG autoantibodies attach to the receptor sites, block the attachment of acetylcholine, and eventually destroy the receptor sites. Blockage and destruction of the receptor sites lead to weakness and easy fatigability.

44. List the three types of myasthenia gravis.

- Ocular myasthenia, which affects the extraocular muscles of the eyes
- Bulbar myasthenia, which affects the muscles innervated by cranial nerves IX, X, XI, and XII
- Generalized myasthenia, which affects the proximal muscles of the body

45. What muscles are potentially affected by bulbar myasthenia?

Cranial nerve (CN) IX (glossopharyngeal nerve) innervates the pharyngeal motor fibers involved with swallowing. Assessing the gag reflex and checking for the soft palate to rise when the patient says "ahh" test the function of CN IX. CN X (vagus nerve) innervates the motor fibers of the palate, pharynx, digestive tract, respiratory tract, and cardiovascular system. CN X is generally tested in the same way as CN IX. The spinal accessory nerve, CN XI, innervates the palate, pharynx, larynx, and sternocleidomastoid and trapezius muscles. Checking strength to resisted rotation of the neck and shoulder shrug generally assesses the spinal accessory nerve. The hypoglossal nerve, CN XII, innervates the muscles of the tongue and is assessed by ensuring that the tongue remains in the midline when protruded.

46. Describe myasthenic crisis.

Myasthenic crisis is characterized by severe muscular weakness. This weakness leads to serious potential complications, including swallowing difficulty, respiratory insufficiency or arrest, and/or quadriplegia.

47. What are the characteristics of neurofibromatosis?

Neurofibromatosis is a congenital genetic disorder that is characterized by the development of café-au-lait spots, cutaneous neurofibroma, and plexiform neurofibroma. In addition, patients may develop optic glioma, nodules on the iris of the eye, and inguinal or axillary freckles. Patients with von Recklinghausen disease (type I neurofibromatosis) frequently have orthopedic disorders such as idiopathic or dystrophic scoliosis, poorly healing fractures, bowing or pseudarthrosis of the tibia or other long bones, and structural abnormalities of the vertebra.

48. How can the orthopedic complications of neurofibromatosis be addressed?

Patients with scoliosis can be treated with observation, bracing, or surgical intervention. Bracing and surgical intervention, including bone grafting, can address pseudarthrosis of the long bones.

49. Define neuropathic arthropathy.

Neuropathic arthropathy is a joint disease that most often affects the foot and ankle. It leads to disruption of a joint characterized by dislocation or subluxation of the joint as well as destruction of the joint bones. The patient exhibits decreased to absent sensation, degeneration of the involved joint, inflammation, and swelling.

50. By what other name is neuropathic arthropathy known? Why?

Charcot neuropathy or Charcot joint. Jean-Martin Charcot performed early research related to neuropathic arthropathy in the mid 1800s.

51. How does surgical intervention address neuropathic arthropathy?

If conservative treatment (bracing, splinting, and custom orthotics) fails and joint deformity ensues, surgical intervention can be considered. Surgical fusion may help to stabilize an unstable joint. The choice of last resort is amputation.

BIBLIOGRAPHY

1. Apley AG, Solomon L: Concise System of Orthopedics and Fractures, 2nd ed. London, Reed Educational and Professional Publishing, 1996.
2. Huether S, McCance K: Understanding Pathophysiology, 2nd ed. St. Louis, Mosby, 2000.
3. Lewis SM, Heitkemper MM, Dirksen SR: Medical Surgical Nursing: Assessment and Management of Clinical Problems, 5th ed. St Louis, Mosby, 2000.
4. Maher AB, Salmond SW, Pellino TA: Orthopaedic Nursing, 3rd ed. Philadelphia, W.B. Saunders, 2002.
5. Schoen DC: NAON Core Curriculum for Orthopaedic Nursing, 4th ed. Pittman, NJ, Anthony J. Jannetti, 2001.

11. ORTHOPEDIC ONCOLOGY

Cindy Jo Horrell, RN, MS, AOCN

1. Are all bone tumors malignant?

Bone tumors may be malignant or benign. The benign tumors are more common. Both can grow, apply pressure, and destroy healthy tissue. Benign bone tumors do not metastasize and rarely are life-threatening.

2. What is the incidence of bone and joint cancers?

The American Cancer Society estimates 2,900 new cases of bone and joint cancers in the United States in 2001.[13]

3. What are risk factors for cancers of the bone?

Researchers are uncertain of the cause of many bone cancers. The following factors are thought to place a person at risk: younger age, previous radiotherapy or chemotherapy for other diseases, and Paget's disease.

4. What are the common symptoms of bone cancer?

Pain is the usual presenting symptom of most bone cancers. Other symptoms depend on the site of the cancer. For instance, if the cancer appears near a joint, it may cause swelling and limitation of movement. Occasionally the cancer can weaken the bone, causing pathologic fractures.

5. What information about a bone tumor can an x-ray provide?

Plain film radiographs demonstrate the extent of tumor involvement and tumor location. Cortical destruction may be seen along with bony expansion, calcification, or pathologic fractures. Soft tissue shadows or outlines, such as those seen with erosion through the bone cortex by sarcomas, also are visualized.

6. What information can computed tomography (CT) give about a bone tumor?

CT scans provide cross-sectional views of tumor involvement and delineate tumor invasion into bone, soft tissues, and neurovascular structures. They are particularly beneficial for diagnosing intraosseous tumors and tumors of the trunk.

7. Magnetic resonance imaging (MRI) is effective in evaluation of what tissues?

MRI is the technique of choice to evaluate the spine, bone marrow, and soft tissue masses because of the multiple coronal and sagittal views of the tumor. It is superior for viewing growth plates, where several bone tumors tend to occur (e.g., chondroblastoma). Compared with CT scanning, MRI is better for extraosseous lesions, including the sciatic nerve and brachial plexus.

8. What is the shortcoming of a bone scan?

Bone scans are sensitive but not specific in detecting the skeletal extent of the disease process.

9. Describe useful laboratory data in the assessment of a bone lesion.

To rule out infection, a complete blood count (CBC), sedimentation rate, and levels of glycoprotein fibrinogen and C-reactive protein are ordered. An elevated white blood cell (WBC) count suggests inflammation, hematologic malignancy, and myeloproliferative disorder. Decreased WBC count suggests replacement of the bone marrow by tumor. A serum calcium level is elevated in malignancies with bone involvement. Alkaline phosphatase is elevated with osteoblastic tumors. Elevated levels of acid phosphatase are seen with metastatic prostate cancer to the bone.

10. What is staging?

Staging is a method of classifying a cancer according to the pathologic diagnoses, size, anatomic structural involvement, and absence or presence of metastases.

11. Why is staging important?

Staging is important because it directs the medical and surgical treatment and predicts prognosis. Staging also contributes to cancer research by ensuring reliable comparisons.

12. What is the most widely accepted system for staging?

The most widely used staging system is the T (tumor), N (lymph node), and M (metastases) system. The use of numbers after each letter indicates the extent of disease. The higher the number, the more advanced the disease.

13. What is histologic grading of tumors?

For most cancer sites, the anatomic extent of the disease is considered the most important factor. In the instance of soft tissue sarcomas, however, histologic grade assumes greater significance and has been seen to influence prognosis.

The histopathologic grade is a qualitative assessment of the differentiation of a tumor. It is expressed as the extent to which a tumor resembles the normal tissue type or cell type at the site. Based on the microscopic appearance of cancer cells, pathologists commonly describe tumor grade by four degrees of severity: grades 1, 2, 3, and 4. The cells of grade 1 tumors are often well-differentiated or low-grade tumors and are generally considered the least aggressive. Conversely, the cells of grade 3 or grade 4 tumors are usually poorly differentiated or undifferentiated high-grade tumors and are generally the most aggressive.

14. What is the objective of histologic grading of tumors?

The objective of a grading system is to provide information about the probable growth rate of the tumor and its tendency to spread. The systems used to grade tumors vary with each type of cancer. Grading plays a role in treatment decisions.

15. What is the most common primary cancer of the bone?

Osteosarcoma, which is characterized by production of neoplastic osteoid bone directly from anaplastic osteoblast-like cells. It usually occurs between the ages of 10 and 25 years, although it can be seen in older adults.

16. What are the prognostic factors for bone cancer?

Prognostic factors for bone cancer include T-classification (T1 tumors have a better prognosis than T2 tumors), histopathologic grade (the lower the better), location and size of the primary tumor, whether the primary tumor is localized, and the degree of histologic response after chemotherapy.

17. Where are osteosarcomas found?

Osteosarcomas occur in metaphyseal regions of the large, long bones, such as the distal femur, proximal tibia, and humerus. In older adults they can be found after osteomyelitis, in association with Paget's disease, or with prior radiotherapy to the bone.

18. What are the initial symptoms and clinical features of osteosarcoma?

The initial symptom is intermittent pain that progresses, as the tumor grows, to constant and incapacitating pain. A palpable mass with venous distension and associated warmth may be seen. With tumor growth the patient experiences weight loss, limitation of motion, and fatigue.

19. What are the radiologic findings?

Plain x-rays show cortical destruction, bony expansion, calcification, and a "sunburst" appearance. CT or MRI demonstrates cortical and medullary irregularities and possible bone mass extending outward into the soft tissue.

20. What is the differential diagnosis?

Differential diagnoses of such lesions include infection, aneursymal bone cyst, Ewing's sarcoma, chondrosarcoma, and metastatic bony tumor.

21. If left untreated, what is the natural course of osteosarcoma?

It rapidly destroys bone and soft tissues and metastasizes to the lungs within 2 years of diagnosis. Most patients live only 2–3 months after discovery of lung metastases.

22. Does osteosarcoma differ in children?

It accounts for about 5% of all childhood cancers. In children about half of these tumors arise from the bones around the knee.

23. How is osteosarcoma treated?

Because nearly all patients have microscopic metastases at the time of diagnoses, successful outcomes mandate use of systemic chemotherapy. Since the addition of chemotherapy in a multimodality approach to treatment, long-term survival has increased. Most centers use chemotherapy intra-arterially or intravenously before surgery to shrink the tumor. The surgeon then removes the affected area. Often more chemotherapy is given after surgical intervention.

24. What chemotherapy drugs are used?

The most effective agents include doxorubicin (Adriamycin), high-dose methotrexate with leucovorin rescue, cisplatin and ifosfamide, cyclophosphamide (Cytoxan), etoposide, and carboplatin.

25. When is amputation a justifiable surgical intervention?

Limb-sparing surgery offers similar local control rates as amputation and has a positive effect on quality of life. However, if it provides inadequate margins for local control or if reconstruction after resection would give less satisfactory function than the use of prostheses, amputation is a viable option. In general, about 80% of extremity osteosarcomas can be treated by limb-sparing surgery.

26. Nursing care of the patient undergoing amputation should address which concerns?
Issues surrounding self-concept, grieving, pain, skin integrity, and mobility.

27. What is the possibility of recurrence?
Incidence of local recurrence is highest in patients with primary sites in the femur; amputation is associated with lower rates of local recurrence than limb-sparing procedures.

28. What is parosteal osteosarcoma?
This relatively low-grade sarcoma usually occurs on the bone surface, particularly the posterior aspect of the distal femur. Patients present with a painless swelling. Treatment is surgical resection. The cure rate is > 90% with complete excision.

29. What factors have prognostic significance in localized osteosarcoma?
• Site of tumor (axial tumors have greatest risk of progression and death)
• Age of patient
• Size of tumor
• Skip lesions
• Lactate dehydrogenase (LDH) levels (elevated LDH levels = poor prognosis)

30. What factors affect prognosis in metastatic disease?
In metastatic disease, prognosis seems determined for the most part by site(s), number of metastasis, and surgical resectability.

31. Compare chondroma (enchondroma) and chondrosarcoma.
Chondromas (enchondromas) are a benign mature hyaline cartilage growth within the medullary cavity of a single bone. They present in young adults in the appendicular skeleton, particularly the hands. They are also found in the proximal humerus, distal femur, and proximal tibia.
Chondrosarcomas are primary malignant bone tumors that produce cartilage. They occur at the point where muscles attach to bones, near a joint, and at sites where cartilage formation continues throughout life (knee, shoulder, pelvis). Nearly always associated with pain, they may result from malignant degeneration of a benign chondroma. They are often seen in the axial skeleton and are the most common primary malignant tumor of the chest wall.

32. How do chondromas and chondrosarcomas differ in presentation?
• Different sites of origin (chondromas originate in hands, chondrosarcomas in central skeleton).
• Pain is present with chondrosarcomas and tends to worsen at night.
• Chondromas are seen more often in young adults.

33. What is Ollier's disease?
Ollier's disease is the presence of multiple chondromas that can cause deformity and stunting of growth. People with this disease are predisposed to develop malignant transformation to chondrosarcomas.

34. Describe the treatment of chondrosarcomas.

The histologic diagnoses of chondrosarcomas are quite challenging because many tumors tend to be low-grade and therefore difficult to distinguish from chondromas (benign tumors). Chondrosarcomas are notorious for seeding the soft tissue after biopsy or inadequate resection. Although they are relatively radioresistant with conventional radiotherapy dosing, new research shows promise with the use of fractionated proton radiation therapy. For the most part, they are managed with aggressive surgical intervention. A recent study by Bergh et al.[3] identified the following factors as indicating a poor prognosis in terms of local control and survival in pelvic, sacral, and spinal chondrosarcomas: high histologic grade, increasing patient age, primary surgery outside a tumor center, incisional biopsy vs. a noninvasive diagnostic procedure, and inadequate surgical margins.

35. Describe the chondroblastoma.

Chondroblastoma is an uncommon benign bone tumor that characteristically presents at the epiphyseal location of the long bones. The cell of origin is the epiphyseal plate or its remnant.

36. What age groups develop chondroblastoma?

Typically chondroblastomas are seen between the ages of 15 and 20 years. Males are affected more frequently than females (3:2 male-to-female ratio).

37. Describe presenting complaints and current treatment for chondroblastomas.

Most patients complain of limitation of joint movement and pain, which may be severe. The current treatment consists of curettage and packing with bone graft.

38. List the risk factors for recurrence.

A significant risk factor for recurrence has been identified as the location of the tumor.[27] Investigators found that the most common sites of recurrence were the proximal part of the femur and the greater trochanter.

39. What benign bone tumor is seen during periods of rapid bone growth?

Osteochondroma, a benign bone tumor, is seen during the first and second decade of life. It represents a hyperplastic/dysplastic proliferation of bone, appearing and growing during periods of rapid bone growth. The growth causes progressive symptoms of pain and development of a palpable mass.

40. What are the complications of osteochondromas?

Osteochondromas can promote bursa formation, pathologic fracture, or osteomyelitis. Joint motion may be limited, or weakness and deformity may result. Vascular sequelae may include arterial occlusion, embolism, and phlebitis. Malignant transformation may occur, particularly in the pelvic or shoulder girdles.

41. Define hereditary multiple exostoses (HME).

HME, an autosomal dominant syndrome, consists of multiple osteochondromas. Complications are more frequent and include significant deformity, neurologic sequelae, and increased risk of malignant transformation.

42. Describe the recommended treatment for osteochondroma.

Treatment is indicated when the tumor interferes with joint function, when bone fracture is present, or when malignant transformation is suspected. Excision of the tumor is the usual treatment.

43. What are osteomas?

Seen most frequently in men aged 5–25 years, osteomas are benign tumors composed of vascular fibrous tissue, proliferating fibroblasts, and osteoid. They are thought to be caused by malformed embryologic tissue, trauma, or infection.

44. What are the usual presenting features of osteomas?

Patients complain of mild pain, especially at night, which is relieved by aspirin. Swelling becomes palpable, and, if the osteoma is located near a synovial joint, stiffness and effusion of the joint may occur.

45. What is the differential diagnosis of suspected osteoma?

Radiographic differential diagnoses include osteochondroma, myositis ossificans, and parosteal osteosarcoma. Osteomas appear as dense exophytic growths from the diaphyseal or metadiaphyseal cortex of the long bone. Osteochondromas have a cartilaginous cap, and the medullary space is continuous with the bone. In myositis ossificans, which occurs after trauma, ossification proceeds from the periphery toward the inside. Osteosarcomas commonly present with swelling and pain. They grow outward into the surrounding tissue and often demonstrate radiolucent foci within the tumor mass.

46. How are the osteomas treated?

The growth rate of the osteoma is very slow. Asymptomatic tumors can be observed clinically and radiographically. Complete resection removes underlying cortex and involves allograft reconstruction that may result in permanent disability.

47. Contrast aneursymal and unicameral (simple) bone cysts.

The aneursymal bone cyst is a blood-filled cavity, whereas the unicameral bone cyst is fluid-filled. Unicameral cysts are benign; they occur within the bone and are contained by a thin layer of fibrous tissue. Unicameral bone cysts are common in children and adolescents. Aneursymal bone cysts are common between 20 and 30 years of age. Both types of cysts cause expansion of the bone and may cause pathologic fractures. Common sites are similar and include long bones, flat bones, and vertebrae. Most unicameral bone cysts are found at the proximal end of the humerus.

48. How does the treatment differ for aneurysmal and unicameral cysts?

For the **unicameral cyst**, treatment consists of aspiration and/or restriction of activity until the cyst heals. Steroid injections (methylprednisolone) or curettage with bone grafting may be used for patients with pain or limited motion.

Treatment of the **aneursymal cyst** consists of curettage or resection with bone grafting. According to a recent study[10] of patients with recurrent or inoperable cysts, radiotherapy to a tumor dose of 26–30Gy was effective with no evidence of local recurrence (median follow-up: 17 years).

49. Describe the distinctive clinical, radiologic, and pathologic features of giant-cell tumors of the bone.

Clinically, females are affected slightly more often than males (1.5:1 female-to-male ratio). The usual age at presentation is 20–50 years. The tumor is typically locally aggressive. The patient complains of chronic pain in the region of the affected joint, which increases at night and with activity. There may also be stretching of the overlying skin. Radiographically, the giant cell tumor commonly appears in the epiphyses of the long, tubular bones as a radiolucent lesion. It is an expansile lesion, causing thinning or fracture of the cortex. On pathologic examination it is composed of oval and spindle mononuclear cells and evenly distributed multinucleated osteoclast-like giant cells.

50. What are the options for treatment of giant-cell bone tumors?

The first treatment options include curettage with bone graft, cryotherapy of the cavity, application of phenol in the cavity, or insertion of methylmethacrylate cement in the cavity. En bloc resection with reconstruction of the joint is another option for giant cell tumors. Radiotherapy is an option in patients in whom resection is not feasible because of tumor location or medical reasons.

51. What are soft tissue sarcomas?

Malignant tumors that develop in muscles, tendons, synovial tissues, fibrous tissues, and nerves are known as soft tissue sarcomas. They can spread locally and metastasize to other distant organs. Some soft tissue tumors are benign. They do not spread and are rarely life-threatening. They can, however, compress and hinder normal organ functioning.

52. List the risk factors for development of soft tissue sarcomas.

Researchers are unsure of the cause of soft tissue sarcomas. Some studies have identified exposure to certain chemicals and herbicides in some people with soft tissue sarcomas. People with certain inherited conditions (e.g., von Recklinghausen's disease [neurofibromatosis]) have an increased risk for developing soft tissue sarcomas.

53. What is the incidence of soft tissue sarcomas?

Soft tissue sarcomas are a relatively rare form of cancer. In 2001 there is estimated to be 8,700 new cases in the United States. About 1,000 cases are estimated to occur in persons under the age of 20 years.

54. What are the presenting symptoms of soft tissue sarcomas?

In the early stages, soft tissue sarcomas rarely cause symptoms because soft tissue is flexible and can stretch to accommodate the tumor growth. Normally the first sign is swelling or a mass.

55. What is the cell of origin in rhabdomyosarcomas (RMS)?

A rare malignant neoplasm of mesenchymal origin, RMS arises from cells committed to the skeletal muscle lineage.

56. What are the common sites of RMS?

RMS is often seen in areas of striated muscles of the head and neck region, genitourinary tract, and extremities.

57. What chromosome abnormality is seen in many patients with RMS?

Translocation t(2;13)(q35;q14) on the short arm of chromosome 3 is found in many of the alveolar-type tumors that are associated with adolescence, metastatic disease at presentation, and poor prognosis.

58. Which soft tissue sarcomas are most common in children and adults?

Embryonal RMS occurs more often in children, whereas leiomyosarcoma is more likely to be found in older patients.

59. Describe the clinical picture of RMS at presentation.

The clinical picture depends on the site of the tumor. Orbital tumors present with proptosis, periorbital edema, and ptosis. Patients with tumors of the ear may complain of ear pain, hemorrhagic discharge from the ear canal, or recurrent middle ear infections. Tumors of the extremities present with swelling or a mass. Genitourinary tumors may manifest as hematuria, incontinence, recurrent urinary tract infections, or obstruction. Vaginal or uterine RMS may appear as a grape-like cluster or mass growing through the vaginal orifice.

60. Identify poor prognostic factors in RMS.

The Intergroup Rhabdomyosarcoma Studies identified the following as poor prognostic factors:
- Tumor size > 5 cm
- Positive node status
- Alveolar or undifferentiated histology
- Primary sites other than genitourinary tract

61. Describe the currently recommended treatment of RMS.

Initial surgical resection is generally recommended if it is believed to be feasible without loss of organ function. If this option is not realistic, initial biopsy is followed by intensive chemotherapy and radiotherapy. Residual disease should be resected once optimal response to adjuvant therapy has been achieved. For tumors of the orbit, vagina, and bladder, chemotherapy with or without radiotherapy or limited surgery after multiagent chemotherapy treatment offers the same survival outcome as aggressive initial resection.

62. What imaging modality is indicated for following patients with pelvic RMS?

MRI detects residual pelvic RMS better than CT scanning. Tissue planes are well delineated. MRI allows accurate assessment of tumor invasion into adjacent structures.

63. What are leiomyosarcomas? Where do they occur?

Leiomyosarcoma is a cancer of the smooth muscle and is seen mainly in the gastrointestinal tract and retroperitoneum. In adults visceral metastases are most common in the liver, whereas in children metastases are rare. The stomach is the most common site, followed by the small bowel. Discovery of the tumor is usually delayed until the size has become considerable. Usual presenting complaints include abdominal pain, weight loss, early satiety, nausea, and vomiting. Over one-half of patients have a palpable mass at presentation.

64. Why is the histologic grade important in sarcomas?

Histologic grade evaluates the aggressiveness of the tumor. High-grade tumors are the most aggressive, have a poorer prognosis, and often present with distant metastases. Histologic grade is the single best prognostic indicator for the development of recurrent disease and eventual outcome.

65. Describe the outcome for nonmetastatic and metastatic leiomyosarcoma.

The general prognosis is good for tumors arising outside the gastrointestinal tract. Prognosis for children with metastatic disease is poor. Children with pulmonary metastases should undergo thoracotomy to resect all gross disease. The estimated 5-year survival rate after thoracotomy for pulmonary metastases in adults ranges from 10% to 58%. Locoregional recurrence after complete surgical resection is the most common pattern of failure. Current pediatric clinical trials are evaluating chemotherapy with doxorubicin and ifosfamide, based on several adult trials suggesting that ifosfamide-based regimens are superior for soft-tissue sarcomas.

66. Compare Ewing's sarcoma with osteosarcoma.

Ewing's sarcoma belongs to a group of neoplasms known as small, round, blue cell tumors. Often occurring in the extremities and pelvis, 50% of osteosarcomas arise from the bones around the knee. When the long bones are involved, Ewing's sarcoma usually presents in the midshaft, whereas osteosarcomas begin in the ends of the bone. Similar characteristics include patient age (young people), patient gender (males are affected more often than females), and presenting symptoms (pain with swelling or a mass). Both neoplasms have a propensity to metastasize to the lungs

67. What cytogenetic abnormalities are seen in Ewing's sarcoma?

Studies have identified consistent alteration of the EWS locus on chromosome 22 band q12; gains of chromosomes 2,5,7,8,9, and 12; nonreciprocal translocation t(1;16)(q12;q11.2); and deletions at the short arm of chromosome 1.

68. What factors demonstrate favorable prognostic significance in Ewing's sarcoma?

Major favorable factors include site (distal extremities, central location), small tumor volume, and absence of metastases. Other favorable factors include younger age, gender (girls have better prognoses), absence of systemic findings (e.g., anemia, fever, increased LDH), massive tumor necrosis after induction chemotherapy, and minimal or no residual tumor after presurgical chemotherapy.

69. How is Ewing's sarcoma treated?

Successful treatment requires collaboration among the orthopedic surgeon, radiation oncologist, pathologist, and medical oncologist. Multidrug chemotherapy and control of local disease with surgery and/or radiotherapy are indicated in the treatment of all patients.

70. What chemotherapy agents are commonly used in the treatment of Ewing's sarcoma?

Current chemotherapy includes vincristine, doxorubicin, cyclophosphamide, ifosfamide, and etoposide.

71. When is radiotherapy used in the treatment of Ewing's sarcoma?
Radiotherapy is used when no surgical option can preserve function, in patients with inadequate margins, and in patients with gross residual disease after surgery. In patients with metastatic disease, radiotherapy may be given to the primary tumor site as will as sites of metastases. Patients with pulmonary metastases should undergo whole-lung radiation.

72. Does intensive therapy have a role in the treatment of Ewing's sarcoma?
Approaches that incorporate high-dose chemotherapy with or without total-body irradiation in combination with stem cell transplant have not yet demonstrated an advantage in terms of disease-free survival. Secondary leukemias and the development of osteosarcomas within the radiation field are risk factors.

BIBLIOGRAPHY

1. American Joint Committee on Cancer: AJCC Cancer Staging Manual. Philadelphia, J.B. Lippincott, 1997.
2. Bacci G, et al: Prognostic factors in nonmetastatic Ewing's sarcoma of bone treated with adjuvant chemotherapy: Analysis of 359 patients at the Instituto Ortopedico Rizzoli. J Clin Oncol 18: 4–11, 2000.
3. Bergh P, Gunterberg B, Mer-Kindblom JM, Kindblom LG: Prognostic factors and outcome of pelvis, sacral and spinal chondrosarcomas: A center-based study of 69 cases. Cancer 91:1201–1212, 2001.
4. Blackley HR, Wunder JS, Davis AM, et al: Treatment of giant-cell tumors of long bones with curettage and bone grafting. J Bone Joint 81A:811–820, 1999.
5. Carnesale PG: Tumors, part IV. In Canale St (ed): Campbell's Operative Orthopaedics, 9th ed. St. Louis, Mosby, 1998.
6. Chakravarti A, Spiro IJ, Hig EB, et al: Megavoltage radiation therapy for axial and inoperable giant-cell tumor of bone. J Bone Joint Surg 81A:1566–1573, 1999.
7. Chin KR, Kharrazi FD, Miller BS, et al: Osteochondromas of the distal aspect of the tibia or fibula: Natural history and treatment. J Bone Joint Surg 82A:1269–1278, 2000.
8. Conlon KC, Brennan MF: Soft tissue sarcomas. In Murphy GP, Lawrence W Jr, Lenhard RE Jr (eds): Clinical Oncology, 2nd ed. Atlanta, American Cancer Society, 1995, pp 435–450.
9. Copley L, Dorman JP: Benign pediatric bone tumors: Evaluation and treatment. Pediatr Clin North Am 43:949–966, 1996.
10. Feigenberg SJ, Marcus RB Jr, Zlotecki RA, et al: Megavoltage radiotherapy for aneursymal bone cysts. Int J Radiat Oncol Biol Physics 49:1243–1247, 2001.
11. Flemming DJ, Murphy MD: Enchondroma and chondrosarcoma. Semin Musculoskel Radiol 14:59–71, 2000.
12. Finelli A, Babyn P, Lorie GA, et al: The use of magnetic resonance imaging in the diagnosis and follow-up of pediatric pelvic rhabdomyosarcoma. J Urol 163:1952–1953, 2000.
13. Greenlee RT, Hill-Harmon MB, Murray T, Thun M: Cancer statistics 2001. Cancer J Clin 51: 15–36, 2001.
14. Grier HE: The Ewing family of tumors. Pediatr Clin North Am 44:991–1001, 1997.
15. Haynes K: Neoplasms of the musculoskeletal system. In Maher AB, Salmond SW, Pellino TA (eds): Orthopaedic Nursing, 2nd ed. Philadelphia, W. B. Saunders, 1998, pp 769–803.
16. Himelstein BP, Dormans JP: Malignant bone tumors of childhood. Pediatr Clin North Am 43: 967–984, 1996.
17. Hug EB, Slater JD: Proton radiation therapy for chordomas and chondrosarcomas of the skull base. Neurosurg Clin North Am 11:627–638, 2000.
18. Lambiase RE, Levine SM, Terek RM, Wyman JJ: Long bone surface osteomas: Imaging features that may help avoid unnecessary biopsies. Am J Roentgenol 171:775–778, 1998.
19. Marina NM, Bowman LC, Ching-Hou P, Crist WM: Pediatric solid tumors. In Murphy GP,

Lawrence W Jr, Lenhard RE Jr (eds). Clinical Oncology, 2nd ed. Atlanta, American Cancer Society, 1995, pp 524–530, 540–545.

20. McGrory JE, Pritchard DJ, Arndt CS, et al: Nonrhabdomyosarcoma soft tissue sarcomas in children. Clin Orthop Rel Res 374:247–258, 2000.

21. Meyers PA, Gorlick R: Osteosarcoma. Pediatr Clin North Am 44:973–987, 1997.

22. Murphy MD, Choi JJ, Kransdorf MJ, et al: Imaging of osteochondroma: Variants and complications with radiologic-pathologic correlation. Radiographics 20:1407–1434, 2000.

23. NCIs CancerNet PDQ Summaries: Ewing's Family of Tumors Including PNET; Osteosarcoma/ Malignant Fibrous Histiocytoma of Bone; Childhood Rhabdomyosarcoma; Adult Soft Tissue Sarcoma; Childhood Soft Tissue Sarcoma. Retrieved August 8, 2001, from <http://cancernet.nci.nih.gov/pdq.html>.

24. Neville HL, et al: Preoperative staging, prognostic factors, and outcome for extremity rhabdomyosarcoma: A preliminary report from the Intergroup Rhabdomyosarcoma Study IV (1991-1997). J Pediatr Surg 35:317–321, 2000.

25. Pappo AS, Shapiro DN, Crist W: Rhabdomyosarcoma: Biology and treatment. Pediatr Clin North Am 44:953–949, 1997.

26. Pritchard DJ: Malignant tumors of bone. In Murphy GP, Lawrence W Jr, Lenhard RE Jr (eds): Clinical Oncology, 2nd ed. Atlanta, American Cancer Society, 1995, pp 428–434.

27. Ramappa AJ, Lee FY, Tang P, et al: Chondroblastoma of bone. J Bone Joint Surg 82A:1140–1145, 2000.

28. Russell EC, Dunn NL, Massey GV: Lymphomas and bone tumors: Clinical presentation, management and potential late effects of current treatment strategies. Adolesc Med State Art Rev 10:423–429, 1999.

29. Schoen DC: Adult Orthopaedic Nursing. Philadelphia, J.B. Lippincott, 2000.

30. Somers J, Faber LP: Chondroma and chondrosarcoma. Semin Thorac Cardiovasc Surg 11:270–277, 1999.

31. Wilche B, Widhe T: Initial symptoms and clinical features in osteosarcoma and Ewing's sarcoma. J Bone Joint Surg 82A:667–674, 2000.

32. Wolden SL, et al: Indications for radiotherapy and chemotherapy after complete resection in rhabdomyosarcoma: A report from the Intergroup Rhabdomyosarcoma Studies I to III. J Clin Oncol 17:3468–3475, 1999.

33. Zheng MH, Robbins P, Xu J, et al: The histogenesis of giant-cell tumor of bone: A model of interaction between neoplastic cells and osteoclasts. Histol Histopathol 16:297–307, 2001.

12. PEDIATRIC ORTHOPEDIC CONDITIONS

Sandra B. Van Dyke, RN, MS

1. What is congenital hip dysplasia or, to use the more recent term, developmental dysplasia of the hip (DDH)?

DDH refers to a variety of conditions in which the head of the femur is displaced in relation to the acetabulum. The most common form is posterior dislocation, which causes the lower extremity to be flexed, adducted, and internally rotated at the hip.

2. What is the incidence of DDH?

DDH occurs in 1–2 cases per 1000 births and is 4–6 times more common in females than males.

3. What causes DDH?

DDH is multifactorial in origin. Physiologic factors include a positive family history (20%); maternal pelvic laxity related to hormone secretion, especially estrogen; and the laxity of fetal points. Mechanical factors include breech presentation, first-born infants, twinning, and large infant size.

4. How is DDH diagnosed?

Ultrasonography is done in the newborn period to assess hip stability and acetabular development. In older children, x-ray evaluation is useful.

5. What are the clinical features of DDH in newborns and infants?
- Limitation of hip adduction
- Allis sign (uneven knee height when the thighs are flexed to a 90° angle toward the abdomen)
- Asymmetric thigh and gluteal folds
- Broad perineum in bilateral dislocation
- Positive Barlow test (the femoral head is felt to slip out over the posterior lip of the acetabulum when pressure is applied to the front)
- Positive Ortolani test (After placing the infant in a supine position and flexing the knee to 90°, the examiner grasps the thigh with the middle finger over the greater trochanter. The thigh is lifted anteriorly into the acetabulum while it is adducted. In a positive finding a palpable, possibly audible "clunk" is felt as reduction occurs.)

6. What are the clinical features of DDH in older children?
- Affected leg is shorter than the other leg
- Limping
- Waddling (bilateral DDH)
- Increased lordosis (bilateral DDH)
- Toe walking
- Trendelenburg's sign (when the child bears weight on the affected side, the pelvis tilts downward instead of upward on the normal side)

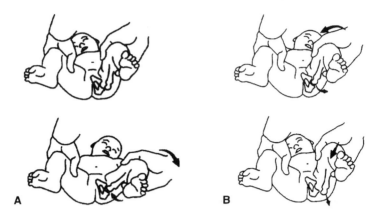

A, The Ortolani test. This maneuver reduces a posteriorly dislocated hip. The affected hip is gently abducted while the femoral head is reduced with an anteriorly directed forced provided by the fingers placed over the great trochanter. *B*, The Barlow test. This maneuver tests for dislocation or subluxation of a reduced hip. The test is done by gently adducting the examined hip while directing a posterior force across the hip. (From Staheli LT (ed): Pediatric Orthopedic Secrets. Philadelphia, Hanley & Belfus, 1998, with permission.)

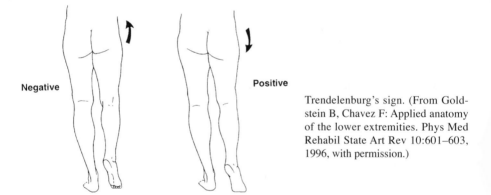

Trendelenburg's sign. (From Goldstein B, Chavez F: Applied anatomy of the lower extremities. Phys Med Rehabil State Art Rev 10:601–603, 1996, with permission.)

7. Describe the therapeutic management of children with DDH.

The major goal of treatment is to place the femoral head against the acetabulum. The earlier that successful management is implemented, the more positive the prognosis. From birth to 6 months of age, splinting is used to maintain the proximal femur in the acetabulum. The most common mode of treatment is the Pavlik harness. The harness is worn continuously until the hip is clinically and radiographically stable, usually 3–6 months. In children 6–18 months of age, treatment includes shortening of the limb and contractions of the hip flexor, and adduction muscles may be widened. In such children traction is used for about 3 weeks; then operative reduction is performed, followed by a spica cast. In older children, open reduction and casting are done, followed by a period of rehabilitation.

8. What are the nursing implications of DDH?

The child in a reduction device (such as the Pavlik harness) must be observed for proper application and skin integrity. The skin beneath the harness should be protected with clothing. Gentle massage is valuable. The parents must be taught modification of car seats and the proper positions for nursing and eating. In older children, care of traction, casts, and braces must be explained. The parents and the child need support throughout the treatment period. Appropriate referrals should be made as necessary to promote a positive outcome. The normal growth and development needs of the child must be encouraged at all times.

9. What is talipes equinovarus (TEV)?
TEV, or clubfoot, is a congenital deformity of the foot that occurs in 1 per 1000 live births. Males are affected twice as often as females. The foot is twisted inward and flexed in a downward position, with bone deformity and soft tissue contracture.

10. What causes TEV?
The exact cause is unknown, but a genetic tendency may be present.

11. How is TEV diagnosed?
The deformity of the foot is readily apparent at birth. Foot flexibility is variable. The foot is usually smaller and shorter, with an empty and possibly transverse heel pad. The affected limb is usually shorter with mild atrophy of the calf muscles. The child should be assessed for any associated muscle deformities or other neuromuscular dysfunctions. Early diagnosis and intervention are important for the most positive outcome because the small bones of the foot begin to ossify shortly after birth. If necessary, radiographs may be ordered.

12. Describe the therapeutic management of the child with TEV.
Manipulation and casting are begun shortly after diagnosis. The casts are changed every 2–3 weeks because of the rapid growth in early infancy. A thermoplastic brace may be applied after the cast is removed to hold the correction. If correction is not achieved by 3 months of age, surgical intervention involving fixation and the release of tight joints and tendons is performed.

13. What is the prognosis for the child with TEV?
The outcome depends on the age of the child when treatment is started, the severity of the deformity, and compliance with treatment protocols.

14. What are the nursing implications of TEV?
In the initial period after casting, the nurse must perform neurovascular assessments, check for drainage from the cast, and observe for any signs of swelling. Discharge teaching should include cast care, the need for passive range of motion exercises, and careful observation of the infant for any signs of pain.

15. What is metatarsus adductus varus?
Metatarsus adductus (MTA) is one of the most common foot deformities in children. The foot is adducted and occasionally supinated. MTA may occur bilaterally, and 50% of cases are associated with developmental dysplasia of the hip. Unlike TEV, the deformity occurs at the tarsometatarsal joint while the heel and ankle remain in a neutral position.

16. What causes MTA?
It is most frequently associated with intrauterine positioning.

17. Describe the therapeutic management of MTA.

The postural form of MTA usually resolves in 6–12 weeks. In a small percentage of children, the foot does not improve and treatment must be initiated. The family is given a series of stretching exercises. If the foot does not improve, a series of corrective shoes, casts, and exercises is implemented.

18. What are the nursing implications of MTA?

Early identification of the deformity is important for the best prognosis. Reinforcement of the exercises is needed. If casting is done, cast care education must be implemented.

19. What is hypermobile pes planus (flexible flatfeet)?

Ligamentous laxity and fat in the area of medial longitudinal arch.

20. How is pes planus diagnosed?

When the child is in a weight-bearing position, the medial longitudinal arch is not evident.

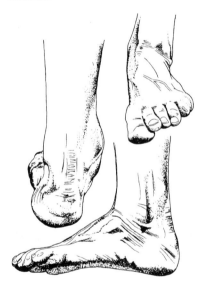

Pes planus (flat foot). (From Mellion MB, Walsh WM, Shelton GL: The Team Physician's Handbook, 2nd ed. Philadelphia, Hanley & Belfus, 1997, with permission.)

21. Describe the therapeutic management of pes planus.

Treatment is conservative and begins after the age of 6 years. If pain is present, it usually can be managed with a medial longitudinal arch support.

22. What is internal tibial torsion (ITT)?

Tibial torsion is an inward twisting of the tibia that causes the child's feet to turn inward as he or she walks. ITT causes a bowed-leg stance and helps children achieve better balance as they learn to walk. With walking, ITT resolves and should not persist after 18–24 months. It is found more frequently in females.

23. What causes ITT?

The cause is controversial. It may be congenital due to persistent infantile femoral anteversion or uterine position, or it may be acquired secondary to abnormal sitting habits.

24. How is ITT diagnosed?

The major characteristic of ITT is an in-toed ("pigeon-toed") stance. On assessment, the examiner notes that the entire leg is internally rotated. Generalized ligamentous laxity is often seen, and the child may seem to "trip and fall" more than normal. The thigh-foot angle (TF angle) is measured. An angle less than 10° is positive for ITT.

25. Describe the therapeutic management of ITT.

ITT usually resolves with age. Occasionally braces or special shoes may be used. The child is taught to avoid sitting in the "W" position or sleeping in a knee–chest position. In rare cases, persistent ITT may require surgical intervention to straighten the tibia.

26. What are the nursing implications of ITT?

Reassure the family that in most cases ITT resolves by itself. Teach the family to help the child correct abnormal sitting habits and/or sleeping positions.

27. What is external tibial torsion?

External tibial torsion is associated with abduction/external rotation and soft tissue contraction due to uterine position. It produces an externally rotated or out-toed appearance. Like ITT, it usually resolves with age and minimal intervention.

28. What is femoral anteversion?

Femoral anteversion is defined as excessive medial rotation of the femur that causes the neck and head of the femur to point inward with a slight forward inclination. It is a common cause of toeing-in in children.

29. What causes femoral anteversion?

Femoral anteversion is often familial. Femoral anteversion is twice as common in females and is considered a developmental abnormality.

30. List the clinical features of femoral anteversion.

- Positive Reeder test (on assessment the examiner notes a prominence of the greater trochanter)
- Ambulation with the patella medially rotated and running in an awkward position
- Sitting in the "W" position
- Inward rotation of femur, knees, patellae, and feet
- Clumsy gait

31. Describe the therapeutic management of femoral anteversion.

The normal child is born with 40° of femoral anteversion, which gradually decreases to 10°–15° at adolescence. In 99% of all cases, therefore, no further treatment is needed. In rare cases, surgery may be done if the anteversion is over 50° and the child is at least 8 years of age.

32. What are the nursing implications of femoral anteversion?

Assure the parents that the prognosis is very good and that the child is not at risk for arthritis or other related physical impairments later in life.

33. What is Osgood-Schlatter disease (OSD)?

OSD is osteochondritis involving a disturbance of the patellar tendon attachment to the tibial tuberosity and resulting in knee pain and swelling. It is one of the overuse disorders seen in adolescents.

34. What causes OSD?

OSD results from repeated pulling of the patellar tendon. Repetitive overuse injuries by active young athletic people cause microtrauma at the tibial tuberosity. Ultrasound and magnetic resonance imaging (MRI) scans reveal changes in the patellar tendon and the adjacent soft tissues.[14]

35. How is OSD diagnosed?

The physical exam indicates knee tenderness, localized over the tibial tubercle. There should be no limitation of range of motion in the knee or hip. Typically the patient points to the tibial tuberosity as the source of pain and states that the pain occurs with activity and eases with rest. Radiographs may be normal or show changes in the patellar tendon. Other causes of knee pain must be ruled out.

36. Describe the therapeutic management of OSD.

OSD is a self-limiting condition that normally resolves in 6–18 months with rest. Limited activity, use of a mild analgesic when needed for pain and swelling, and local application of ice after periods of activity are useful. Cortisone injections are not indicated. The use of a knee sleeve that pads the tubercle tuberosity or occasionally a dual-hinged knee brace may be recommended. An isometric exercise program is also beneficial.

37. What are the long-term implications of OSD?

OSD is generally benign but may result in a bony enlargement of the tibial tuberosity and/or painful kneeling as an adult.

38. What are the nursing implications of OSD?

The nurse should assess the knee for swelling, areas of tenderness, and any limitations in range of motion. Education includes the use of ice, mild analgesics, and the application of knee immobilizers. Resting the area should be stressed as well as limiting athletics. The nurse can also reinforce the stretching and strengthening exercises that the young athlete has been taught.

39. What is congenital dislocation/subluxation of the knee (CDK)?

CDK is a descriptive term indicating recurvation of the knees at birth.

40. What is the incidence of CDK?

CDK is a rare condition, occurring in about 1 in 40,000–80,000 live births. It is often associated with other congenital deformities, especially developmental dysplasia of the hip.

41. What causes CDK?

CDK appears to be both mechanical and genetic in origin, although views are conflicting.

42. How is CDK diagnosed?

A history of oligohydramnios and positional abnormalities may have been present in utero. Physical examination may show the following:

- Irreducibly hyperextended knees
- Patella that is difficult to palpate or small and/or dislocated
- Anteriorly displaced hamstrings
- Presence of transverse creases over the front of the knee
- Presence of developmental dysplasia of the hip
- Fibroses of the quadriceps
- Other congenital anomalies, such as talipes equinovarus and Larson's syndrome[11]

43. Describe the therapeutic management of CDK.

The major goal of treatment is to provide as much range of motion as possible so that patients are able to perform activities of daily living adequately. If the deformities are mild, early intervention consists of serial casting and/or splinting. Physical therapy is initiated to encourage range of motion. If adequate flexion is obtained, the child is placed in a Pavlik harness. Surgical treatment is initiated when conservative methods fail. The long-term outlook varies, but accomplishment of full function is not common.

44. What are the nursing implications of CDK?

Teach parents the necessary care of the child in a cast, splint, and/or brace. Assessment of the child undergoing conservative treatment should include observation for signs of fractures of the distal femur and/or tibia. Assess the child's range of motion, and reinforce exercises that have been taught to the parents. If surgery is performed, the child is assessed for postoperative complications. Observation of active and passive exercises is an important part of postoperative care, in both the short and long term, to determine the success of treatment.

45. What is leg length discrepancy (LLD)?

LLD is defined as unequal lengths of the lower limbs. The discrepancy may be in the femur, tibia, or both. It may be accompanied by shortening of the upper limbs. One side of the body may grow faster than the other.

46. What are the common causes of LLD?

The many contributing causes of LLD include the following:

- Congenital (e.g., coxa vara)
- Developmental (e.g., Legg-Calvé-Perthes disease)
- Neuromuscular (e.g., cerebral palsy)
- Infectious (e.g., pyogenicosteomyelitis)
- Trauma (e.g., physical injury with premature growth plate closure)
- Tumor (e.g., radiation-induced injury)[2]

47. How is LLD diagnosed?

LLD of 2 cm or less is often undetected. If LLD is over 3 cm, a limp becomes evident. Measurements of the limb are taken. The most accurate clinical measurement is from the superior iliac spine to the medial malleolus. The most accurate diagnosis of LLD is done via a scanogram. A radiolucent ruler is placed next to the limb and accurate measurements are taken by x-ray.

48. Describe the therapeutic management of LLD.

It is important to determine the extent of the discrepancy at skeletal maturity. If it is predicted to be less than 2 cm, no intervention may be necessary. For discrepancies up to 3 cm, a small lift may be adequate. For discrepancies over 3 cm, intervention is often necessary. Surgical interventions are aimed at shortening the longer extremity, lengthening the shorter extremity, or both. One leg-shortening procedure is called epiphysiodesis. In the child whose growth plates have not closed, this procedure stops growth in the longer leg and allows the shorter leg to grow to the same length or stops the length discrepancy from becoming greater. Lengthening the shorter limb is performed by partially cutting and distracting the leg slowly, using an external device such as an Illizarov or Orthofix apparatus. The slow lengthening enables the bone to heal as lengthening is done. Lengthening procedures can make corrections greater than 5 cm.

49. What are the nursing implications of LLD?

Successful outcome of surgery requires a team approach. Education of the family is important because the treatment takes from 6 months to 1 year for completion. Monitoring for complications and supporting the family and child are important aspects of care.

50. What is osteogenesis imperfecta (OI)?

OI is a group of inherited disorders of connective tissue and bone defects characterized by pathologic fractures at birth or during childhood. The incidence is 1 per 10,000 live births.

51. What causes OI?

The severe forms of OI (types II and III) are autosomal recessive genetic disorders, whereas the milder forms (types I and IV) are autosomal dominant.

52. Describe the signs and symptoms of OI.

The abnormal formation of type I collagen is found in bones, teeth, sclera, and ligaments. In bones the results are severe osteoporosis and therefore fractures. In the more severe forms, fractures may be seen at birth. Signs and symptoms vary greatly and may include:

- Genetic history
- Bones that fracture easily
- Very small in stature to near normal
- Blue sclera
- Dental problems
- Hearing loss
- Tendency to have scoliosis
- Laxity of joints
- Easy bruising
- Hypoplastic teeth with bluish-brown discoloration

The incidence of fractures tends to decrease in puberty when the high hormone levels help strengthen bones. OI must be differentiated from child abuse.

53. How is OI diagnosed?

In most cases, diagnosis is based on clinical manifestations, genetic history, and radiographs. When the diagnosis is not clear, a skin biopsy may be done for collagen testing.

54. Describe the therapeutic management of OI.

The goal of care is to provide as normal a level of growth and development as possible. Care is primarily supportive and aimed at preventing fractures, contractures, deformities, and malalignments. Medications have limited benefit, but calcitonin may be used to aid bone healing and growth hormone may be given to stimulate growth. Care is usually supportive and requires a team approach. Lightweight braces and splints support limbs, prevent fractures, and aid in ambulation. Walkers may also be used to facilitate ambulation. The physical therapist plays an important role in helping to strengthen muscles and thus improving bone density. Exercises are geared to light resistance and include such activities as swimming. Surgery may be done to correct deformities, and intramedullary rods may be inserted to give the bones stability. Longer rods are inserted as the child grows.

55. What are the nursing considerations of OI?

The family must be encouraged to provide the child with every opportunity for normal growth and development. Infants and children require careful handling when they are moved to prevent fractures. Teach the family how to bathe, dress, diaper, and change the child. For example, when diapering a severely affected infant, the parent should lift the infant at the buttocks rather than the ankles. The parents may want to carry a letter certifying the child's condition to prevent accusations of abuse. Involvement in support groups is useful, and the nurse can refer the family to the Osteogenesis Imperfecta Foundation at <www.oif.org>. Long-term goals should include genetic counseling and career planning.

56. What is Legg-Calvé-Perthes disease (LCPD)?

LCPD, also known as osteochondritis deformans juvenilis, is a self-limiting disorder characterized by aseptic necrosis of the femoral head. It is most common in children 4–8 years of age and in white males. It occurs in 1 per 1200 births. Involvement is usually unilateral but can be bilateral.

57. Discuss the cause and pathophysiology of LCPD.

Research has shown a familial predisposition, but the basic cause is unknown. During middle childhood the blood supply to the femoral head is most tenuous and may become obstructed by trauma, inflammation, and other conditions. This obstruction leads to aseptic necrosis of the femoral head. A study of 344 children at Shriner's Hospital for Crippled Children in St. Louis showed a strong statistical correlation between parents who smoke at home and children with LCPD.[13] The frequency climbed from 1 per 1,200 people to 1 in 100 among youngsters subjected to passive smoke at home.

58. Describe the clinical manifestations of LCPD.

Onset is insidious. The child may limp and complain of pain in the hip or anterior thigh. Activity aggravates the symptoms, and rest eases the pain. As the disease progresses, range of motion is limited with weakness and muscle wasting in the affected limb.

59. How is LCPD diagnosed?

Radiographic examinations, combined with the history of the present illness confirm the diagnosis.

60. Describe the therapeutic management of LCPD.

The aim of treatment is to keep the head of the femur contained in the acetabulum to prevent deformities. Treatment modalities vary with the severity of the symptoms and include measures to reduce pain and inflammation and to restore motion. The initial therapy is usually conservative and includes a period of rest and non–weight-bearing. Traction, leg casts, leather harness slings, and/or abduction braces may be used. Conservative therapy may be continued for 2–3 years. If surgical intervention is done, the child may return to normal function in 3–4 months.

61. What is the usual outcome for LCPD?

LCPD is a self-limiting condition with an excellent prognosis as long as parents and child comply with the therapeutic regimen.

62. What are the nursing implications of LCPD?

The nurse plays an important role in referring a child with LCPD. The parents and the child may rely on the nurse to help them adjust to the prescribed therapy. The family needs to be taught the purpose, function, application, and care of any corrective device, and the nurse should provide follow-up care to ensure compliance with the therapeutic regimen. Because therapy is often long-term, the nurse should assist the child to select appropriate activities. If surgery is carried out, the nurse needs to assess the child postoperatively. Neurovascular checks, pain management, and appropriate activities are included in nursing functions.

63. What is slipped capital femoral epiphysis (SCFE)?

SCFE is a well-known disorder of the hip that is characterized by the displacement of the capital femoral epiphysis in a posterior and inferior direction out of its functional position. It occurs most frequently during the rapid growth spurt of adolescence: 13–16 years of age for males and 11–14 years of age for females.

64. What causes SCFE?

The cause is basically unknown, but SCFE is more common in rapidly growing children, suggesting that growth hormone trauma from excessive weight may play a role. It is also more common in children with a known endocrine disorder, renal failure, osteodystrophy, or previous radiation. SCFE may be acute or chronic, but the chronic form is far more common, accounting for 85% of all cases.

65. Describe the clinical manifestations of SCFE.

Children generally present with persistent hip pain that affects the groin, thigh, and knee. A limp is evident, along with decreased range of motion on the affected side. The examiner may notice the child holding the leg in an externally rotated position to relieve stress and pain in the hip joint. In an acute slip, the pain is sudden and severe.

66. How is SCFE classified?

SCFE is classified by both clinical signs and radiographic exam. Clinically it is important to note whether the child can walk. SCFE is considered stable if the child can walk with or without crutches and unstable if the child cannot tolerate any weight-bearing. Ultrasonography is also useful in classification. If effusion is present and no remodeling of the metaphyseal plate is seen, the child is likely to have had an acute event and unstable SCFE. If there is no effusion and evidence of remodeling is seen,

SCFE is considered stable. This classification is considered predictive of the outcome. A stable SCFE has a much better outcome.[10]

67. Describe the therapeutic management of SCFE.

The immediate goal of treatment is to prevent a further slip. The initial treatment is to put the child on bed rest until surgery and/or to have the child use crutches with no weight-bearing on the affected leg. The child is then prepared for hip pinning or external fixation to stabilize the femoral head.

68. What are the nursing implications of SCFE?

In the preoperative period the nurse needs to encourage the child to comply with non–weight-bearing restrictions and to prepare the child and family for the operative procedure. In the immediate postoperative period, neurovascular checks and pain management are the two most important nursing interventions. As healing occurs, it is most important for the nurse to teach the child and family the progression of ambulation and weight-bearing as ordered by the physician. Contact sports are avoided until growth is complete. Compliance with the regimen is essential, and follow-up care is needed until the epiphyseal plates are closed.

69. What is the prognosis of SCFE?

The prognosis depends on the initial diagnosis of stable or unstable SCFE, the occurrence of complications, and compliance with the medical regimen.

70. What is torticollis?

Torticollis (wryneck) is a congenital or acquired condition of limited neck motion in which the neck is flexed and turned to the side due to the shortening of the sternocleidomastoid muscle on the affected side. It may occur alone or with other defects.

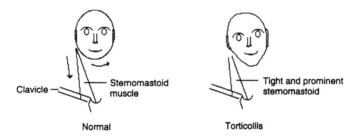

Comparison of normal anatomy and torticollis. (From Mehta A: Common Musculoskeletal Problems. Philadelphia, Hanley & Belfus, 1997, with permission.)

71. What causes torticollis?

Torticollis may result from fetal malposition, birth trauma, sternocleidomastoid muscle compartment syndrome, and heredity. Torticollis may be acquired as a result of central nervous system lesions, infections in the area of the neck, and abnormalities of the cervical spine.

72. How is torticollis diagnosed?

The child with torticollis persistently holds the head in a tilted position. There is no apparent pain. Typically the child holds the head tilted to the right, with the face and chin rotated to the left. In infants less than 3 months of age, a "tumor" may be felt on the sternocleidomastoid muscle; in reality, it is a swelling of the central portion of the muscle. After 3 months of age, a contracture of the muscle appears. If the problem is not corrected, facial asymmetry may become permanent. Examination of the child should include a thorough neurologic examination and anteroposterior and lateral radiographs of the cervical spine. A CT scan or MRI may be indicated if pain is present. It is imperative to rule out associated conditions. Ultrasound of the hips should be performed because developmental dysplasia of the hip may be seen with torticollis.

73. Describe the therapeutic management of torticollis.

The mainstay of treatment for torticollis complicated by tumors or other abnormalities in the cervical region is gentle stretching exercises to increase the range of motion of the muscle. Exercises are done 4–6 times per day, 15–20 times each session. Exercises are most effective in children younger than 1 year who have no complications and show a positive response to the stretching exercises. If exercise is not successful or the child is older, surgical release of the sternocleidomastoid muscle may be indicated.

74. What is the prognosis for a child with torticollis?

When treatment is begun early and the stretching exercises are done consistently, most children with uncomplicated torticollis recover completely. Surgery is done if the child does not respond to the exercises.

75. Describe the nursing management of torticollis.

Case finding and referrals are important roles for the nurse. Once a diagnosis is made, the nurse works with the doctor and the physical therapist to implement an exercise program for the child. The parents are taught to work together as often as possible so that one person can stabilize the torso while the other performs the exercises. The parents can also be taught techniques that encourage the child to move his or her head. Toys can be placed on the opposite side so that the child must turn to see them. The infant may be held so that the head is positioned in the opposite direction or in a side-lying position so that the affected side is up and the child must stretch the neck muscles to look down. If surgery is done, physical therapy is begun again within 2 weeks. Because therapy is a long-term commitment, the nurse can provide needed support for the family.

BIBLIOGRAPHY

1. Aldegheri R: Distraction osteogenesis for lengthening of the tibia in patients who have limb length discrepancy or short stature. J Bone Joint Surg 81A:624–634, 1999.
2. Behrman RE, Kliegman RM: Nelson Essentials of Pediatrics, 3rd ed. Philadelphia, W.B. Saunders, 1998.
3. Femoral anteversion. Retrieved June 4, 2002, from <http://www.condata.com/health/pedbase/file/femoralA.htm>.
4. Femoral anteversion. In Textbook of Orthopedics on the World Wide Web. Retrieved June 4, 2002 from <http://www.medmedia.com/lib4/64.httm>.
5. Femoral torsion. Retrieved August 21, 2001, from <http://www.orthoseek.com/articles/femtorsion.html>.
6. Hip dysplasia. Retrieved August 21, 2001, from <http://www.orthseek.com/artilces/hipdys.html>.
7. Hogan MA, White JE: Child Health Nursing: Reviews and Rationales. New Jersey, Prentice Hall, 2003.

8. Internal tibial torsion. Retrieved August 21, 2001, from <http://www.orthoseek.com/articles/int-tibtor.html>.

9. Leg length discrepancy. Retrieved August 21, 2001, from <http://www.orthoseek.com/artilces/leglength.html>.

10. Loder R, Aronsson D, Dobbs M, Weinstein S: Slipped capital and femoral epiphysis. J Bone Joint Surg 82A:1170, 2000.

11. Muhammad [initial}, Kernitt [initial], Koman [initial], et al: Congenital dislocation of the knee: Overview of management options. J South Orthop 8(20):93–97, 2000.

12. Ponseti I: Treatment of congenital clubfoot. Virtual Hospital. Retrieved from <http://www.vh.org/providers/textbooks/clubfoot/clubfoot.html>.

13. Smoking linked to Legg-Perthes disease. Academy News: American Academy of Orthopaedic Surgeons. Retrieved August 10, 2001, from <http://www.aaos.org/wordhtml/aaosnews/legg/htm>.

14. Wall EJ: Osgood-Schlatter disease: Practical treatment for a self-limiting condition. Physician Sports Med 26, 1998. Retrieved from <http://www.physsportmed.com/issues/1998/03mar/wall/htm>.

15. Wong D: Whaley and Wong's Nursing Care of Infants and Children, 6th ed. St. Louis, Mosby, 1999.

13. OPERATIVE ORTHOPEDICS

Michael E. Zychowicz, RN, MS, NP-C, and Tom Bush, MSN, RN, CS, FNP

1. In general, what tasks need to be performed before surgery?
The patient should be educated thoroughly about the surgery, including goals, alternatives, and potential adverse outcomes. Postoperative teaching should begin before surgery. Unless the surgery is emergent, the patient must have a thorough history, physical exam, blood work, diagnostic testing, and medical clearance. All of the appropriate paperwork must be completed, including informed consent for surgery and anesthesia, health care proxy forms, or do-not-resuscitate orders. If outpatient surgery is to be performed, the patient may be given prescriptions before surgery for required splints or pain medications, eliminating the need to visit a pharmacy or surgical supply store postoperatively. Patients planning to use autologous transfusion for the surgery must begin the process within the appropriate timeframe.

2. How much blood can a patient put aside for autologous transfusion?
The answer depends on the amount of time for donation before surgery. The average patient can store 1 unit of blood per week, but the last donation must be made no less than 72 hours before surgery. Frozen blood can be stored for up to 1 year, but unfrozen blood is viable for approximately 5–6 weeks. If the patient's blood is not frozen for storage, smart planning may allow donation of 5 units of blood before surgery in a 5- to 6-week preoperative period.

3. Should all patients donate blood preoperatively for autologous transfusion?
It is not necessary for all patients to set aside blood for themselves preoperatively. Autologous donation and transfusion are recommended options if at least a 10% likelihood exists that the surgical procedure will require a transfusion. This rule generally applies to larger operative cases, such as total hip or knee arthroplasty.

4. List criteria for donation of blood for autologous transfusion.
- No history of seizures since infancy
- No history of severe respiratory disease, including severe asthma
- No history of cardiovascular disease
- Patient age between 12 and 75 years
- Minimum hemoglobin (Hgb) of 11 gm/dl and hematocrit (Hct) of 34%
- No active infection
- If the patient's weight is less than 100 lb, the amount donated will be less than 1 unit and is calculated according to weight.

5. What are the advantages and disadvantages of autologous blood donation?
One clear advantage of preoperative autologous blood donation is significant reduction of the possibility of transfusion reaction. In general, patients find this approach acceptable because the risk of transferring infection (e.g., HIV, hepatitis) is virtually eliminated. Some patients may have an elevated sense that they are participating in their own care by donating blood.

The disadvantages are that the patient must meet the criteria in question 4 and the time investment to go to the draw site and give blood. If the operative dates are changed or cancelled, the blood may expire and be wasted. Blood will also be wasted if it is unused in surgery. Because of donating multiple units of blood, the patient may have a low Hgb and Hct preoperatively.

6. **List basic orthopedic preoperative nursing interventions.**
   - Administer preoperative antibiotics, antianxiety agents, or other medications as ordered.
   - Perform thorough hand washing and maintain aseptic technique when indicated.
   - Assess and educate the patient about adequate nutrition.
   - Maintain adequate preoperative nutritional status.
   - Assess patient anxiety level and implement anxiety reduction techniques.
   - Educate the patient about the operative procedure and planned postoperative course.
   - Begin postoperative teaching, including cough, deep breathing, and use of crutches or walker.
   - Demonstrate and discuss possible postoperative drains, tubes, intravenous (IV) lines, and immobilization.
   - Monitor intake and output, lab work, dietary intake, and vital signs.
   - Initiate and maintain IV site as ordered.
   - Perform a physical assessment and reassess as indicated.

7. **What are the major potential complications of anesthesia administration?**
   - Malignant hyperthermia
   - Hypothermia
   - Aspiration
   - Cardiac arrest, infarction, or ischemia
   - Cardiac arrhythmias
   - Hypovolemia and shock
   - Pseudocholinesterase deficiency, causing prolonged neuromuscular blockage

8. **List interventions in the operating room that decrease the risk of infection.**
   - Proper surgical attire
   - Special airflow and filtration systems
   - Universal precautions and aseptic technique
   - Proper hand washing and surgical hand scrub
   - Operative site preparation techniques
   - Management and control of traffic patterns within the operating room

9. **What potential problems can result from patient positioning during surgery?**
   One of the potential complications due to patient positioning is nerve injury. From prolonged pressure, inadequate padding, and prolonged or excessive stretch on a nerve the patient can develop pain, numbness, tingling, weakness, or paralysis of the area innervated by the affected nerve. Pressure ulcers and clot formation are other potential complications of inadequate or improper patient positioning in the operating room.

10. **Discuss basic nursing considerations during recovery from anesthesia.**
    Whether the patient recovers in the postanesthesia care unit or intensive care unit, some of the major nursing care considerations remain the same:

- Monitor the patient's level of consciousness, immobilization devices, vital signs, operative site, tubes, catheters, IV lines, and drains.
- Monitor the patient's temperature, and keep the patient warm because hypothermia is common after anesthesia.
- Assess pain and provide appropriate management.
- Perform neurovascular assessments.
- Because patients frequently develop nausea and vomiting after anesthesia administration, the nurse should treat nausea and vomiting pharmacologically, provide comfort measures, and position the patient to prevent aspiration.
- Monitor the patient's intake and output, and assess for urinary retention.
- Provide adequate oxygenation.
- Monitor the patient for laryngospasm, bronchospasm, airway obstruction, and respiratory depression.

11. What nursing care should be delivered to the postoperative patient after arrival at the inpatient unit?
- Perform physical assessment, including neurovascular checks.
- Assess and manage pain.
- Provide cast care, pin care, and wound care, and monitor for infection.
- Ensure that proper immobilization methods are used.
- Assist with ambulation, provide range-of-motion exercises, or ensure that physical therapy is started.
- Encourage incentive spirometry and cough/deep-breathing exercises.
- Monitor intake and output and bowel elimination.

12. After outpatient surgery, when is it safe to discharge the patient home?
Patients should be able to ambulate (if not contraindicated) and should be accompanied by someone to assist them in getting home. Written discharge instructions should be given and understood. Pain should be adequately managed with oral medications only, and the patient should not have had any IV sedation or pain medications within the previous hour. The patient should also have minimal-to-no nausea or vomiting and be able to tolerate sipping liquids.

13. What should general outpatient discharge instructions include?
- Instructions about cast care, splint care, wound care, and/or pin care
- Information to assess for infection, wound care, and dressing changes
- Instructions for when to contact the surgeon (e.g., infection, neurovascular compromise)
- Use of medications, including antibiotics, pain medications, and anti-inflammatory drugs
- Activity instructions and restrictions

14. What are the usual causes of carpal tunnel syndrome (CTS)?
CTS is due to compression of the median nerve at the wrist. Compression at the carpal tunnel can result from trauma such as a fractured wrist or inflammation due to repetitive wrist motion (e.g., computer operator or assembly line worker). Pregnancy or birth control pill usage can cause swelling and compression of the median nerve. In addition, soft tissue masses, rheumatoid disease, metabolic disorders, or even the patient's anatomy can produce CTS.

15. What are the typical signs and symptoms of CTS?

The median nerve and flexor tendons pass through the carpal tunnel at the wrist surrounded by the carpal bones, transverse carpal ligament, and flexor retinaculum. The patient with CTS typically complains of pain and/or numbness and tingling along the distribution of the median nerve into the first, second, and third fingers and half of the fourth finger. Patients may give a history of being awakened by symptoms at night, which is usually caused by sleeping with the wrist flexed, exacerbating CTS. Weakness and atrophy of the thenar muscles may be present. Patients usually have positive Phalen's and Tinel's signs at the wrist. In addition, some providers report reproduction of symptoms with an Allen's test at the affected wrist. Electromyography and nerve conduction studies may be ordered to confirm the diagnosis, especially if the clinical picture is ambiguous or if surgical intervention is being considered.

16. What is the usual nonoperative treatment for CTS?

Usual treatment for CTS begins with splinting of the affected wrist at night to prevent prolonged flexion at the wrist during sleep, which may exacerbate the symptoms. In addition, anti-inflammatory medications are helpful. If the patient has symptoms during the daytime, it may also be advisable to wear the splints during the daytime hours as well. Control of any disease process that may contribute to or exacerbate CTS is important. Some providers may choose to inject the carpal tunnel with a steroid medication to obtain some relief of the symptoms.

17. When is surgical intervention indicated for CTS?

When conservative treatment has failed, surgical intervention for carpal tunnel release is considered.

18. How is carpal tunnel release performed?

Carpal tunnel release is usually an outpatient procedure and can be performed both as an open procedure and by endoscopy. During the open procedure, the surgeon makes an incision at the volar surface of the hand/wrist approximately 1.5–2 inches in length. During the endoscopic procedure, an endoscope is introduced into the wrist through a small incision. During both procedures, the transverse carpal ligament and the flexor retinaculum are released, relieving the compression on the median nerve.

19. What is the nurse's role in caring for patients with CTS?

As always, education is a key role. The nurse should educate the patient about the proper fit and wear of the carpal tunnel splint as well as about medication usage. Explanation of what to expect in the postoperative period decreases patient anxiety. The surgeon usually discusses the postoperative protocol with the patient, and the nurse can help to answer any questions that the patient may have. While caring for the patient in the postoperative period, the nurse should assess neurovascular and motor function of the hand and medicate the patient appropriately for pain. Usually the carpal tunnel release is performed on an outpatient basis; thus, the nurse should educate the patient before discharge about signs and symptoms of postoperative infection. The patient should be instructed to call the surgeon's office if circulatory problems develop, including coolness of the skin and skin color changes or signs of infection, such as fever, chills, or wound drainage. In addition, the patient should be instructed to keep the surgical dressing dry and to elevate the hand to reduce swelling. Active range of motion of the fingers should be encouraged.

20. Describe the usual course of recovery after carpal tunnel release.

Postoperative protocols vary from surgeon to surgeon, but the patient can expect to return to full activities without restrictions in approximately 4 weeks. Patients usually have a bulky dressing and/or wrist splint in place for a few days. Sutures are removed in 1–2 weeks. Some patients may enter into occupational therapy for range-of-motion exercises.

21. What is a mallet finger?

A mallet finger is an extensor mechanism injury to the distal interphalangeal (DIP) joint of a finger, usually due to jamming or spraining the finger. This disorder involves rupture of the extensor tendon or avulsion of the bony insertion of the extensor tendon. Either mechanism leads to an inability to actively extend the DIP joint of the involved finger (also called an extensor lag).

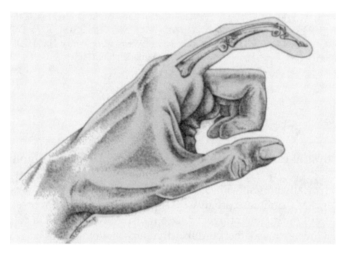

Mallet finger. The extensor tendon is usually torn near its insertion. (From Mellion MB: Office Sports Medicine, 2nd ed. Philadelphia, Hanley & Belfus, 1996, with permission.)

22. How is a mallet finger typically treated?

A mallet finger injury is initially treated with splinting of the injured DIP joint in extension for 6 weeks to allow the extensor mechanism to heal. The injured DIP joint should not be allowed to flex, because flexion tears the healing that is taking place. If the patient continues to have an extensor lag after the 6 weeks of splinting, surgical repair of the ruptured tendon is considered. Surgical repair is not absolutely necessary. Some patients choose not to have surgical repair because extensor lag at the DIP joint is mostly a cosmetic deformity and usually does not cause difficulty with performing activities of daily living (ADLs).

23. What complications of mallet finger should the nurse discuss with the patient?
- DIP instability
- Inadequate healing of the tendon rupture or avulsion fracture
- Continued extensor lag after splinting
- Potential difficulty with ADLs
- Potential postsurgical infection

24. How does Dupuytren's contracture develop?

Dupuytren's contracture develops when the palmar fascia, usually of both hands, becomes progressively thicker and more fibrotic. Palmar fibrosis consists primarily of collagen and connective tissue, which develop into a cordlike organization. These cords eventually shrink, causing contractures of the fingers as they are attached to soft tissue skin, tendons, fascia, and periosteum.

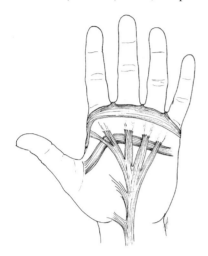

The normal parts of the palmar fascia that become diseased. (From McFarlane RM, Ross DC: Dupuytren's disease. In Weinzweig J (ed): Hand and Wrist Surgery Secrets, Philadelphia, Hanley & Belfus, 2000, with permission.)

25. What physical exam findings are typically associated with Dupuytren's contracture?

Patients typically present with decreased range of motion, which advances to flexion contractures as the disease progresses. A patient may have skin breakdown in the flexion creases of the affected fingers due to moisture collection. On palpation of the palmar fascia, the nurse may feel cordlike structures and/or nodules.

26. How is Dupuytren's contracture treated surgically?

The surgical intervention for Dupuytren's contracture involves palmar fascia resection. The patient participates in physical or occupational therapy after being immobilized for approximately 1 week.

27. What is the best treatment of a quadriceps or patellar tendon rupture?

For complete rupture to either structure, early surgical repair is indicated. If the patient has only a partial tear of the quadriceps tendon, extension bracing of the knee for 4 weeks is attempted.

28. What is the anterior cruciate ligament (ACL)? How is it injured?

The ACL and the posterior cruciate ligament (PCL) are the primary rotary stabilizers of the knee. Injury to the ACL is much more common. It prevents anterior translation of the tibia on the femur. The most common mechanism of ACL injury includes noncontact deceleration, such as suddenly stopping or pivoting, with a valgus force applied to an externally rotated leg. The athlete often describes a pop with the knee giving way, along with immediate pain and swelling. This initial presentation is typically followed by profound disability with painful or guarded range of motion and an inability to ambulate. Jumping and "cutting" sports place the ACL at risk.

29. Describe the treatment for acute ACL tear.
Stabilization of the knee by a splint or supportive dressing and application of ice are important general measures. Crutches are usually recommended with weight bearing as tolerated. General range of motion is encouraged as soon as comfort allows. Quadriceps-strengthening exercises are begun to prevent quadriceps atrophy. Follow-up is required in 10–14 days for a more thorough exam.

30. How is an ACL tear diagnosed?
An acute ACL tear is often difficult to differentiate from other ligamentous and meniscal injuries. Provocative tests to isolate the ACL can be difficult to perform in a patient with pain and muscle spasm. After 7–10 days pain and spasm subside, and physical exam directed at assessing the ACL can be much more informative. Isolated assessment of the ligamentous structure is performed by stabilizing the femur with one hand and using the other hand to apply anterior distraction force to the tibia (Lachman test). The goal is to evaluate any tibial displacement and compare with the uninvolved knee. Excessive anterior displacement with a soft end-point usually indicates ACL rupture. Plain radiographs are often unremarkable in the acute, isolated ACL tear. Magnetic resonance imaging is the best test for ACL assessment. It is also helpful in identifying fractures, collateral ligament injury, and meniscal tears.

31. Must a torn ACL be repaired?
No. Physiologically young, active patients who wish to continue participation in high-demand activity require reconstruction. Many patients who make fewer demands on the knee and have no associated injuries and mild symptoms may be treated nonoperatively. Younger patients are usually encouraged to undergo reconstruction, because even occasional instability may result in significant damage to articular surfaces and menisci.

32. How is the ACL repaired?
ACL reconstruction involves replacement of the torn ligament with a tendon allograft from the patellar tendon or hamstring tendons. This typically outpatient procedure is performed with an arthroscope.

33. Discuss the role of physical therapy in recovery from ACL rupture.
In both reconstructed and nonreconstructed knees, therapy involves hamstring- and quadriceps-strengthening exercises along with knee range of motion. Physical therapy plays a crucial role in regaining functional mobility after ACL rupture and reconstruction. The patient should know that surgery is only part of the treatment regimen and that participation in physical therapy is critical to obtaining the best outcome.

34. What causes a torn meniscus?
The menisci are c-shaped cartilage structures that sit on the medial and lateral tibial plateau. Sports injuries are a common cause of meniscus tears. Often rotational stress is applied to the knee while the foot is in a fixed position on the ground. Tears of the meniscus can also be due to degeneration, repetitive stress of kneeling and squatting, or direct injuries to the knee.

35. What are the signs and symptoms of a meniscus tear?
Patients with a torn meniscus may have popping, clicking, giving way, or even locking of the affected knee. Swelling and pain may be present. On examination, pa-

tients usually have pain at the knee with rotatory stress of the lower leg with the knee flexed. They may have pain at the injured knee with end-range flexion. Pain on palpation along the joint line and positive McMurray and Apley grind tests are also indicative of a meniscus tear.

36. Is one meniscus torn more frequently than the other?
The lateral meniscus is less fixed in place than the medial meniscus. Thus the medial meniscus is torn more often.

37. What is a meniscectomy?
Meniscectomy is a procedure usually done arthroscopically on an outpatient basis to remove part of the injured meniscus.

38. Does the meniscus ever heal itself without meniscectomy?
Yes. Tears of the outer one-third of the meniscus have the ability to heal spontaneously because of the available blood supply. Large tears of the outer third of the meniscus that do not heal may require arthroscopic repair. The avascularity of the inner two-thirds of the meniscus significantly decreases the ability to heal spontaneously.

39. When is the patient expected to return to full function after arthroscopic meniscectomy?
After uncomplicated arthroscopic meniscectomy, most patients can expect to return to full activities at approximately 4–6 weeks postoperatively. After the procedure patients are typically allowed to bear weight as tolerated within a day or two after surgery. Among the keys to speedy recovery are physical therapy and a structured home exercise program. Patients may need pain medications for only a day or two.

40. What are the potential outcomes if a torn meniscus is not addressed surgically?
Not all meniscus tears need to be addressed surgically. However, a symptomatic tear may lead to chronic synovitis and swelling of the knee due to irritation of the synovial membrane. In addition, there is the potential for degeneration of the articular cartilage.

41. Define chondromalacia patellae.
Chondromalacia patellae refers to softening and degeneration of the patellar cartilage. This condition can result from acute knee injury, chronic biomechanical stress to the patella, knee immobilization, multiple intra-articular steroid injections, or various disease processes.

42. Describe conservative treatment for chondromalacia patellae.
Nonoperative treatment, the usual approach to chondromalacia patellae, typically involves physical therapy and home exercises for quadriceps strengthening. Ice and nonsteroidal anti-inflammatory drugs (NSAIDs) may provide pain relief after activity. The patient may benefit from a knee brace such as a neoprene knee sleeve with patella stabilization. The nurse should reinforce the fact that the patient should not squat or perform activities in which the knee will be placed into flexion greater than 90°. Such activities increase mechanical stress on the patellar cartilage.

43. If conservative treatment fails to resolve the pain from chondromalacia patellae, what can be done surgically?

The surgeon can perform a variety of procedures to address chondromalacia patellae, but they are attempted only if conservative treatment has failed. Examples include autologous chondrocyte transplant, shaving the patella cartilage arthroscopically, release of the lateral retinaculum to align the patella, elevating the tibial tuberosity to decrease the mechanical force at the patellofemoral joint, and patellectomy.

44. How is rupture of an Achilles tendon treated?

Patients with an incomplete Achilles tendon rupture can be treated conservatively with a heel cup, ice, and NSAIDs. They may benefit from the use of crutches or a cane to assist with ambulation. Complete rupture of the Achilles tendon can be treated conservatively with avoidance of weight bearing and casting in plantar flexion. The ankle is gradually brought into neutral position with multiple recasting over a period of weeks, followed by progressive stretching.

Surgical intervention is an option for a complete Achilles tendon rupture, especially if the tendon ends have retracted or if the patient is a competitive athlete. After surgical repair, the patient is treated with casting of the lower extremity, followed by progressive stretching.

45. What are the indications for arthroplasty?

Arthroplasty is joint surgery that includes resection, reconstruction, and partial or total joint replacement. One of the primary indications for arthroplasty is a painful joint with failure of conservative treatment. The patient with a painful joint, such as the knee, shoulder, or hip, may have a significant inability to perform ADLs. Other reasons to perform arthroplasty include correction of deformities and maintaining or improving range of motion at a joint. Arthroplasty is performed on patients with varying conditions, including fractures, rheumatoid and osteoarthritis, avascular necrosis, and congenital deformities. Absolute and relative contraindications for joint replacement include inability to perform the necessary rehabilitation postoperatively, active or past joint infection, and neuropathic arthropathy.

46. Are the hips and knees the only joints that can undergo arthroplasty?

No. In addition to the hips and knees, arthroplasty can be performed on the joints at the fingers, wrists, shoulders, ankles, and elbows. Spine surgery for intervertebral disc replacement is performed in a few medical centers.

47. What is the difference between cemented and noncemented prostheses?

The noncemented prosthesis is held in place by ingrowth of bone into the rough or porous surface of the prosthetic shaft. The patient with a noncemented prosthesis must avoid full weight bearing until the prosthesis is fixed in place with new bone growth, which may take as long as 6 weeks. The cemented prosthesis allows relatively fast fixation with polymethyl methacrylate, which cements the prosthesis to the bone and allows the patient to bear weight when able. Although patients with a cemented prosthesis are able to bear weight early after surgery, they typically use a walker until they regain muscle strength and coordination. Patients with poor bone stock, usually the elderly with osteoporosis, should have a cemented prosthesis. In patients who are more active and younger with good bone stock, a noncemented prosthesis is implanted.

48. Summarize the postoperative nursing care of patients after total hip arthroplasty (THA).

The nurse can assist and remind the patient to avoid excessive abduction, rotation, and flexion, which may lead to dislocation of the prosthesis. The patient can use an abduction pillow and an elevated toilet seat. Skin care, effective pain management, sleep, and rest are essential components of postoperative care. The surgeon may order compression stockings. The nurse should perform the usual neurologic, cardiovascular, gastrointestinal, pulmonary, and urinary assessments. Physical assessments must encompass identification of alterations, including pulmonary edema, pulmonary emboli, heart failure, infection, deep vein thrombosis, and altered mental status. Incentive spirometry, patient mobilization, and wound care must be addressed. Patient teaching should be reinforced. Family education and assistance in care should be encouraged. Discharge planning should be developed in conjunction with the physical therapist, surgeon, home care provider, case manager, and a rehabilitation facility, if applicable. Lab values, including complete blood count, prothrombin/partial thromboplastin time, and international normalized ratio (INR) must be monitored

49. Do all patients require a stay at a rehabilitation facility after THA?

No. Many patients are able to recover at home with home care and physical therapy visits if they have the family support as well as physical and mental capacity.

50. What should be the focus of preoperative nursing care for patients undergoing THA?

Education is a key component in preoperative nursing care aimed at decreasing adverse outcomes. Ensure that the patient has the necessary preoperative medical clearance. The nurse can provide education about incentive spirometry. Discussion of home modification for postoperative recovery should address the installation of ramps or rails. All throw rugs should be removed.

51. Summarize the nursing considerations for the various surgical approaches to THA.

The three surgical approaches to hip replacement are the transtrochanteric (direct lateral), anterolateral, and posterolateral approach. Surgeons rarely use the transtrochanteric (direct lateral) approach to THA; the anterolateral and posterolateral approaches are far more common and preferred. The patient undergoing an anterolateral approach should avoid external rotation, extension, and active abduction of the hip. The patient who has undergone a posterolateral approach should avoid flexion of the hip past 90°, internal rotation, and adduction of the leg, especially past midline.

52. Describe the postoperative care of patients who undergo total knee arthroplasty (TKA).

Cryocuff, pain management, continuous passive motion (CPM), urinary output, diet of clear liquids that progresses as tolerated, pain management, mobilization, skin and wound care, incentive spirometry, and physical therapy are crucial components. The nurse also should monitor any IV lines and wound drains.

53. Why would an arthroplasty need revision?

One of the primary reasons for revision of an arthroplasty is hardware failure. Other reasons include joint stiffness and loosening of the hardware at the joint.

54. Define osteotomy.
An osteotomy is a procedure used to correct the angle of a particular bone. An osteotomy can be performed either by removing a wedge of bone with a bone saw or by inserting a bone wedge into a cut made through the bone.

55. When is an osteotomy performed?
The angle correction obtained from an osteotomy is beneficial in treating many orthopedic problems. One application for an osteotomy is treatment of pain from osteoarthritis. The proximal tibial osteotomy is used primarily in younger patients with significant osteoarthritis of the knee. This procedure realigns the knee angle, allowing the patient to delay TKA. Another application of osteotomy is realignment of a deformed or misshapen bone. This procedure may be useful in correcting an angulated fracture that has healed with a malunion or a hallux valgus deformity (bunion) of the great toe.

56. What are the common reasons for amputation?
Traumatic amputation is the most common reason for upper extremity amputations, whereas the most common reason for amputations overall is ischemia due to peripheral vascular disease. Other indications for amputation include severe frostbite or burns, gangrene, malignancy, and necrosis.

57. Do all amputees experience phantom limb pain?
No. About 60–85% of amputees experience phantom limb pain, which is a sensation of aching or itching in the amputated limb. This sensation is reported to diminish over time. Severe pain occurs only in a small percentage of patients. Both phantom limb sensation and pain may occur immediately postoperatively. The patient can also have a delayed onset of pain up to 3 months or an onset of sensation up to several months after amputation. Several studies support the use of epidural analgesia 24–48 hours before amputation to reduce the incidence of phantom limb pain and suggest that postoperative efforts alone have no effect.

58. Summarize the major postoperative nursing concerns in caring for the patient who has had an amputation.
- Pain management after amputation is a major nursing concern. The nurse must address the pain from the stump, any pain from associated trauma, and phantom limb pain.
- Good skin care is always a nursing concern. Impaired mobility may contribute to impaired skin integrity. The nurse should monitor the patient for evidence of infection or bleeding.
- The hip is a common site for development of a flexion contracture. This complication can be avoided after amputation with a few nursing interventions. The patient should avoid lying in bed with the stump elevated as well as sitting with the stump flexed at the hip for extended periods. The patient should lie prone for approximately half an hour up to 4 times per day.
- Elastic or compression bandages can assist with edema control. The surgeon may apply a plaster cast to the stump immediately after surgery to assist with edema control.
- The nurse needs to be attentive to the patient's underlying medical problems, such as diabetes, as well as new traumatic injuries, if present.
- Last, but not least, the patient may need a great deal of assistance in coping with the loss.

59. How is the stump shaped for prosthetic fitting?
The stump is shaped to allow prosthetic fitting through the use of shrinker or compression bandages,

60. How might the nurse's approach to patients with traumatic amputation differ from the approach to patients with elective amputation?
Although physically the end state is essentially the same with traumatic and elective amputation, there are some clear differences in the nurse's approach to the patient and family. The patient with a traumatic amputation may have additional acute traumatic injuries that complicate care. The patient with an elective amputation usually has an associated chronic disease, such as diabetes, that needs additional attention. Elective amputation offers the opportunity for the nurse to deliver solid teaching. In addition, the elective patient may have an adequate amount of time before surgery to begin strengthening for the postoperative period as well as to work through issues related to body image disturbance.

61. Discuss patient education after a lower extremity amputation.
The nurse should be sure to educate the patient about phantom limb pain and phantom limb sensation. The patient should be taught to massage the end of the stump to decrease or prevent scar tissue formation as well as to desensitize the stump. Inspect the stump daily for any signs of infection or irritation. The stump and any shrinker or compression wraps must be washed daily. Meticulous foot care should be taught or reviewed with the patient, especially if he or she has diabetes or peripheral vascular disease. The patient should also be encouraged to use the over-bed trapeze to move instead of pushing with the remaining foot.

62. What is the purpose of arthrodesis surgery?
Arthrodesis is a surgical procedure that induces bony growth across a joint, leading to a fused joint. An arthrodesis can also occur spontaneously as a result of an infected joint. The main reasons for patients to undergo an arthrodesis are to eliminate movement at a painful joint and to produce stability at an unstable joint. Indications for arthrodesis of a joint include avascular necrosis, arthritis, neuropathic joint, infection, and failure of arthroplasty.

63. On which joints can an arthrodesis be performed?
An arthrodesis can be performed on almost any joint. Common sites include the spine, wrist, knee, ankle, toes, elbow, shoulder, and hip.

64. How is the arthrodesis performed?
No matter which joint is involved, the essence of the procedure remains the same. The articular cartilage is removed from the joint ends to be fused. The bone ends are placed together, and the joint is placed in the appropriate position for fusion. Typically, bone graft is used in addition to internal or external fixation.

65. Summarize the nursing assessment of patients who have had spine surgery.
- The nurse should know the patient's preoperative level of function and disability. The assessment should be performed approximately every 2-4 hours for the first 48 hours after surgery and compared with the preoperative assessment.

- The patient's level of pain should be assessed and addressed. The nurse should distinguish between operative pain and the usual pain that the patient has experienced in the back and/or legs.
- The operative site is monitored for drainage and evidence of infection.
- Movement and strength of the extremities are assessed and compared with preoperative findings.
- The nurse should also assess sensation along dermatomes as well as deep tendon reflexes.

66. Should the nurse be concerned if a patient continues to have symptoms of pain, numbness, tingling, and/or weakness in the postoperative period?

No. The nurse should continue to assess the patient for new or worsening pain, numbness, tingling, and muscle weakness and notify the surgeon if they occur. The patient's usual symptoms may take a few weeks to a few months to dissipate. The nurse should notify the surgeon if the patient develops postoperative bowel or bladder dysfunction.

67. When is surgical intervention indicated for an ankle sprain?

Surgical intervention is considered for a grade III ankle sprain (complete ligament rupture) if the ankle is severely unstable. Ligament reconstruction can be considered when repetitive sprains have led to ligament laxity and chronic instability.

68. Define osteochondritis dissecans (OCD).

Osteochondritis refers to a group of lesions to the osteochondral portion of bones where crushing, pulling, or splitting (dissecans) has occurred. OCD usually results from repetitive microtrauma and injury to arterioles and capillaries, leading to avascular necrosis. The avascular section of bone may fracture and/or detach, causing symptoms of locking or catching at the joint. OCD typically occurs in the medial femoral condyle; however, it can also occur at the talar dome or capitellum.

69. When is surgical intervention considered for OCD?

Surgical intervention is usually indicated to address a large or unstable OCD lesion. The procedure involves either arthroscopic removal or stabilization of the lesion with screws or wires. Rest, activity reduction, or immobilization is the usual course of conservative treatment if the OCD lesion is not loose or is too small to fix surgically. A stable lesion may also be addressed arthroscopically by drilling into the core of the lesion in an attempt to stimulate healing.

70. Explain open reduction and internal fixation (ORIF) of a fracture.

ORIF is exactly what the name implies. The fracture is reduced through an open surgical incision. Reduction is followed by internal fixation to stabilize the fracture.

71. What methods are commonly used for internal fixation?

- Kirschner wires (K-wires) and pins
- Metal plates
- Various screws (e.g., cancellous or cortical, self-tapping, fully or partially threaded)
- Intramedullary rod or nail
- Nail and sliding screw-plate devices (fixed nail/plate, sliding nail/plate, and sliding screw plate)

72. When is ORIF of a fracture indicated?
- Nonunion of a fracture
- In conjunction with reattachment of an amputated body part
- Displaced epiphyseal or intra-articular fractures
- Significant tendon or ligament avulsion fractures
- Inability to reduce or maintain closed reduction of a fracture
- Pathologic fractures

73. List the contraindications to ORIF.
- Overall poor surgical candidate (not medically cleared)
- Poor bone stock (e.g., osteoporosis)
- Fracture fragments too small to secure with fixation methods
- Osteomyelitis or other infection
- Burns or other soft tissue problems at the proposed operative site

74. What are the advantages to ORIF of a fracture?
The clear advantage to ORIF is early mobilization due to fracture stabilization. In addition, the bony anatomy is restored to a relatively normal shape, contributing to cosmetic and functional benefits.

75. What are the purposes for performing a bone graft?
A bone graft is a surgical procedure in which additional bony material is used to fill a bony void, replace missing bone and add stability, or stimulate bone growth at a fracture or arthrodesis site.

76. What are the two types of bone graft material?
Bone graft material is either autograft or allograft. **Autograft** bone graft is taken from the patient's bone stock—frequently from the iliac crest. **Allograft** bone graft is obtained from another human, usually a cadaver.

77. What is the most common form of shoulder dislocation?
More than 95% of all shoulder dislocations are anterior to the glenoid cavity of the scapula. This injury is usually caused by an indirect force applied to the upper extremity with a combination of external rotation, abduction, and hyperextension of the shoulder. An anterior blow to the shoulder is a less common cause. A force applied indirectly to the arm with the shoulder internally rotated, adducted, and flexed causes posterior dislocations. Seizures, electrocutions, and lightening strikes are also associated with posterior dislocations of the shoulder.

78. What factors increase the risk of shoulder dislocation?
Shoulder instability encompasses both subluxation and dislocation. Repetitive overhead activities and extremes of external rotation stretch the anterior joint capsule and may lead to instability. Swimming, throwing, and high-contact/high-velocity sports increase the risk of shoulder instability and dislocation. Generalized ligamentous laxity may create serious performance problems in throwing, swimming, and paddle sports. The patient's age at initial dislocation dramatically affects risk of subsequent dislocations, with a recurrence rate more than 50% in patients aged 12–22 years. Subtle primary instability of the shoulder may cause secondary impingement of the rotator cuff and lead to rotator cuff tear.

79. Describe the signs and symptoms of an anterior shoulder dislocation.
This condition is acutely painful. The patient may be immobilized by pain and unable to move the shoulder. The affected shoulder may have a sulcus below the acromion, and the patient may hold the arm in an internally rotated position with the elbow flexed and supported by the contralateral arm.

80. What injuries are most often associated with anterior shoulder dislocation?
The axillary nerve and radial artery can become impinged, requiring prompt neurovascular assessment of distal pulses and sensation over the deltoid muscle (axillary patch). Bony injury to the anterior glenoid rim is strongly associated with recurrence of dislocation. Rotator cuff tear is more common in people over 40 years of age. Fractures of the humeral head that are significantly displaced may be a contraindication to attempts at closed reduction. Repeated dislocations may result in a depression fracture of the posterolateral humeral head, called a Hill-Sachs lesion.

81. Summarize important nursing considerations after shoulder reduction.
Reassess the neurovascular status and rotator cuff strength. Postreduction axillary radiographs are the best way to evaluate success of reduction. Immobilization in a sling and swathe is required only until pain improves and for no more than 3 weeks. Patients over 40 should be immobilized no more than 10 days because they have a lower incidence of recurrence and increased risk of stiffness from prolonged immobilization. Extremes of shoulder abduction and external rotation should be avoided for 6 weeks. Rotator cuff-strengthening exercises help maintain dynamic stability. With appropriate therapy, the patient should regain full pain-free range of motion.

82. Define impingement syndrome. How does it contribute to rotator cuff tear?
Impingement syndrome is an overuse injury caused by chronic overload of the muscles of the rotator cuff (supraspinatus, infraspinatus, teres minor, and subscapularis). This overload leads to rotator cuff tendinitis and inflammation of the subacromial bursa, which contribute to impingement of the cuff muscles and tendons between the acromion and humeral head, causing pain with overhead arm motion. Swelling and repeated microtrauma of the cuff muscles reduce the stability of the shoulder and lead to further impingement and rupture of the rotator cuff.

83. Which muscles are most commonly torn?
The supraspinatus and infraspinatus muscle-tendon complexes are most commonly torn. Rotator cuff tears are uncommon in people under 40. Repetitive overhead use and previous trauma increase the risk of cuff tear.

84. Describe the signs and symptoms of a rotator cuff tear.
Pain and weakness are seen through the arc of 80°–120° of abduction or with internal rotation and the arm abducted at 90°. Pain is produced as the inflamed structures are impinged between the acromion and the head of the humerus. Chronic overuse presents with gradual onset of pain, nocturnal pain, and pain with overhead activity. Massive cuff tear can result in an inability to externally rotate or abduct the arm.

85. What modalities are most helpful in diagnosing shoulder pathology?
Plain radiographs may show calcification of the tendons of the rotator cuff, subacromial osteophytes, and position of the humeral head. Magnetic resonance imaging

is most helpful in identifying muscle and tendon tears. An arthrogram can help identify tears of the labrum from its bony attachment on the glenoid rim.

86. How is a rotator cuff tear treated?

Incomplete tears are treated with rest, NSAIDs, and supervised rehabilitation. Subacromial injection with lidocaine and a corticosteroid may provide temporary pain relief and help distinguish impingement from cuff tear (pain and strength remain unchanged after injection). Complete tears usually require surgical intervention. Early operative repair provides the best chance of functional recovery. Arthroscopy alone or an arthroscopy-assisted procedure aid in direct examination and debridement of the cuff. Subacromial debridement and resection of the distal clavicle may also be performed to increase the subacromial space and to prevent recurrence. Large tears often require an open surgical procedure and several months of intense rehabilitation.

87. Discuss the role of physical therapy in recovery from a rotator cuff tear.

Physical therapy plays an important role in the active treatment of partial rotator cuff tears and a more significant role in the postoperative recovery of surgically repaired tears. After operative repair, the patient is usually required to remain in a specialized sling for up to 6 weeks with daily removal for gentle passive range-of-motion exercises. Active shoulder range-of-motion exercises can begin after the repair has begun to heal. Several months are required to regain full active range of motion. These exercises are important to the overall success of the surgical repair of complete rotator cuff tears. Partial tears of the rotator cuff are treated with daily isometric toning exercises of shoulder abduction and external rotation. These exercises are typically performed with low tension and high repetition, using a large rubber band.

88. Describe adhesive capsulitis.

Patients can develop adhesive capsulitis after immobilization of the shoulder. The patient may be immobilized as part of the treatment after an injury such as a fracture, dislocation, or rotator cuff tear. The patient may also immobilize himself or herself because of pain due to arthritis or subacromial bursitis. The patient gradually develops stiffness and decreasing range of motion at the glenohumoral joint due to fibrosis of the joint capsule. Adhesive capsulitis has an increased incidence in patients with diabetes mellitus and people over 50 years of age.

89. Is adhesive capsulitis treated surgically?

Adhesive capsulitis can be treated with manipulation under anesthesia or even by releasing the adhesions, if conservative treatment fails to improve range of motion. Initial treatment usually includes physical therapy, home stretching, moist heat, steroid injections into the shoulder, NSAIDs, and pain medications.

BIBLIOGRAPHY

1. Apley AG, Solomon L: Concise System of Orthopedics and Fractures, 2nd ed. London, Reed Educational and Professional Publishing, 1996.
2. Campbell WC: Campbell's Operative Orthopaedics, 9th ed. St. Louis, Mosby, 1992.
3. Huether S, McCance K: Understanding Pathophysiology, 2nd ed. St. Louis, Mosby, 2000.
4. Hulstyn MJ, Paddale PD: Shoulder injuries in the athlete. Clin Sports Med 16:663–679. 1997.
5. Larson RL, Taillon M: Anterior cruciate ligament insufficiency: Principles of treatment. J Am Acad of Orthop Surg 2:26–35. 1994.

6. Lewis SM, Heitkemper MM, Dirksen SR: Medical Surgical Nursing: Assessment and Management of Clinical Problems, 5th ed. St. Louis, Mosby, 2000.

7. Maher AB, Salmond SW, Pellino TA: Orthopaedic Nursing, 3rd ed. Philadelphia, W.B. Saunders, 2002.

8. Schoen DC: NAON Core Curriculum for Orthopaedic Nursing, 4th ed. Pittman, NJ, Anthony J. Jannetti, 2001.

9. Wen DY: Current concepts in the treatment of anterior shoulder dislocations. Am J Emerg Med 17:401–407, 1999.

14. IMMOBILIZATION

Andrea Dodge Ackermann, MS, RN, CCRN

1. What is the purpose of orthopedic immobilization?

The purposes of orthopedic immobilization are to secure, correct, align, promote healing, relieve pain, and prevent injury to alterations in the musculoskeletal system. Immobilization is used to treat injuries such as sprains, strains, fractures, soft tissue injuries, congenital abnormalities, and dislocations.

2. What types of immobilization are available for orthopedic alterations?

The types of immobilization are traction, casts, braces, splints, and external fixation.

3. Define traction.

Traction is the application of a pulling force, either directly or indirectly, to areas of the body in order to treat alterations to the bones.

4. When is traction used?

It is used to treat fractures for reduction, immobilization, and alignment; to relieve muscle spasms and pain; to treat dislocated joints; to overcome deformities; to prevent soft tissue damage; to promote rest; and to maintain position of the injured area.

5. What are the mechanical components of traction?

Traction is applied using one or more components to provide the proper mechanical forces needed to optimize the outcome. The components of traction include countertraction, weights, angles, and pulleys. Countertraction is a pulling force in the opposite direction provided by body weight, elevation of the bed, or weights. It provides a point from which the traction can pull. Weights are attached to a rope or weight holder. The physician orders the amount of weight needed for the individual patient. The weight determines the pulling force. The weights must hang freely. Angles determine the line of pull of the traction along the axis of the bone. The physician determines the angles used. Pulleys are attached to the bed frame and are used to adjust the amount of pull exerted on the affected area. Multiple pulleys increase the amount of pull exerted by the weights.

6. How is traction classified?

There are three basic types of traction: skin traction, skeletal traction, and manual traction.

7. How is skin traction maintained? Why is it used?

Skin traction is maintained by applying the force directly to the patient's skin and soft tissue. It is generally used to provide alignment and immobility before surgery; short-term traction; intermittent traction; relief of muscle spasms; and assistance in decreasing muscle contraction.

8. What types of skin traction are used?

Many types of skin traction exist in clinical practice. Some are more widely used than others. Examples include Bryant's, Buck's, Dunlop's, Russell's, pelvic, cervical, and Cotrel's traction.

9. When is Bryant's traction applied?

Bryant's traction is used in children under the age of 3 years who weigh less than 40 lb to treat fractures of the femur or developmental dysplasia of the hip. Adhesive strips are attached to both legs and secured with elastic bandages. Weight is applied to raise both legs upward until the buttocks are slightly raised above the mattress. Bryant's traction is used to immobilize and relieve muscle spasms.

10. How is Buck's traction applied?

Buck's traction is applied to the lateral surfaces of one or more extremities by adhesive straps or foam boots attached with Velcro straps. Weights are attached to a spreader with ropes and pulleys to provide countertraction. It is used to provide immobilization of hip fractures, reduce muscle spasms, treat arthritic conditions, and ensure preoperative immobilization.

11. What modifications of Buck's traction are used?

Dunlop's traction and Russell's traction are essentially modifications of Buck's traction. Dunlop's traction is Buck's traction with both horizontal and vertical extension of the humerus and forearm. It is used to treat fractures of the humerus and to maintain position of the forearm. Russell's traction is Buck's traction with the addition of a sling under the affected limb. This addition doubles the force of traction without the need for extra weight by utilizing Newton's third law of thermodynamics (for each force in one direction, there is an equal force in the opposite direction). Russell's traction may also be used with skeletal traction.

12. What types of pelvic traction are available?

The pelvic belt uses a girdle-like belt attached around the abdominal/lumbosacral area. Straps extend down each side to a spreader bar beyond the feet. A rope is attached to the spreader and, with the use of a pulley and weights, applies countertraction to the lower back. The pelvic belt is used to relieve muscle spasms and lower back pain and to treat a herniated or ruptured disk.

The pelvic sling is actually a suspension system rather than traction. A sling (belt) is placed under the pelvis, lower back, and buttocks and raised slightly off the bed by ropes and weights attached to metal bars and spreaders fed through the sling. It is used to treat pelvic fractures, although its use has become rare since the use of external fixation.

13. When is skin traction applied to the head and neck?

The cervical halter is a specially designed halter placed on the head and chin with openings for the face, ears, and top of the head. Ropes are attached to a spreader, and weights provide countertraction. The cervical halter is used to treat arthritic and degenerative conditions as well as strains, sprains, spasm, and cervical nerve root compression. It is not safe to use in the setting of actual or potential cervical vertebral fractures.

14. What is the purpose of Cotrel's traction?

Cotrel's traction consists of the combination of a head halter and pelvic belt. It pulls in opposite directions to help straighten spinal curvatures before surgical correction.

15. When is skeletal traction used instead of skin traction?
Skeletal traction is attached directly to the bone by pins, wires, screws, or tongs. It provides direct pulling force on the affected bone or area of the body. It is used for long-term traction of fractures or soft tissue injuries, treatment of deformities, and suspension of a particular body part in the treatment of burns, fractures, or congenital abnormalities.

16. What types of skeletal traction are used?
Various types of skeletal traction are used for varying purposes. Examples include skull tongs, halo traction, halo vest, side-arm or overhead traction, and balanced suspension.

17. What types of traction can be used for patients with a cervical or high thoracic fracture?
Skull tongs are used to stabilize cervical vertebral fractures. The various types include Gardner-Wells, Cruchfield, Vinke, and Barton tongs. Tongs are drilled into the skull or under the scalp and attached to ropes, pulleys, and weights. They are used to immobilize and/or reduce both cervical and high thoracic vertebral fractures or dislocations.

Halo traction is a metal ring that encircles the head and is attached to the skull with pins. It is used much like skull tongs. Halo traction helps to prevent further spinal damage in neurologically intact patients.

Halo vests use the same type of metal ring around the head attached to the skull with pins. The halo is attached to a plastic sheepskin-lined vest by four lightweight metal bars. This device provides stability to the spine and allows early mobilization after spinal cord injury.

18. Are humerus fractures treated with skeletal traction?
Humerus fractures can be treated with skeletal traction when indicated. Side-arm or overhead traction is used for severe fractures of the humerus. The technique is similar to Dunlop's traction except that a pin is drilled into the lower humerus or a wire is placed through the olecranon process of the ulna and attached to ropes, pulleys, and wires to provide countertraction. It is often used in conjunction with skin traction and slings to suspend the arm to the side or above the body at a 90° angle.

19. How can femur fractures be treated with skeletal traction?
Balanced-suspension skeletal traction uses Kirschner wires or Steinmann pins that are drilled through the upper tibia and attached to a spreader that is connected to rope, pulleys, and weights to provide countertraction. Splints under the thigh and leg, which suspend the limb off the bed, also support the leg. This form of traction is used for displaced supracondylar femur fractures.

20. What is a Thomas splint?
A Thomas splint is used to provide alignment and to promote an effective line of pull. It also allows flexion of the knee. A half ring is placed as high as possible under the thigh without causing skin breakdown in the groin area. It is mainly used with skeletal pins to treat femur fractures and hip and knee contracture and to ensure pre- and postoperative immobilization.

21. When is a Boehler-Braun frame used?

The Boehler-Braun frame supports the leg in position while a pin or wire is placed in the calcaneus. Ropes, pulley, and weights are used to align the lower leg. This device is used for compound fractures of the tibia and complex ankle fractures.

22. When is manual traction applied?

Manual traction is applied by hand for temporary immobilization to provide a firm, steady pull of traction during casting, reduction of fracture or dislocation, or application of skin or skeletal traction.

23. What are the nursing responsibilities before traction application?

Before the application of traction, the nurse assesses the patient's underlying medical condition to identify any preexisting health alterations that may affect mobility, healing, and coping. This assessment is necessary to tailor care to the specific needs of individual patients. The knowledge level of the patient and family, with respect to the traction device, is assessed to identify any teaching needs. Application of the traction device may be painful or uncomfortable, especially in light of the patient's reason for traction (e.g., fracture). The nurse takes time to assess the patient's baseline pain level and provides analgesics or pain-relieving interventions. A baseline neurovascular assessment should be performed before application of traction. Assessment of the condition of the skin on the area in contact with the traction apparatus is important. The nurse should clean the area where the traction is to be applied, removing hair if necessary, and identify and document any open areas, rashes, or bruises. The patient also should be positioned for proper application of traction, and the nurse should assist with application of the traction device as needed. Skin traction and some skeletal traction may be done at the bedside; however the patient may have to go to the operating room for certain application procedures. Such patients should be prepared according to facility protocol and guidelines.

24. What are the nursing responsibilities while the patient is in traction?

The nurse should assess patient and family understanding of traction and its implications and provide follow-up teaching as needed. The nurse should monitor the patient's vital signs according to hospital or department policy. Lung sounds should be monitored for signs of complications due to immobility, including atelectasis. Neurovascular checks should be performed every 15 minutes after the traction is applied for 1–2 hours and then every 4 hours for the first 24 hours or according to facility protocol. Any abnormal changes should be reported immediately to the physician. Monitoring the level and location of pain and/or muscles spasm and providing treatment as needed are essential elements in providing optimal comfort. The nurse must check for signs of deep vein thrombosis (DVT), including pain in the calf, coolness or pallor of extremity, redness at the location of thrombosis, or a positive Homan's sign. Assessment of the skin at all pressure points, with treatment as needed, is an essential component of nursing care. The pin sites are assessed for drainage, redness, and pain. The nurse is responsible for providing pin care according to facility protocol. Ropes, pulleys, and weights are maintained in their proper position, and the nurse must watch for knots or fraying in the ropes. The weights must be free-hanging and off the floor. The correct position of the patient in bed and of the patient's extremities is maintained as ordered by the physician. The nurse observes the patient's self-care and provides assistance when necessary. Skin traction is released and skin care is performed according to orders or facility policy—usually every 4–8 hours. Finally, the patient's and family's coping skills are assessed, and support is provided as needed.

25. How are neurovascular checks performed?

Neurovascular checks are performed to assess for improvement or compromise of a patient's limb for multiple reasons. As the name implies, blood flow and nerve function are evaluated. The reasons for this evaluation include assessment before and/or after surgery, assessment of trauma, cast application, and traction application.

26. What are the components of a neurovascular evaluation?

The usual components of a neurovascular evaluation include assessment of skin temperature and color, capillary refill, edema, sensation, deep tendon reflexes, muscle strength, and movement. The patient is also asked about pain. The neurovascular assessment, like any other examination, is performed bilaterally for comparison.

27. What is pin care?

Pin care is a procedure to clean the pins used for a skeletal fixation device. Although procedures vary from facility to facility, the basics of washing hands and applying gloves always apply. After hand washing and explaining the procedure to the patient, the dressings are removed from around the pins. The insertion sites are observed for drainage and other obvious signs of infection, including erythema, induration, and fluctuance. The nurse assesses the condition of the skin around the pin or wire.

The nurse then applies a new set of clean gloves. Each pin site is cleaned using a sterile cotton-tipped applicator dipped in a solution of half saline and half hydrogen peroxide. The pin is cleansed in a circular, outward motion with a new applicator dipped in saline for each site. If ordered, place antibiotic ointment on the pin site and/or cover with a 2×2 gauze pad that has been split to fit around the pin. Perform this procedure on each pin, one at a time, to prevent possible cross-contamination.

28. What nursing interventions should be performed to avoid or address the potential complications of traction?

1. Problems with skin integrity can be avoided by repositioning the patient as needed, assessing pressure points and providing padding as needed, and keeping the skin clean and dry. Adequate skin care, pin care, and aseptic technique help to avoid infection. In addition, the nurse can monitor for signs of infection, such as redness, warmth, drainage, or pain. The nurse can also monitor the white blood cell count.

2. Neurovascular compromise may be avoided by monitoring pressure on major nerves. The nurse can also assess pulses, color, temperature, and sensation. Monitoring for compartment syndrome is also essential.

3. Inadequate bone alignment can be avoided by maintaining proper position of the patient. The patient should be taught the proper techniques in moving and using the trapeze.

4. Pain should obviously be assessed and treated as needed, in addition to encouraging the optimal level of self-care.

5. Maintenance of adequate nutrition and fluid intake helps to avoid alterations in bowel function. The nurse should monitor the patient's bowel sounds, flatus, and bowel movements. The patient should be provided privacy for elimination.

6. Impaired gas exchange may be caused by atelectasis. The nurse should monitor the patient for signs of pulmonary embolism, agitation, dyspnea, and hypoxia. Lung sounds, temperature, and sputum must be monitored. The patient should be encouraged to breathe deeply and cough. Chest x-rays are ordered as needed.

7. The patient's urine output should be monitored. Signs of urinary retention must be addressed. The patient should maintain adequate fluid intake.

8. Assessment of the knowledge level and teaching needs of patient and family is an essential nursing intervention. The nurse also assesses and provides support to patient and family, addressing comfort and fears as well as concerns about privacy and loss of control.

29. What kinds of casting materials are available?

Casts are made of the traditional plaster of Paris and of synthetic materials such as polyurethane, fiberglass, or thermoplast. The use of plaster casts has diminished significantly because of the advantages of lightweight synthetic materials. The most common material used in casting is fiberglass.

30. What are the differences between plaster and synthetic casting materials?

Plaster of Paris casts are inexpensive and easy to mold, with smooth surfaces, and can be effective in immobilizing severely displaced fractures after reduction. On the other hand, the application can be quite messy, and the cast can take a long time to dry (24–48 hours). The cast must be kept dry, or the outer shell will disintegrate.

Synthetic casts, typically fiberglass, are lighter in weight, set very fast (in 7–30 minutes), and are easy to mold. The actual cast material is not affected by water and will not crumble after contact with water. Although the outer synthetic shell of the cast is not affected by water, the inner padding, usually of cotton, will hold water and cause skin breakdown. Gore-Tex inner padding, which may be used instead of cotton lining, allows the patient to get the cast wet. The synthetic cast can tolerate weight-bearing within 15–30 minutes and is less restrictive. The synthetic materials are usually more expensive than plaster of Paris casts, especially if the Gore-Tex inner lining is applied.

31. What types of casts are used for the upper and lower extremities?

The type of cast applied depends on the location and severity of the injury, the age and developmental level of the patient, and physician preference. Casts types that can be applied to the lower extremities include the short and long leg casts, total contact cast, abduction cast, short and long abduction boots, and the leg cylinder. Casts for the upper extremity include the short and long arm casts, thumb spica cast, and the long arm cylinder.

32. What types of whole body casts exist?

Several types of whole body casts can be applied, including the hip spica (unilateral, bilateral, one and a half, or short leg), turnbuckle, Risser cast, shoulder spica, spinal body vest, Minerva jacket, and the English walking cast.

33. Why are casts used?

Casts are used to maintain bone alignment, to prevent deformity, and to immobilize the affected limb for a sufficient amount of time to allow bone union. Casts are also used to realign malformed structures, as in congenital disorders. Patients may be able to recuperate at home and ambulate while protecting the fracture or injured soft tissue.

34. As a nurse, am I expected to be able to put a cast on the patient?

The answer depends on the setting and the training that the nurse has received. While working in the inpatient setting, emergency department, or outpatient surgical center, the nurse may not have the opportunity to apply casts. Lack of opportunity may be due to physician preference, training limitations, and/or hospital policy. It is not uncommon, and almost expected, for the nurse and or medical technician to apply and remove casts in the outpatient orthopedic office.

35. What equipment is needed to apply a cast?

Several rolls of cast material in the appropriate width for the body part to be casted are required. The nurse also needs several other supplies, no matter what type of cast is applied, including the appropriate length of stockinet to place against the skin. Stockinet is available in various widths. Next, the nurse needs several rolls of cast padding in the width appropriate for the body area to be covered. A bucket or basin with water can be used to wet the cast material. The cast material sets faster with warmer water. Faster setting, however, is not always better. The cast material may harden before it is completely applied to the patient, leading to increased waste. Scissors are used to cut the stockinet, padding, cast tape, and old cast padding on removal. The person applying the cast should wear gloves and gown or apron. In addition, a gown or covering may be placed over the patient's clothing in the outpatient setting. A floor covering is useful. A cast saw is necessary if an old cast is to be removed. A chair or table for the proper positioning and comfort of the patient is essential.

36. What are the nursing responsibilities before cast application?

Before the cast application, the nurse should review the patient's history to identify any previous health alterations that may affect wound healing. The nurse also should assess the skin and any wounds, rashes, or bruises that will be covered by the cast to allow cleaning or interventions before cast application. The patient's pain and/or anxiety level should be assessed to determine the need for education, diversion activities, or medication. The patient's level of understanding and the extent to which the cast will affect the patient's ambulation and lifestyle also should be assessed. The nurse should determine patient and family education needs before cast application. The patient's vital signs should be assessed as needed, and medications should be administered as needed (e.g., analgesic, muscle relaxant, sedation). After gathering all of the required materials, the nurse positions the patient appropriately for cast application.

37. What are the nursing responsibilities during cast application?

Immediately before cast application, the nurse should instruct the patient and any other assistants in the proper positioning of limbs and tissues for application. The nurse also should offer information and comfort to the patient and family as needed. The person applying the cast and all assistants should wash their hands and apply gloves. The skin is prepared for cast application by washing the affected area and applying dressings as indicated. The patient's hair should be trimmed as needed.

After stockinet is applied to the extremity, adequate cast padding must be ensured. The nurse should apply or assist in the application of the cast material. For casting, the nurse should open one packaged roll of cast material at a time, wet the material, squeeze out the excessive water, and roll the material onto the area to be casted. If assisting in the application, the nurse should ensure that the needed supplies are available, comfort the patient, and position the affected area as needed. The nurse should ensure that the cast edges are smooth and that the stockinet and other materials are correctly placed for the comfort and protection of the patient's skin. Finally, the nurse should remain with the patient while casting material is applied, molded, and hardened.

38. What are the nursing responsibilities after cast application?

The nurse is responsible for placing the casted limb comfortably on pillows or letting it hang freely in the air. This approach allows the cast to dry with no indentations created by pressure points. The nurse assesses the patient's vital signs as needed, comforts the patient, and answers any questions and concerns posed by the patient or family. A neurovascular assessment of the casted limb should be performed. The nurse should use caution in handling the cast, holding it only with the palms of the hands rather than the fingertips. This approach prevents indentation of the cast material before it is fully dry. The cast should be kept uncovered until it is fully dry. The nurse should assist the patient with discharge or transfer, including reviewing patient and family education and assessing the patient and family member's response to instructions.

39. What should the patient and family be taught about cast care?

The limb should be elevated no higher than heart level to control edema. The patient should be taught to check and report drainage, edema that does not resolve with elevation, and neurovascular changes. The patient should leave the cast uncovered until it is dry. The nurse or even a physical therapist should teach the proper use of slings and crutches. Proper application of ice bags should be taught to reduce itch and pain and to control edema. The patient should be instructed to use a hair dryer (on cool setting) or medication to treat itching. Sticking objects down the cast to scratch can lead to skin breakdown and infection and should be avoided.

Bathing and self-performance of activities of daily living with a cast in place can be a challenge. The patient may need assistance from a home health aid, friend, or family member. The nurse should ensure that the patient knows how to use a cast cover or plastic bag over the cast for bathing. If the cast becomes wet, the patient should try to dry it with a hairdryer on cool setting. If the cast does not dry, is completely soaked, becomes loose, or begins to deteriorate, the patient should contact the health care provider.

Caregivers should be taught how to address the specific needs of children in casts, including feeding, positioning, pain assessment and treatment, diversion activities, and anxiety-reducing activities.

40. When does the cast need to be removed or changed?

A cast needs to be changed if the material becomes wet and does not dry adequately or if the cast material deteriorates and does not provide adequate support. A new cast should also be applied if the original cast becomes loose, particularly when edema of the limb decreases. A loose cast may fall off or provide inadequate support for the limb. If a foreign object is placed in the cast, the cast should be changed to remove the object and assess the skin. The examiner may also remove and change a cast to assess a wound under the cast or to replace a cast that becomes too tight or painful. If the original cast is applied with poor technique or positioning, it may be replaced.

41. What should the nurse do if drainage is observed in the cast?

Drainage may be present on the surface of a cast if there are any open wounds, particularly if there is a surgical site beneath the cast. Early drainage may be bright red to brown. This drainage may be absorbed by the padding inside the cast or wicked to areas of the cast not directly over the drainage source. For the postoperative patient or the patient with drainage, the drainage must be assessed and documented at least every 4 hours. Casts may be marked by circling the drainage and indicating the time and date directly on the cast. Patients need to be educated about wound drainage and instructed when to call the physician in the outpatient setting.

42. How can compromised nerve function result from cast application?

Casts and immobilizers or improper positioning of the limb may compromise nerve function by compressing nerves under the cast. Edema can increase the pressure within the cast. Ice and elevation of limb (no higher than heart level) may help to relieve edema. Neurologic assessment includes checking for pain, tingling, numbness, and movement distal to the cast.

43. What can cause circulatory compromise in patients with a cast?

Pressure on blood vessels can compromise the circulation and tissue perfusion in the casted limb. Pulses may be assessed by palpation, or, if they are not accessible, a Doppler device may be needed. Temperature, color, capillary refill, and edema of the area distal to the immobilizer or cast must be assessed to identify circulatory insufficiency. This assessment can be compared with the opposite limb, assuming that it does not have a deficit. Any lack of tissue perfusion may lead to pressure ulcers, skin breakdown, and infection. Cast splitting may be necessary for the patient with signs of impaired circulation or compartment syndrome. Neurologic and vascular status are assessed together.

44. What is cast splitting?

To relieve the possible effects of circumferential constriction caused by casts, the physician may need to split the cast anteriorly, medially, and/or laterally. Signs that the cast may need to be split include increased pain, swelling, or pressure; compartment syndrome; or decreased circulation.

45. What equipment is needed to remove a cast?

Basic equipment needed for cast removal includes gloves, cast saw, cast splitter, blunt-end scissors, and a dust vacuum.

46. What is needed for skin care after cast removal?

After the cast is removed, the patient will want to scratch the skin. The nurse should instruct the patient not to do so, because scratching increases skin irritation and possibly injures the skin. The patient may gently cleanse the skin with warm water and soap or with a skin cleanser. The patient should gently pat dry the skin and apply a soothing skin lotion.

47. What are the nursing responsibilities during cast removal?

The nurse should assess the patient's readiness for cast removal, including the patient's knowledge level, x-ray reports, and physician orders. The nurse should explain the procedure to the patient and family and prepare the patient by explaining the sound and sensation of the saw, reassuring the patient that the saw will cut only the outer cast layer and not the skin. The patient should be instructed to tell the nurse if the cast saw becomes hot during removal. The nurse should apply gloves before the cast is removed, place the patient in a comfortable position, and hold the cast to assist the person cutting it off.

After the cast is removed, the nurse should assess the condition of the skin for breakdown, drainage, temperature, and color. If used, apply the cold-water enzyme wash to help dissolve the layers of dead skin and crusty lesions. Leave the enzyme wash on the skin for approximately 15–20 minutes. Gently wash the affected area with soap and water. Rinse the area with clear warm water, and gently pat it dry. Do not rub or scrub the skin because such actions may lead to skin breakdown. A skin lotion should be applied to the affected area. If ordered, perform gentle range of motion to affected limbs.

48. What instructions should be given for care of the limb after cast removal?

Nursing education for the patient about care of the limb after cast removal should include the following:

- Wash the affected area in 24 hours with soap and water.
- Remember to pat dry.
- Do not rub the skin.
- Apply skin lotion.
- Explain range of motion exercises and use of limb as ordered by the physician.
- Explain that edema may occur after the cast is removed.
- Elevate the affected area no higher than the level of the heart.
- Apply ice to the area, if necessary.
- Evaluate the patient's response to teaching and reinforce as necessary.

49. What are the complications of immobilization with casts?

Nonunion of the casted fracture may result from many causes, including poor bone healing, poor nutrition, smoking, and loosely fitting cast. The nurse should assess the cast for looseness. Proper nutrition, control of diabetes if indicated, and infection control are essential for optimal bone healing.

Infection is a possible complication of cast immobilization. The nurse should monitor vital signs as well as signs of lethargy and increased pain. Osteomyelitis should be considered in patients with open wounds or surgery prior to cast application. A "window" can be maintained by removing a piece of cast for treatment of an infected area. The patient's response to any treatment should be monitored.

All efforts should be made to avoid development of **pressure ulcers**. All pressure points at high risk for developing ulcers should be identified, and the skin around the cast should be inspected for evidence of breakdown. Do not allow scratching with any objects placed into the cast. The nurse should monitor the edge of the cast, ensuring that it does not rub against adjacent areas of skin. Vital signs, pain, and signs of infection should be monitored as needed. The nurse may need to assist in removal, splitting, or window placement in the cast. Prevention during cast application and with limb positioning is a crucial nursing intervention.

Muscle weakness occurs with immobilization of an extremity. The patient should exercise the nonimmobilized joints while in the cast as instructed by the physician. Physical therapy may be necessary after cast removal because of muscle weakness and stiffness of the previously immobilized joint.

The nurse should be aware of **decreased circulation** or **impaired neurologic status** of the limb, which may be complications of a tight cast. Assessment for compartment syndrome should be ongoing. The physician should be notified immediately of any evidence of neurovascular compromise that does not respond to ice and elevation. The cast may need to be removed or split.

50. What is cast syndrome?

Cast syndrome may be seen in any patient in a cast but occurs most often with a body or spica cast. This serious condition results in severe ileus caused by decreased blood flow through the mesenteric artery. Signs and symptoms include anxiety, nausea, inability to take a deep breath, and decreases in blood pressure and heart rate. Treatment includes nothing by mouth, nasogastric suctioning, intravenous fluid administration, repositioning, sedation, and splitting of the cast to relieve pressure.

51. What is external fixation?

External fixation is used to stabilize a fracture with pins and external hardware while providing early mobility and active exercise of the unaffected joints.

52. How does external fixation work?

Pins are placed above and below the fracture or affected area and attached to a frame parallel with the body part. Clamps and screws hold the hardware in place. External fixation uses immobilization, reduction, and compression rather than traction by weights.

53. What are the indications for external fixation?

External fixation is indicated for unstable or open humerus and/or radius fractures. Nonunion, comminution, and open fractures of the lower extremities are also indications for an external fixator. External fixation for pelvic injuries includes open-book fractures, vertical shear fractures, and lateral compression fractures.

54. Discuss the nursing implications for care of external fixation devices.

The nurse should assist the patient with mobility and encourage independence in activities of daily living. The patient's level of pain should be assessed and treated appropriately with elevation of the limb (no higher than heart level), ice, and medication. The pin sites should be assessed and cleaned according to facility protocol. Neurovascular status of the limb must be monitored, including pulses distal to the affected area, color, temperature, and sensation. Vital signs should be monitored for evidence of alterations due to infection or other complications, and DVT prevention should be continued. The nurse should assess the patient's coping ability and provide support to patient and family. The patient's educational needs also should be assessed, and the nurse should provide teaching to the patient and family as needed.

55. What are the complications of external fixation?

Alterations in patient mobility can be addressed by providing assistance as needed, educating the patient and family, and encouraging maximal level of independence. Edema can be controlled by instructing the patient to elevate the extremity. Pain should be assessed on a regular basis and treated with positioning, ice, and medication, as ordered. The use of aseptic technique with open areas and surgical sites helps to avoid infection. The nurse or patient should perform proper pin care. Mobilization and deep breathing with cough should be encouraged to prevent pneumonia. The nurse should assess the patient for adventitious lung sounds and monitor the complete blood count as ordered by the physician. The patient's bowel sounds, flatus, and bowel movements also should be monitored as well as any complaints of nausea and bloating. Signs of an ileus or bowel obstruction should be reported immediately to the physician. Venous stasis can lead to DVTs and complications such as pulmonary emboli. The nurse should monitor for and report any signs of DVT as well as respiratory and neurologic dysfunction.

BIBLIOGRAPHY

1. Folick MA, Carini-Garcia B, Birmingham JJ: Traction: Assessment and Management. St. Louis, Mosby, 1994.
2. Maher AB, Salmond SW, Pellino TA: Orthopedic Nursing, 3rd ed. Philadelphia, W. B. Saunders, 2002.
3. Mourad LA, Droste MM: The Nursing Process in the Care of Adults with Orthopaedic Conditions, 3rd ed. Albany, NY, Delmar Publisher, 1993.
4. Perry AG, Potter PA: Clinical Nursing Skills and Techniques, 5th ed. St. Louis, Mosby, 2002.
5. Smith SF, Duell DJ, Martin BC: Photo Guide of Nursing Skills. Upper Saddle River, NJ, Prentice Hall, 2002.

15. ORTHOPEDIC COMPLICATIONS

Dianne Murphy, RN, MS, CCRN, and Michael E. Zychowicz, RN, MS, NP-C

1. What orthopedic injuries have a high incidence of infection?

Soft tissue injuries and open fractures have a high incidence of infection because any break in the integrity of the skin allows the entrance of pathogens. The extent of soft tissue trauma and the contamination of the wound with dirt, bone fragments, and foreign material add to the risk of infection in patients with open fractures. In addition, patients with open fractures may have drains, packing, external fixation devices, or a closed suction drainage system, all of which increase infection risk.

2. What other risk factors predispose orthopedic patients to infection?

- Diabetes
- Immunosuppression (chemotherapy, steroid use, HIV/AIDS)
- Obesity
- Malnutrition
- Inactivity
- Age less than 1 year or advanced age with poor blood perfusion
- Preexisting or latent infection
- Inadequate aseptic technique during the perioperative period
- Inappropriate use of antibiotics.

3. Describe the assessment findings in patients with infection.

The classic signs and symptoms of infection (redness, tenderness, and swelling) are evident around the wound or incision. Patients also may have a purulent discharge, foul odor, and poor wound healing. They may develop increased pain at the site, chills, and fever. Lab work may show an increase in white blood cell (WBC) count, sedimentation rate, and C-reactive protein; wound cultures may be positive.

4. Discuss the nursing care for patients with an infected orthopedic injury.

In caring for patients with a wound infection from a fracture, aseptic technique is imperative during the performance of wound care. Adherence to standard precautions is necessary to decrease the risk for infection. Administer antibiotics as ordered, and monitor their effectiveness by assessment of the wound for healing as well as decreases in WBC count, sedimentation rate, temperature, and pain. Check culture and sensitivity reports for sensitivity of the pathogen to specific antibiotics. The patient or caregiver should be taught the signs and symptoms of infection, the importance of hand washing and wound care, and the action and side effects of medications. Assess the patient for pain; give analgesics and use nonpharmacologic techniques such as repositioning and controlling environmental factors that may influence the patient's discomfort. Optimal nutritional intake is also important because increased protein and calories are needed for wound healing. The patient's nutritional intake should be monitored for increased protein and vitamin C as well as adequate intake of calories and fiber.

5. What complications may result from infection?

Infection may lead to delayed healing, repeated surgical debridement, and increased length of hospital stay. Osteomyelitis, septicemia, and death may also occur.

6. What are muscle compartments?

Compartments are groups of muscle, nerves, blood vessels, and lymphatics that are enclosed and separated into groups by fascia and bone. Although skin is relatively elastic and stretches with underlying edema and swelling, the fascia that surrounds the compartments is relatively inelastic. Thus, swelling within the compartment can lead to significant problems. Most people have a total of 46 muscular compartments. Thirty-six of the compartments are located in the arms and legs.

7. Define compartment syndrome.

Compartment syndrome results from significantly increased pressure within muscle compartments. The increased pressure is due either to external compression of the compartment or increased contents of the compartment. If significant enough, the increased pressure can lead to vascular, nerve, and soft tissue impairment as well as tissue hypoxia within the compartment. Compounding the effects of the initial injury is the body's response to tissue hypoxia. Degranulation of mast cells releasing histamine causes vasodilation and increased vascular permeability, which in turn cause increased pressure within the compartment. Compartment pressure is also increased by decreased venous return and additional vasodilation due to lactic acid production with anaerobic metabolism. This downward spiral of events leads to continued tissue hypoxia and/or ischemia.

8. What area of the body is most frequently affected by compartment syndrome?

Compartment syndrome can affect any of the 46 muscle compartments in the body, including the paraspinal muscles of the back and the extraocular muscles of the eyes. The most frequently affected compartments are the four compartments of the lower leg.

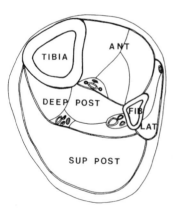

The four compartments of the leg. ANT = anterior compartment, DEEP POST = deep posterior compartment, LAT = lateral compartment, SUP POST = superficial posterior compartment, FIB = fibula. (From Brown DE: Ankle and leg injuries. In Mellion MB, Walsh WM, Shelton GL (eds): The Team Physician's Handbook, 2nd ed. Philadelphia, Hanley & Belfus, 1997, pp 50-51, with permission.)

9. List the types of compartment syndrome.

- Acute compartment syndrome
- Chronic compartment syndrome
- Crush syndrome

10. Describe acute compartment syndrome.

Acute compartment syndrome is a surgical emergency because it can be limb-threatening. Generally it follows some type of acute trauma to an extremity. Other causes of acute compartment syndrome include casts, tight dressings, burn eschar, contusions, intravenous infiltrate, and vein obstruction.

11. How is chronic different from acute compartment syndrome?

Chronic compartment syndrome results from swelling within the compartment after exercise and overuse injury. Increases in capillary flow and hydrostatic pressure with exercise lead to filtering of an increased amount of fluid from the circulation into the tissues. This increased capillary filtration can contribute to a 20% increase in muscle volume during exercise. As mentioned above, the fascia is relatively nondistendible, leading to increased compartment pressure and symptoms due to increased muscular volume. Key features of chronic compartment syndrome are relief of symptoms with rest and rare involvement of neurologic deficit.

12. What other names are used for chronic compartment syndrome?

Chronic compartment syndrome is sometimes called recurrent compartment syndrome, exertional compartment syndrome, exercise ischemia, or exercise myopathy.

13. Can chronic compartment syndrome develop into acute compartment syndrome?

Yes—especially if the patient does not stop activity and rest when symptoms develop. Examples include long-distance runners and people in the military who are "forced" to march long distances.

14. Explain crush syndrome.

Crush syndrome can result from muscle necrosis due to prolonged compartment syndrome. Patients develop systemic effects of muscular necrosis, which may lead to multisystem organ failure or even death. They exhibit myoglobinuria due to the release of myoglobin from ischemic muscle, which is filtered out in the urine. Myoglobinuria may lead to renal failure. Patients can also develop hypovolemia due to edema and third spacing as well as hyperkalemia due to release of potassium from injured muscle.

15. What are the earliest signs of compartment syndrome?

- Pain distal to the injury that is out of proportion to the injury sustained
- Pain on passive stretch of muscle in the affected extremity

16. List the six Ps of compartment syndrome.

The **six Ps** summarize the typical signs and symptoms of compartment syndrome:

• Pain	• Pressure
• Pallor	• Paralysis
• Paresthesia	• Pulselessness

Pulselessness is a late and ominous sign because it indicates severe interference with circulation.

17. What testing can be done in patients with suspected compartment syndrome?

Pressure monitoring of the muscle compartment is performed with a pressure transducer and a catheter inserted into the muscle. Pressures greater than 30 mmHg are typical of compartment syndrome. Urine myoglobin should be evaluated to monitor for muscle necrosis. Creatine phosphokinase (CPK), lactate dehydrogenase (LDH), aspartate aminotransferase (AST), and electrolytes should also be monitored. A magnetic resonance imaging (MRI) scan may be useful to investigate changes in muscular density. A biopsy of muscle tissue may be useful for further assessment of muscle damage.

18. Describe the treatment for compartment syndrome.

- For acute compartment syndrome treatment should address any cause that can be corrected, including decreasing or releasing traction, bivalving a tight cast, removing constricting splints or loosening tight bandages. Necessary treatment may include a fasciotomy, or release of the compartment with a surgical scalpel or cautery tool through the skin and fascia to restore the blood flow and tissue perfusion that were completely stopped by increased pressure.
- The patient with crush syndrome should receive essentially the same care as the patient with acute compartment syndrome. In addition, monitor and provide supportive treatment for potential renal failure, rhabdomyolysis, and any systemic problem that may develop.
- For chronic compartment syndrome, the treatment is cessation of activities until the symptoms have subsided. The patient can enter formal physical therapy as well as use anti-inflammatory medications and orthotics. A high-level competitive (professional or Olympic) athlete may choose to undergo fasciotomy or fasciectomy for surgical release if the symptoms hinder performance.

19. What are the usual nursing interventions for compartment syndrome?

- Educate the patient about compartment syndrome as well as any interventions performed.
- Perform frequent neurovascular exams according to institutional protocol.
- Provide adequate pain management.
- Elevate the affected extremity to the level of the heart.
- Monitor for signs of infection.
- Assess and care for the surgical sites according to institutional protocol.

20. What are the potential consequences of untreated compartment syndrome?

Volkmann's contracture is the most common consequence of delayed or untreated compartment syndrome, resulting in flexion contracture of the affected area. The patient also may develop renal failure, motor and sensory deficits, rhabdomyolysis, and infection.

21. How do pressure ulcers develop?

Pressure ulcers develop from prolonged, sustained pressure over an area of body tissue or from shearing forces on the tissues. Increased pressure is usually due to the body weight of patients who have decreased mobility or are immobile (e.g., patients with a significant spinal fracture). Sustained pressure causes a decrease or cessation of vascular flow to the tissues, leading to ischemia and eventually necrosis. Shearing forces can damage the microvasculature of the affected tissues. For example, shearing forces are applied to the skin, primarily of the back and buttocks, when a patient slowly but continuously slides downward toward the foot of the bed. The shearing forces, like sustained pressure, cause decreased blood flow to the injured tissues, leading to ischemia and possibly necrosis.

22. Why are orthopedic patients usually at an increased risk for developing pressure ulcers?

Restrictions are imposed on the mobility of many orthopedic patients by casting, splinting, and traction. Because of their limited mobility orthopedic patients are at an increased risk for pressure ulcers.

23. How are pressure ulcers properly graded?

Pressure ulcers are graded on a scale of I–IV, depending on the severity of the tissue damage:
- **Stage I** pressure ulcers are not true ulcers, because the skin remains intact. They are characterized by erythema of the skin that does not blanch.
- **Stage II** pressure ulcers consist of epidermal and dermal tissue damage.
- **Stage III** pressure ulcers involve the epidermis, dermis, and subcutaneous layer. The tissue damage may even involve the fascia layer.
- In **stage IV** pressure ulcers, necrosis extends downward to the bone and muscle.

24. Discuss the risk factors for developing pressure ulcers.

Risk factors for the development of pressure ulcers include immobility, moisture, obesity, incontinence, increased age, and malnutrition. Systemic illnesses such as diabetes mellitus and neurologic disorders that alter sensory perception, tissue perfusion, and level of consciousness also predispose to the development of pressure ulcers.

25. What orthopedic injuries place the patient at higher risk for the development of pressure ulcers?

Orthopedic patients with casts, traction, and slings are at high risk for the development of pressure ulcers. Depending on the injury, different sites have the potential for skin breakdown.

26. Do specific immobilization devices increase the risk for developing specific areas of skin ulceration?

Yes. Orthopedic patients are treated with a wide variety of immobilization devices. Each of these devices places the patient at risk for specific areas of skin irritation or ulceration. The following table correlates immobilization devices with areas of potential skin ulceration.

Type of Immobilization	Potential Pressure Ulcer Areas
Cervical traction	Occipital area, pin sites
Head halter	Over ears and mandibular joint, under chin and occipital area
Buck's traction	Bony prominences of anterior tibial border, fibular head, maleoli, Achilles tendon, calcaneous and dorsum of foot, also sacrum
Russell's traction	Same as Buck's traction, also popliteal space where hamstring tendon is located
Bryant's traction	Outer head and neck of fibula, dorsum of foot, Achilles tendon, scapulae and shoulders
Pelvic sling traction	Iliac crest, intergluteal fold, greater trochanter
Pelvic belt	Iliac crest and intergluteal fold
Balanced suspension traction—Thomas splint and Pearson attachment	Greater trochanter, ischial tuberosity, hamstring tendons, fibular head and maleoli, also pin sites and sacrum

(*Table continued on next page*)

Type of Immobilization	Potential Pressure Ulcer Areas
Overhead arm traction	Under the sling over the bony prominences
Casts	Edges of cast, areas inside the cast where crumbs may have fallen
Slings	Skin near the ends of the sling

27. What is the Braden scale?
The Braden scale is a tool used to predict the likelihood that a patient will develop a pressure ulcer. The scale assesses many factors, including sensory perception, skin moisture, degree of activity, mobility, nutrition, and friction/shearing forces.

28. What strategies can help prevent the development of pressure ulcers in orthopedic patients?
- Assess the patient for adequate nutritional status, encouraging adequate intake of protein, vitamins, fiber, and fluids.
- Assess neurovascular status every 4 hours.
- Instruct patients to notify the nurse of changes in color, temperature, pain, sensation, or strength.
- Assess areas under elastic wrapping, at bony prominences, and at the edges of casts or slings.
- Keep skin clean and dry.
- Avoid massaging bony prominences.
- Use a protective or moisturized barrier on intact skin.
- Turn and position the patient every 2 hours
- Have patients shift in their chair every 15 minutes.
- Use a draw sheet for positioning patients to avoid shearing pressure.
- Use pressure-relief devices (i.e., wheelchair cushions, specialized mattresses and beds).
- Keep the patient's heels off the bed.
- Handle a wet cast only with the palms of your hand to prevent pressure areas.
- Prevent crumbs from falling into the cast.
- Instruct patients to avoid putting objects into the cast to scratch the skin.

29. If a patient develops a pressure ulcer, what additional nursing interventions are necessary?
- The size, length, and depth of the ulcer must be documented.
- Cleanse the area with normal saline.
- Avoid hydrogen peroxide, betadine, acetic acid, and Dakin's solution when performing wound care.
- Select a dressing that maintains a moist healing environment.
- Consult a dermatologist or wound care service.
- Assess the wound for signs and symptoms of infection.
- Reassess the pressure ulcer according to institutional protocol.

30. How does immobility lead to constipation?
Patients who are immobile may develop constipation due to decreased activity of the colon.

31. What nursing interventions can be implemented to prevent and/or treat constipation?
- Encourage a high-fiber diet.
- Promote adequate fluid intake.
- Use stool softeners as ordered.
- Promote mobility as indicated, ordered, or tolerated.
- Avoid medications with constipating qualities, such as narcotics.

32. Define paralytic ileus.
A paralytic ileus is a nonmechanical intestinal obstruction.

33. In what orthopedic injury does paralytic ileus occur?
In addition to surgery, inflammation, and electrolyte imbalance, a paralytic ileus may result from neurologic damage in a spinal cord transection above the level of T5.

34. What assessment findings may be seen with paralytic ileus?
Assessment findings related to hypomobility of the gastrointestinal tract include decreased or absent bowel sounds and abdominal distention. A flat-plate radiograph of the abdomen confirms the diagnosis.

35. Describe the usual treatment for paralytic ileus.
A nasogastric (NG) tube at low intermittent suction helps relieve gastric distention.

36. For preoperative patients, what can be done to prevent hemorrhage?
Laboratory parameters such as complete blood count (CBC), partial thromboplastin time (PTT), prothrombin time (PT), international normalized ratio (INR), fibrinogen assay, platelet count, and liver function studies should be evaluated. Patients should discontinue aspirin, nonsteroidal anti-inflammatory drugs (NSAIDs), vitamin E, and warfarin (Coumadin) preoperatively. Vitamin K can be given to reverse anticoagulated patients.

37. How can preoperative patients assist with the treatment of potential blood loss?
Patients undergoing elective surgery can participate in autologus blood donation.

38. What are the common causes of hypovolemic shock?
- Traumatic or surgical blood loss
- Excessive perspiration
- Inadequate fluid intake
- Persistent vomiting

39. List the three stages of hypovolemic shock.
- **Stage I**: compensated stage
- **Stage II**: progressive stage
- **Stage III**: irreversible stage

40. Describe the clinical manifestations for the three stages of shock.
Stage I (compensated)
- Symptoms may be minimal
- Normal to increased heart rate
- Normal to decreased blood pressure

Stage II (progressive)
- Confusion, restless, anxiety, or disorientation
- Possibly chest pain/myocardial ischemia
- Decreased urinary output
- Increased urine specific gravity
- Cyanotic, cold, clammy skin
- Decreased blood pressure
- Increased pulse pressure
- Increased heart rate
- Increased respiratory rate and depth

Stage III (irreversible)
- Fatally low blood pressure
- Unresponsiveness
- Cyanotic, mottled, diaphoretic skin
- Absent peripheral pulses
- Severe tachycardia
- Decreased or absent urinary output
- Organ ischemia (e.g., heart, bowel, kidneys, brain)
- Death

41. Describe the physiologic response during the compensated stage of shock.

The body attempts to elevate blood volume and cardiac output by release of antidiuretic hormone (ADH) and activation of the renin-angiotensin-aldosterone (RAA) system. ADH causes increased water retention in the kidneys, whereas RAA activation causes renal sodium and water retention. In addition, the release of epinephrine and norepinephrine stimulates heart rate and causes peripheral vasoconstriction. Interstitial fluid shifts into the vascular space because of a decrease in capillary hydrostatic pressure. The liver and spleen return sequestered blood to the circulation to increase blood volume. If hypovolemia lasts for days, the kidneys release erythropoietin to stimulate red cell maturation and release, causing increased blood volume and oxygen-carrying capacity. The above compensatory mechanisms are attempts to maintain normal blood pressure and volume.

42. What physiologic events occur during the progressive stage of shock?

The body is unable to maintain homeostasis with the compensatory mechanisms described in the previous answer. This decompensation centers on three vicious cycles stemming from significantly decreased cardiac output and blood volume:
- The myocardial ischemia/infarction due to decreased myocardial blood flow causes continued reductions in cardiac output.
- As a result of diminished peripheral blood flow, tissue hypoxia develops, leading to lactic acidosis and hypercapnia. The result is intravascular clotting, which leads to decreases in venous return and cardiac output and further diminishes peripheral blood flow.
- Blood volume is further reduced because capillary permeability is increased as a result of lactic acidosis and hypercapnia.

43. What is the central ischemic response during the progressive stage of shock?

The central ischemic response occurs during shock when the systemic blood pressure falls below 50 mmHg as the body activates a significant sympathetic response to decreased blood pressure. The result is minimal peripheral blood flow and an attempt to retain cerebral blood flow. The body diverts the blood centrally, leading to ischemia of other tissues.

44. Summarize the physiologic steps that lead to death in the irreversible stage of shock.

Cardiac output continues to decrease as myocardial infarction ensues. The patient is unable to maintain cerebral blood flow, which leads to further cerebral ischemia and infarction. Impaired cellular metabolism and tissue injury cause failure of the precapillary sphincters and arteriolar smooth muscles, leading to generalized peripheral vasodilation and circulatory collapse. Death results from circulatory collapse and widespread tissue death.

45. What factors increase the risk for hemorrhage with orthopedic injuries?
- Low platelet count
- Coagulation disorders
- Use of anti-inflammatory or anticoagulant medications
- History of hepatic disease
- History of tumors near blood vessels
- Trauma in which fractures, foreign bodies, or penetrating objects interrupt blood vessels
- Injuries with a large amount of soft tissue damage
- Surgical procedures

46. What nursing interventions are indicated for hemorrhaging patients?
- Maintain a patent airway and give oxygen.
- Apply direct pressure or a sterile pressure dressing on the bleeding site, and elevate the extremity above the heart.
- Do not remove any impaled object; simply stabilize it with a dressing.
- Surgery or suturing may also be indicated.
- Restore blood volume with blood transfusions or intravenous fluids such as lactated Ringer's solution, normal saline, or colloids (e.g., albumin, dextran).
- Monitor vital signs, urinary output, neurovascular status (pulses, edema, color, sensation, temperature of skin, capillary refill), intake and output, and lab studies (hematocrit and hemoglobin, electrolytes, blood urea nitrogen, creatinine, coagulation studies).

47. List the complications of hemorrhage.
- Shock
- Edema of subcutaneous tissue
- Poor perfusion to organs
- Disseminated intravascular coagulation (DIC)
- Death

48. After a fracture, which veins are susceptible to deep vein thrombosis (DVT)? What are the predisposing factors?

The pelvic veins and veins in the lower extremities—namely the anterior and posterior tibial vein, peroneal veins, popliteal vein, saphenous vein, and femoral vein—are highly susceptible to developing DVT. They are especially prone to DVT after a hip fracture or knee surgery. Because venous stasis is a precipitating factor, inactive patients, patients with a history of varicose veins, immobile patients on bed rest, and patients with traction are also at risk. Trauma to a vein from a fracture or local pressure on a vein from casts or traction can also lead to DVT. Hypercoagulation due to polycythemia vera, sickle cell disease, estrogen therapy, smoking, pregnancy, and clotting deficiencies are additional predisposing factors.

49. How can DVT be prevented?

Prevention strategies include compression gradient stockings, sequential compression devices, range-of-motion exercises, and ambulation. Immobile patients may receive prophylactic anticoagulants such as enoxaparin (Lovenox), aspirin, heparin, or warfarin (Coumadin).

50. Describe the clinical manifestations of DVT.

The signs and symptoms of DVT in an extremity include unilateral edema, constant tenderness or pain, and redness and warmth of the affected leg. Homan's sign may or may not be present, and the patient's temperature may be 100.4°F or above.

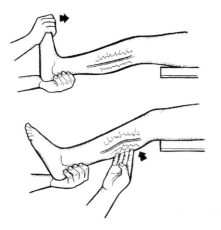

Tests for deep vein thrombosis. *Top*, Homan's sign. *Bottom*, Tenderness elicited by deep palpation of the calf muscle indicates deep vein thrombosis. (From Knight R: Deep vein thrombosis. In Frontera WR, Silver JK (eds): Essentials of Physical Medicine and Rehabilitation. Philadelphia, Hanley & Belfus, 2002, with permission.)

51. What tests are used to diagnose DVT?

- Venous Doppler evaluation
- Duplex scanning
- Venogram

52. Describe the treatment and nursing care of patients with DVT.

Anticoagulant therapy is started with a heparin bolus, followed by a continuous heparin drip for up to 7 days. The patient is placed on bed rest with the leg elevated above the heart until the pain and swelling decrease. Moist heat may also be applied to the extremity. Medications for the relief of pain are given as needed. The circulatory status of the extremity should be monitored by assessing pulses, capillary refill, edema, temperature, and color. Therapeutic levels of heparin are monitored by the activated partial thromboplastin time (aPTT), which should be 1.5–2 times the reference value. Monitor for adverse effects of heparin, such as bleeding, hematoma, hemorrhage, or thrombocytopenia. The oral anticoagulant warfarin (Coumadin) is given for 48–72 hours before heparin is discontinued. Warfarin requires 48–72 hours before it affects prothrombin time (PT). PT and INR are monitored when the patient is taking warfarin. The PT should be 1.5–2 times the reference value, and the INR should be 2.0–3.0. The patient takes warfarin for 3–6 months. Because warfarin is contraindicated in pregnancy, enoxaparin (Lovenox) may be given. Because enoxaparin is a low-molecular-weight heparin, there is no need to monitor coagulation studies. The patient should be taught the importance of follow-up care and told that a diet high in vitamin K foods, such as green leafy vegetables, will interact with the warfarin.

53. What are the complications of DVT?
The complications of DVT include pulmonary emboli, chronic venous insufficiency, and phlegmasia cerulea dolens, which is a sudden, painful swelling with a bluish discoloration of the leg.

54. What are pulmonary emboli?
Pulmonary emboli (PE) are blood clots, air bubbles, or fat globules that have traveled to the pulmonary circulation. They may lodge in a blood vessel of the pulmonary vasculature, causing decreased or absent blood flow and leading to hypoxia, ischemia, and infarction.

55. Which orthopedic patients are at risk for pulmonary emboli?
Patients at risk for pulmonary emboli include postoperative patients, trauma victims, and patients with previous pulmonary emboli. Patients with a hypercoaguability state and those that are immobilized are also at greater risk for pulmonary emboli. Hypercoaguability states include sickle cell disease, pregnancy, oral contraceptive use, and dehydration.

56. Where do pulmonary emboli originate in orthopedic patients?
Pulmonary emboli may originate from the right side of the heart (in a patient with atrial fibrillation), pelvic veins, fat embolism from a long bone fracture, air in an IV line, or tumors. Most often pulmonary emboli originate from a DVT in the femoral or iliac veins.

57. Describe the clinical manifestations of pulmonary emboli.
Patients suddenly develop dyspnea, tachypnea, tachycardia, and hypoxemia. They may also present with chest pain, cough, hemoptysis, crackles in the lungs, restlessness, or change in mental status.

58. What diagnostic studies can be performed in patients with suspected pulmonary embolism?
A ventilation/perfusion (V/Q) scan and pulmonary angiography confirm the diagnosis. Another test to aid the diagnosis of PE is a spiral computed tomography (CT) scan of the chest. CT is noninvasive and, compared with the pulmonary angiogram, has an equivalent sensitivity and specificity. In addition, it has a greater sensitivity and specificity than the V/Q scan. Arterial blood gases (ABGs) show a low partial arterial oxygen tension (PaO_2) due to inadequate oxygenation as well as a low partial pressure of carbon dioxide in arterial blood ($PaCO_2$) due to hyperventilation. The ABGs also reflect underlying pulmonary or cardiac disease. A chest x-ray should be performed. An electrocardiogram (EKG) is not particularly valuable in confirming PE but may show

any associated cardiac ischemia or infarction. If the patient has a PE, nonspecific changes in ST and T waves may be appreciated on the EKG, reflecting right heart strain.

59. Describe the proper management of a patient with pulmonary emboli.

PE requires immediate treatment with oxygen, a heparin bolus and continuous heparin drip, thrombolytics (in the absence of contraindications such as trauma or recent surgery), pain relief with narcotics, and bed rest. If the pulmonary artery is occluded by more than 50% and the patient does not respond to therapy, an embolectomy may be performed. In patients with chronic DVT, a Greenfield filter may be inserted into the inferior vena cava to prevent further pulmonary emboli.

60. What are the complications of pulmonary emboli?

One of the complications of PE is pulmonary infarction, which is associated with hemorrhage, necrosis, and death of the alveolar tissue. PE may develop into an abscess, but more commonly a pleural effusion develops. Another complication is pulmonary hypertension, which may lead to death, depending on the degree of hypertension and how rapidly it develops.

61. How do fat emboli originate?

Two theories have been proposed to explain the origin of fat emboli. An increase in intramedullary pressure from trauma to the bone may release the fat from the bone marrow. The fat is transported by the venous system as emboli. A second theory suggests that free fatty acids in the adipose tissue are mobilized by catecholamines released by the body's reaction to trauma; the result is formation of large fat globules, which become emboli.

62. What factors place patients at risk for fat embolism syndrome?

- Fractures of the long bones (e.g., femur, tibia)
- Multiple fracture and pelvic injuries
- Fractured ribs
- Total joint replacement
- Spinal fusion
- Crushing injuries
- Liposuction
- Bone marrow transplant

63. What are the target organs for the fat emboli?

Target organs for the fat emboli include the lungs, heart, brain, kidneys, and skin.

64. Describe the clinical signs and symptoms of fat emboli syndrome.

The signs and symptoms usually occur within 24–48 hours but may occur within only a few hours after trauma. If the fat emboli reach the lung, the patient may present with chest pain, cyanosis, tachypnea, dyspnea, tachycardia, decreased PaO_2, restlessness, and apprehension. In a trauma patient, central nervous system (CNS) changes can be wrongly attributed to head injury. CNS symptoms include confusion, restlessness, memory loss, headache, decreasing level of consciousness, and temperature elevation. Signs and symptoms that differentiate cerebral fat emboli syndrome from head injury include petechiae around the chest, neck, anterior chest wall, axilla, buccal mucosa, and conjunctiva.

65. What abnormalities aid in the diagnosis of fat embolism syndrome?
ABGs show a PaO_2 less than 60 mmHg, and the EKG shows ST-segment changes. Abnormal lab work includes decreased platelets and hematocrit, prolonged PT, and fat cells in the urine, sputum, and blood. The "snowstorm effect" seen on chest x-ray is characterized by areas of pulmonary infiltrate or areas of consolidation.

66. How can fat embolism syndrome be prevented?
Before stabilization or immobilization of a fracture, the patient should be moved as little as possible to prevent fat droplet emboli.

67. How is fat emboli syndrome treated?
Treatment is based on the patient's symptoms and includes oxygen therapy or possible intubation and mechanical ventilation, correction of acidosis, and fluid and blood loss replacement.

68. What are the complications of fat embolism syndrome?
• Adult respiratory distress syndrome (ARDS)
• Pulmonary edema
• Disseminated intravascular coagulation (DIC)
• Coma
• Death

69. Define malunion.
Malunion occurs when fractures heal in improper alignment. It may result from unequal muscle pull or gravity, improper fracture reduction and in patients who bear weight too soon on an injured extremity. Malunion appears as a deformity on x-ray and can be corrected by traction adjustments or remobilization.

70. How can malunion be prevented?
Patient education about the importance of restricted activity and proper fracture reduction and immobilization can prevent malunion.

71. Define delayed union.
Delayed union is slowed healing beyond the expected period, accompanied by tenderness and bone pain.

72. What causes delayed union?
Delayed union may result from infection, distraction of fracture fragments, or conditions that decrease bone healing, including smoking. The fracture may heal if the cause is corrected or treated.

73. Define nonunion.
Nonunion occurs when a fracture has not healed by 4–6 months after injury and probably will not heal. Radiographs show a persistent fracture line with absent or inadequate callous formation.

74. What factors may influence nonunion?
Causes include poor blood supply, repetitive stress on the fracture site, infection, and inadequate internal fixation or immobilization that allows movement at the fracture site.

75. How can nonunion be treated?
Nonunion can be treated by bone graft, internal or external fixation, electrical bone stimulation or pulsed, low-density ultrasound.

76. Define arthrodesis.
Athrodesis is surgical fusion of joints. Commonly fused joints include the wrist, ankle, cervical spine, lumbar spine, and great toe.

77. Why is arthrodesis performed?
Arthrodesis is indicated only if joint reconstruction cannot be performed because of badly damaged or infected joints.

78. Define pseudarthrosis.
A pseudarthrosis, or false joint, is a type of nonunion in which the bone develops a fibrous connection instead of a bony connection at the fracture site. For many patients, painless passive movement of varying degrees is present at the affected joint. Refracture through the fibrous union is certainly possible.

79. Define myositis ossificans.
Myositis ossificans is a complication of orthopedic injury that involves calcification and ossification of a soft tissue injury with hematoma. The patient may have continued discomfort at the site of myositis ossificans.

80. What causes nerve injury in orthopedic patients?
Bone fragments and edema can cause nerve damage after an orthopedic injury. If compartment syndrome is not recognized or treated, nerve damage results.

81. Describe the clinical manifestations of nerve damage.
Clinical manifestations include increased pain, paresthesia, cool and pale skin, changes in the ability to move, and paralysis.

82. Why does avascular necrosis (AVN) occur?
Bone that is temporarily or permanently without blood flow can develop AVN. The disrupted blood supply can lead to ischemia or infarction of the bone and subsequent collapse of the microscopic structure of the bone due to necrosis.

83. Who is at risk for developing AVN?
Any patient with a fracture can develop AVN. Femoral head fractures develop AVN at a relatively high rate, as do scaphoid, talus, and humeral head fractures. In addition, patients who have undergone chemotherapy or radiation are at risk. Patients taking corticosteroids and patients with sickle cell disease, pancreatitis, alcohol or drug abuse, or decompression sickness are also at risk for developing AVN.

84. How is AVN diagnosed?
A patient may complain of decreased range of motion or continued pain for an abnormally prolonged period after a fracture. Many patients have pain at rest or at night. A patient with AVN of the hip typically complains of pain in the groin. Radiographs, MRI, and CT scan are useful in assessing and diagnosing AVN.

85. Discuss the prevention and treatment of avascular necrosis.

Depending on the orthopedist's recommendation and the extent of bone damage, patients with AVN may undergo conservative or operative treatment. Conservative treatment consists of non–weight-bearing and NSAIDs. Surgical treatment consists of core decompression, arthroplasty, osteotomy, or bone grafting.

86. What causes rhabdomyolysis?

Rhabdomyolysis occurs after trauma to the skeletal muscles in which myoglobin and intracellular substances are released into the blood, resulting in acute renal failure.

87. Which patients are at risk for the development of rhabdomyolysis?

Patients who sustained crush injuries or large soft tissue contusions and patients who were thrown from or dragged by a vehicle or hit with a heavy object are at risk for the development of rhabdomyolysis.

88. Describe the diagnostic studies and clinical manifestations of rhabdomyolysis.

The symptoms include pain, swelling, bruising over the injured muscles, cola-colored urine, fever, nausea, vomiting, confusion, and agitation. The main laboratory indicator is creatinine kinase (CK) that is 5 times or more above the normal value. Since myoglobin may appear in the urine only in the first two days after injury, it is not the best or most reliable laboratory indicator of rhabdomyolysis. Urine myoglobin may not be seen later when the patient's signs and symptoms appear and CK elevation may be present. Hyperkalemia, hyperphosphatemia, hyperuricemia, and hypocalcemia are present initially, but as renal failure progresses, hypercalcemia develops.

89. Describe the treatment and prognosis for rhabdomyolysis.

Immediate hydration of the patient is important in the prevention of renal failure. Intravenous normal saline is given to maintain urine output of at least 300cc/hour or mannitol and sodium bicarbonate to raise the pH of urine and promote diuresis until the CK is under 1000. Dialysis may also be necessary. In patients without preexisting comorbidities, prognosis is good for return to normal renal function.

BIBLIOGRAPHY

1. Black JM, Hawks JH, Keene AM: Medical Surgical Nursing: Clinical Management for Positive Outcomes, 6th ed. Philadelphia, W.B. Saunders, 2001.
2. Huether S, McCance K: Understanding Pathophysiology, 2nd ed. St Louis, Mosby, 2000.
3. Lewis SM, Heitkemper, MM, Dirksen SR: Medical Surgical Nursing: Assessment and Management of Clinical Problems, 5th ed. St Louis, Mosby, 2000.
4. Maher AB, Salmond SW, Pellino TA: Orthopaedic Nursing, 3rd ed. Philadelphia, W.B. Saunders, 2002.
5. Schoen DC: NAON Core Curriculum for Orthopaedic Nursing, 4th ed. Pittman, NJ, Anthony J. Jannetti, 2001.
6. Walls M: Orthopedic trauma. Regist Nurse 65(7):52–56, 2001.

16. PAIN ASSESSMENT AND MANAGEMENT

Suzanne Waters, RN, MS, FNP, and Michael E. Zychowicz, RN, MS, NP-C

1. What is the significance of pain assessment and management for the orthopedic nurse?

Pain assessment and treatment by the orthopedic nurse are significant because most, if not all, orthopedic patients have pain.

2. Distinguish among acute, malignant, and chronic nonmalignant pain.

Acute pain is brief and subsides as healing occurs. In orthopedic patients, acute pain typically is due to some type of trauma, such as fracture, sprain, dislocation, or contusion. The orthopedic patient may present with pain of a cancerous origin, with or without bony metastasis, which is called **malignant pain**. Back pain that wakes the patient from sleep may be a symptom of cancer, in addition to the usual cancer red flags such as blood in the stool, changes in bowel habit, and unexpected weight loss. **Chronic nonmalignant pain** is non–cancer-related pain that lasts for a prolonged period, typically longer than 6 months. An example of chronic pain is the patient who develops an acute onset of low back pain due to a lumbar strain and an annular tear of a lumbar disc after a motor vehicle accident. The pain is treated conservatively and decreases somewhat. The lumbar strain improves, but the patient has constant mild low back pain due to the annular tear.

3. Distinguish among somatic, visceral, and neuropathic pain.

Pain with a **somatic** origin arises from general body structures, such as bone, joint, muscle, and connective tissue. Somatic pain is usually throbbing and well localized. Pain of a **visceral** origin arises from autonomic nervous system fibers of visceral organs, such as the gastrointestinal tract. Tumors usually cause aching and well-localized pain, whereas an intestinal obstruction causes cramping and is poorly localized. **Neuropathic** pain is transmitted by nervous tissue that is damaged or injured by crushing, laceration, compression, or exposure to chemical or viral agents. It results in abnormal processing of sensory input and can originate from either the central or peripheral nervous system. Neuropathic pain is usually described as burning, shooting, or electrical in nature. Examples of disorders that cause neuropathic pain include nerve root compression (tumor or disc herniation), nerve entrapment (carpal tunnel syndrome), diabetic neuropathy, alcohol-related or nutritional neuropathy, Guillain-Barré syndrome, trigeminal neuralgia, and postherpetic neuropathy.

4. What are the four processes in pain physiology?

After an injury, the sensory noxious stimuli are changed to nerve impulses in a process called **transduction**. By way of **transmission**, these nerve impulses move from the point of origin to the brain. **Perception** and **recognition** by the brain define and determine further response to the pain.

5. What is pain modulation?

Pain modulation causes inhibitory effects on pain transmission.

6. How can a person alter pain perception?

Pain perception occurs in the cortical structures of the brain and can be altered with cognitive-behavioral strategies, including distraction, relaxation, and guided imagery. These techniques distract the patient from focusing on the painful stimulus, and fewer pain signals can be transmitted to the brain.

7. What chemicals and receptors are involved in pain transmission?

After tissue injury, important chemical mediators affect pain transmission. Prostaglandin E is one chemical mediator responsible for pain. Leukotrienes and prostaglandins maintain and prolong the inflammatory process. Bradykinin is responsible for triggering pain or perception of pain by the brain via the dorsal nerve root of the spinal cord. C-PMN nocireceptors are pain nerve fibers that transmit pain impulses to the brain and are irritated by bradykinin, prostaglandins, histamine, and substance P. C-PMN also causes the release of substance P, a pain transmitter, resulting in degranulation of mast cells. The release of histamine from the mast cells causes a positive feedback, stimulating further inflammation and further stimuli of C-PMN.

8. Give examples of clinical conditions that stimulate C-PMNs and lead to pain.

- C-PMNs are stimulated when a tumor stretches tissue, causing increased pressure and mechanical/chemical stimulation of local C-PMNs.
- Herpetic neuralgia stimulates the inflammatory response, which in turn stimulates C-PMNs and thus causes pain.
- Muscle spasms create mechanical stimulation of C-PMNs, leading to pain.
- Traction causes mechanical stimulation of C-PMNs, leading to pain.
- A surgical incision leads to chemical stimulation of C-PMNs, causing pain.

9. List three types of pain transmission.

Three types of pain transmission depolarize primary pain nerve fibers:
- Mechanical (stretching, pushing of body tissue)
- Thermal (increased temperature leads to increased pain)
- Chemical (inflammatory response)

10. Name four causes of persistent pain.

1. Persistent nociception is caused by inflammation or mechanical dysfunction. Examples include cancer pain and inflammation.

2. Autonomic firing of upper neurons causes deafferentation, or interruption of afferent nerve impulses, when lower neurons are damaged. Examples include phantom limb pain and postherpetic neuralgia.

3. Vicious cycles can be caused by muscle spasms or sympathetically mediated pain. Stretch injuries or repetitive use injuries cause mechanical stimulation of nocireceptors and are treated with stretching exercises and relaxation techniques. Sympathetically mediated pain results in dystrophy and complex regional pain, causing shiny, mottled, cool skin in the extremities, and is treated with anesthetic blocks.

4. Behavioral factors are conditioned or learned responses and behaviors that favor pain.

11. What is the difference between the gate control mechanism and the descending inhibitory pathway for pain?

The **gate control mechanism** states that pain signals are inhibited by larger nonpain fibers competing for transmission. These nonpain fibers include vibratory, light touch, pressure, and position sense. Because the brain cannot process and comprehend these competing signals, the nonpain signals can override the pain signals, decreasing pain perception.

With the **descending inhibitory pathway** for pain, impulses are sent downward from the brain and inhibit afferent impulses from going upward to the brain. Endorphins can also act to inhibit pain. Pain treatment includes blocking transmission or promoting modulating mechanisms of pain via the gate control mechanism or the descending inhibitory pathway for pain.

12. Describe drug tolerance.

Tolerance occurs when dosing of opioids must be increased to maintain the same analgesic effect. This effect reflects an involuntary mechanism that occurs after repeated exposure to opioid use. Tolerance is first evidenced by decreased duration of relief, followed by decreased degree of relief. Tolerance does not occur with short-term use of opioids but rather with chronic use of opioids for malignant pain. Lack of pain relief after increased dosing is not synonymous with addiction.

13. What is addiction?

Addiction is an overwhelming obsession with obtaining opioids. It is characterized as a voluntary psychological dependence and evidenced by active, compulsive drug-seeking behavior unrelated to pain control. The patient experiences relapses after withdrawal subsides. The duration of opioid use does not increase the incidence of addiction. This behavior reflects a lack of personal control over drug use.

14. Describe physical dependence.

Physical dependence is an involuntary behavior evidenced by withdrawal symptoms if the opioid is suddenly stopped. It occurs after repeated use of opioids. The patient needs to taper off the drug to avoid withdrawal symptoms. Physical dependence is not synonymous with psychological addiction.

15. What questions should the nurse include in the pain assessment?

The pain assessment includes questions related to the following descriptors:

Intensity. Use a pain scale to measure the pain objectively. Scales for measuring pain intensity include the visual analog scale, graphic rating scale, simple word descriptor scale, numerical rating scale, faces rating scale (Wong-Baker Face Scale), cries scale (neonatal), NIPS scale (neonatal), and FLACC scale (pediatrics).

Location. Ask whether the pain is localized or radiates.

Timing. Ask about onset, duration, frequency, variations, and rhythms of the pain.

Quality. Ask about throbbing, shooting, sharp, cramping, aching, tender, pricking, burning, and pulling descriptors. Note that soreness is typically somatic pain, whereas burning/knifelike pain is usually neuropathic.

Aggravating and alleviating factors. The assessor must recognize distinguishing features and patterns associated with the pain. In addition, relationships associated with underlying pathology and diagnostic information, such as radiologic, neurologic, and laboratory findings, are necessary to complete the picture.

Effects of pain. Does pain interfere with sleep, general activity, mood, work, interpersonal relationships, and enjoyment of life?

16. What pain assessment tools are commonly used for adult and adolescent patients?

One widely used pain assessment tool asks patients to rate their pain on a numerical scale from 0 (no pain) to 10 (excruciating pain). This scale is easily communicated from one health care provider to another. The Visual Analog Scale (VAS) uses a 10-cm line; the patient is asked to mark the point that corresponds to his or her level of pain, ranging from no pain to excruciating pain. Pictures or word clues along the length of the scale usually accompany the VAS. Although it is suggested that the VAS is more sensitive in measuring pain, the score is not as easily communicated between health care providers. The verbal rating scale lists adjectives that the patient may use to describe the pain. This scale may not be easy to use by patients with poor language ability.

Numeric Pain Intensity Scale (5 years and older)

|------ |------ |------ |------ |------ |------ |------ |------ |------ |------ |
 0   1   2   3   4   5   6   7   8   9   10

No pain   Moderate Pain   Worst Possible
                                                                     Pain

---

Visual Analog Scale. (From Ruzicka D, Gates RA, Fink RM: Pain management. In Gates RA, Fink RM (eds): Oncology Nursing Secrets, 2nd ed. Philadelphia, Hanley & Belfus, 2001, with permission.)

17. What is the McGill Questionnaire?

The McGill Questionnaire is a useful tool in evaluating the sensory and affective components of pain. The tool helps with the diagnosis of pain syndromes. The patient can complete the short form of this questionnaire in less than five minutes.

18. What is the Faces Scale for pain assessment?

The Faces Scale is a tool for pain assessment that is easily understood by children and therefore is useful in assessing pain in pediatric patients. This tool consists of faces showing differing degrees of comfort and discomfort, from smiling to crying. The child can simply point to the face that best describes the degree of pain or discomfort. The pediatric patient may not have the capacity to place a numeric value on the pain or to answer the questions asked on a more sophisticated pain inventory.

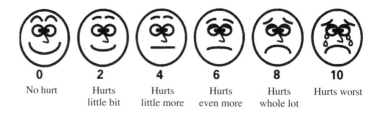

0	2	4	6	8	10
No hurt	Hurts little bit	Hurts little more	Hurts even more	Hurts whole lot	Hurts worst

Faces Scale. (From Wong G, Whaley L: Clinical Handbook of Pediatric Nursing, 2nd ed. St. Louis, Mosby, 1986, p 373, with permission.)

19. How is pain assessed in neonates, infants, and people who cannot express themselves?

One pain assessment tool used in this context is the Behavioral Scales. This somewhat subjective tool evaluates facial expression, movement, and vocalization as indicators of comfort or pain. Other pain assessment tools include the cries scale (neonatal), NIPS scale (neonatal), and FLACC scale (pediatrics).

20. What crucial points should the nurse remember in assessing pain?
Pain is what the patient says it is. Scores of 1–3 points on a 10-point scale indicate mild pain, scores of 4–7 points indicate moderate pain, and scores of 8–10 points suggest severe pain. Studies reveal that pain scored above 3 on a 10-point scale significantly interferes with activities of daily living (ADLs) and requires revision of the pain treatment plan. Pain scores above 4 require intervention, and scores above 6 require immediate intervention. Satisfactory pain relief is a level of pain that is noticeable but not bothersome. A 5-point scale may be used for cognitively impaired patients. Studies reveal that patients feel pain even when unconscious and unable to report it. Clinicians should anticipate the pain based on disease process, diagnostic interventions, facial expressions, body movements, crying, proxy rating of pain, and physiologic measures. Considering these factors, the clinician should treat the pain in the unconscious, noncommunicative patient.

21. How can the health care team and the patient work toward effective pain control?
Treatment for pain must be based on the patient's involvement in his or her own pain management plan. Patients must rate their own acceptable levels of pain, ability to function and perform ADLs, and the number of hours needed for sleep each day. The health care professional must help patients regain control of their own lives using pain control strategies. The underlying causes of pain must be identified to treat the patient correctly. Pain control must be individualized to every patient. The health care professional must identify sources, causes, and contributing factors for pain and then apply pain-reducing interventions, including both pharmacologic and nonpharmacologic adjuncts. The health care professional must modify the treatment plan based on patient input related to effective treatment strategies vs. ineffective treatment strategies.

22. What is the goal of effective pain control?
The goal of effective pain control is pain relief via a knowledgeable, aggressive, and compassionate treatment plan for patients suffering with pain.

23. What are the desired outcomes for managing pain?
Adequate pain management leads to a diminished emotional component of pain, strengthened coping abilities, reduced perceived threat, an increased sense of control, enhanced comfort, decreased fatigue, and restored hope. The outcomes of proper pain management include sleep promotion, improved quality of life, decreased stimulation of the sympathetic nervous system, muscle relaxation, decreased heart rate, improved oxygenation, lower blood pressure, release of endogenous pain-relieving substances, empathetic interpersonal relationships, and reduced stress/tension.

24. What are the major barriers to pain management?
Barriers to pain management include the **health care system's lack of accountability and inadequate education** of physicians and nurse's. Eighty seven percent of graduating nurses did not think that pain management was relevant to their practice. Nursing textbooks also revealed incorrect, irrelevant, and confusing information about

pain management. Fear of regulatory reprisal was evidenced by medical boards that discourage physicians from ordering opioid medication for chronic nonmalignant pain and cancer pain. Professional biases deny patients rightful and appropriate pain management

Social and personal barriers include negative connotations associated with taking pills. In addition, patients believe that physicians overprescribe medications and that natural remedies are preferable to prescription medications. Many people also fear overreliance on pain medications and addiction; in addition, they may fear that medications will lose their effectiveness.

Cultural and religious beliefs, such as stoic or punitive responses to pain, are also barriers. Examples include such attitudes as "Keep a stiff upper lip" or "This is a punishment from God." Other myths about pain control that may act as barriers include proof of one's endurance capability, fear of overdose leading to death, and fear of respiratory depression leading to death.

25. What misconceptions do health care professional have about pain management?

Misconceptions about pain and concerns about opioid use are barriers to effective pain control. Misconceptions about tolerance vs. addiction result in unnecessary withholding of medications from patients who appear to be manipulating the system in effort to obtain more medications. Ashburn, Love, and Pace reported a 0.1% incidence of respiratory depression in patients using intravenous opioids, with no mortality. Portor and Jick investigated the development of substance abuse in patients given postoperative pain medication without knowing that the medication was an opioid. Only 4 of 11,882 patients developed iatrogenic drug abuse. Professionals fear inadequacy in managing intractable pain and not knowing how to handle the situation. This fear results in a perception of personal failure and avoidance of patients with intractable pain. Barriers also include fear of increasing pain by putting too much attention on the issue. Studies support the fact that patient education helps to decrease pain. Many professionals underestimate the severity of a patient's pain. A professional's past experiences with pain management can also represent barriers for proper control of pain.

26. What professional practices are needed to improve pain management?

Health care professionals must examine their own conscience and recognize personal beliefs and biases affecting care delivery. They must be open to establishing new thinking patterns about pain management. Pain is a subjective experience; in other words, it is what the patient says it is. The patient must be part of the pain management team. The patient's self-report of pain is the most reliable indicator for pain. It is important to increase one's knowledge of current research-based strategies and technologic advances for pain relief.

27. How can nurses better incorporate pain management skills into their practice?
Assessment
* Incorporate national standards for pain management into clinical practice.
* Develop organizational pain clinics and pain management teams.
* Utilize standardized pain scales from similar patient populations.
* Have the patient express his or her pain goal.
* Perform initial pain assessment and routine reassessment, including the following factors: pain intensity before and after interventions, the efficacy of both pharmacologic and nonpharmacologic interventions, and modifications added to the plan, if needed.

- Consider pain assessment as the fifth vital sign.

Intervention
- Schedule analgesic dosing around the clock with consideration for breakthrough pain.
- Perform nursing interventions such as distraction or guided imagery.
- Titrate analgesic doses based on the patient's self-report of pain.
- Administer analgesic by the appropriate route.
- Transition the route of delivery from parenteral to oral/enteral as soon as possible.
- Anticipate and manage adverse effects of analgesics.
- Document accurately and completely.

28. What are the national standards and recommendations for pain management?
According to 1997 guidelines, the American Pain Society recommends the use of opioids for nonmalignant pain. The New York State Patient Bill of Rights and the Joint Commission for Accreditation of Hospitals state that pain management is a patient right. The guidelines of the Agency for Health Care Policy and Research (AHCPR) advise consideration of pain management before, during, and after surgery or procedures in an effort to prevent and/or decrease the need for analgesics. The philosophy is that prevention is better than treatment. AHCPR categorizes pain into taxonomy with associated recommendations for treatment strategies:

Pain Level	Severity	Treatment Guideline
Mild pain	1–3 of 10	NSAID, nonopioid, adjuvant medication
Moderate pain	4–7 of 10	Opioid and/or NSAID, combination opioid, adjuvant
Severe pain	8–10 of 10	Strong opioid and/or NSAID adjuvant

NSAID = nonsteroidal anti-inflammatory drug.

The AHCPR guidelines recommend the use of opioids for the treatment of moderate-to-severe pain because opioids bind to pain receptor sites and block pain transmission. Nonsteroidal anti-inflammatory drugs (NSAIDs) are recommended for use with mild-to-moderate pain as well as to decrease inflammation. The use of adjuvant therapy includes tricyclic antidepressants, steroids, antiepileptics, local anesthetics, antihistamines, and antiarrhythmics. Adjuvant agents may be used alone or with another analgesic agent and have been found to increase the effectiveness of opioids in pain control.

29. Summarize the methods that may be used by the management team to treat pain.
Treatment methods are aimed at correcting mechanical irritation and the inflammatory processes by controlling irritable firing of nocireceptors. Various methods for treating pain include:
- Ablating nerve roots that cause recurrent pain
- Reducing muscle spasms
- Enhancing counter-irritants, such as vibration, transcutaneous electrical nerve stimulation (TENS), cold compresses, and warm compresses
- Assessing and treating underlying mechanisms and causes of pain
- Administering pain medication, including combination analgesics

30. Where in this text can the reader find additional pharmacologic information?
In Chapter 17.

31. What is the benefit of combination medications?

Combined preparations allow smaller doses of each analgesic than when it is used alone, thereby reducing side effects. An example of an opioid and nonopioid combination medication is Percocet, which contains oxycodone and acetaminophen.

32. What are endorphins? Discuss their role in pain relief.

Endorphins are endogenous opioid-like substances that bind to receptor sites and block pain transmission. Factors that increase endorphins include brief pain or stress, physical exercise, massive trauma, acupuncture, TENS, and sexual activity. Factors that decrease endorphins include prolonged pain, recurrent stress, and prolonged use of opioids/alcohol. One significant difference between endorphins and opioids is that endogenous endorphins degrade more quickly than exogenous opioids

33. Identify different types of pharmacologic pain relievers used as treatment options for the management of pain?

Opioids, nonopioids, and adjunct analgesics (anticonvulsants, tricyclic antidepressants, steroids, psychostimulants, or anesthetics)

34. What should the nurse know about opioids?

Opioids are the recommended mainstay for treatment of moderate-to-severe pain and cancer-related pain. The clinician should consider alternatives to opioids for patients with chemical dependency, psychiatric history, pregnancy, or unstable social situation. Opioids inhibit the release of neurotransmitters, thereby inhibiting the transmission of pain impulses. They bind to opioid receptor sites in the brain and spinal cord, resulting in pain relief. Common opioids include codeine, morphine sulfate, hydromorphone (Dilaudid), fentanyl, methadone, oxycodone, meperidine (Demerol), and propoxyphene (Darvon). The antagonist is naloxone (Narcan).

If the patient experiences unmanageable or unacceptable side effects, it is necessary to switch to another opioid. The dosage can be increased incrementally by 25-50 % until pain relief occurs or the patient develops unacceptable side effects. The dosage should be decreased by 25% with the consideration of adding an adjunctive analgesic if the patient develops unacceptable side effects.

35. How do anticonvulsants work to decrease pain?

Anticonvulsants inhibit efflux of potassium and influx of sodium at the cell level. This combined action prevents the propagation of impulse conduction and also directly decreases the firing of nocireceptors (C-PMN receptors for pain).

36. How do tricyclic antidepressants work to decrease pain?

Tricyclic antidepressants interfere with the reuptake of serotonin and norepinephrine. As a result, serotonin and norepinephrine are more readily available for analgesia production.

37. How do anesthetics produce pain relief?

Anesthetics are sodium channel-blocking agents that block impulse transmission.

38. What nonpharmacologic strategies are used for the management of pain?

Nondrug pain therapies include relaxation techniques (deep breathing, muscle relaxation, and imagery); distraction (most efficacious if all senses are involved); music therapy; guided imagery (pleasant imaging); meditation; poetry; humor; vibration; hypnosis; and animal therapy. Warm/cold compresses, TENS, and acupuncture are also nonpharmacologic but require a physician order.

39. What are the nursing considerations for nonpharmacologic pain management?
It is important to individualize the pain control plan and to allow the patient to choose the type of strategy that he or she desires. Use nonpharmacologic interventions in addition to pharmacologic interventions. The pain management team can reduce the analgesics gradually and evaluate the efficacy of nonpharmacologic interventions. The involvement of family and friends in the decision-making process may prove useful. Never force the pain management plan onto the patient. Match the intervention to the patient's coping style. Consider any religious or cultural taboos. Consider the patient's condition and the energy expenditure needed to perform the strategy. For example, cancer patients are plagued with fatigue; therefore, it is wise to choose a strategy to which they agree and which they are able to perform.

40. What should the nurse incorporate into patient pain education?
- Explain what pain is.
- Dispel misconceptions.
- State the consequences of unrelieved pain.
- Explain pain intensity rating scales and encourage patient involvement.
- Have patients identify their pain control goals.
- Provide educational materials.

41. What is a disadvantage of using meperidine for pain?
Meperidine has a neurotoxic metabolite that can cause seizures.

42. What are the primary considerations with oral/enteral administration of pain medications?
- When using a nasogastric tube, never crush an extended-release opioid. Crushing concentrates the drug and may cause respiratory depression.
- Oral administration is usually the preferred route.
- In general, oral drugs are less expensive and more convenient.
- Oral drugs have a slower onset and a delayed peak analgesic effect.
- Oral equianalgesic dose is higher than the IV dose.

43. Why is the oral equianalgesic dose higher than the IV dose?
Whereas parenteral medications bypass the GI tract, enteral medications must make their way through the GI tract. After absorption through the GI tract, the medication passes through the liver by way of the portal circulation. This first pass through the liver produces a notable loss of medication due to biotransformation and secretion into the bile. After this initial loss the medication is distributed to the body tissues via the general circulation.

44. Is there a difference between medications given orally and rectally?
Equianalgesic dosing is the same for the oral and rectal routes.

45. What are the nursing considerations in giving IV pain medications?
- The IV route is the first choice for severe pain.

- The IV route has a faster onset of action and more accurate dosing.
- Change to oral medications as soon as possible.
- IV drugs are associated with an increased risk of adverse effects (e.g., respiratory depression).
- Continuous infusion offers steady drug delivery and maintains blood levels through tapering and titrating (patient-controlled analgesia).

46. Is there a difference between intramuscular (IM) and subcutaneous (SQ) administration of pain medication?
- SQ administration has 100% absorption and minimizes circulatory overload.
- IM absorption is erratic, variable, painful, and associated with slow onset of action. It is not recommended for chronic, repetitive analgesic needs and should be avoided in patients with thrombocytopenia, neutropenia, or cachexia.

47. When is epidural or intrathecal administration useful?
- Epidural/intrathecal administration is used for short-term intermediate pain management.
- The equianalgesic dose is as follows: 10 mg morphine = 1 mg epidural = 0.1 mg intrathecal.

48. What are the nursing considerations for using transdermal pain medications?
- Transdermal pain medications can be used for stable, chronic, moderate-to-severe pain.
- Convert to transdermal pain medications only after the pain is controlled with short-acting opioids.
- Onset of action is 8–12 hours.
- Half-life = 16 hours.
- Absorption through the skin forms a deposit of drug under the skin that continues to diffuse even after the patch is removed.
- Absorption is increased by body heat.
- Avoid shaved, broken skin or hairy areas when applying.
- The patient can shower or bathe but should avoid hot tubs or saunas.

49. What positive patient outcomes are associated with successful pain management?
- Shorter recovery time
- Improved patient outcomes and quality of life
- Cost savings in the tens of thousands of dollars
- Decreased incidence of assisted suicide
- Decreased adverse drug reactions from intramuscular injections
- Shorter hospital stay (discharges 2–4 days earlier)
- Decreased readmissions, resulting in a savings of millions of dollars

50. Why is documentation of patient pain and therapy effectiveness necessary?
If it is not documented, it was not done. Incomplete documentation results in a breakdown in the communication process and discontinuity in patient care.

51. Summarize the advantages of complete pain documentation and the disadvantages of incomplete documentation.

Complete Documentation	Incomplete Documentation
Improves pain management	Lack of complete information
Ability to track and trend what is helpful and what is not	Inability to determine medication efficacy
Ability to stay ahead of the pain	Inability to determine maximal ceiling dose
Aids in mobility, healing, and overall comfort and confidence postoperatively	Inability to determine side effect (good vs. undesired)
Allows one to know what to do or try next	Not aware of drug efficacy
Ability to read about side effects	Not aware of teaching efficacy
	Inability to know what to try next

52. What are the physiologic consequences of unrelieved pain?

Unrelieved pain can inhibit the immune system and decrease breathing volume, gastric/bowel function, and mobility. Pain can increase metabolism, fluid retention, blood clotting, muscle tension, and tumor growth; it also triggers stress responses in the body. Cough suppression due to pain may lead to retention of secretions, potentially leading to pneumonia.

53. List the potential psychosocial effects of unrelieved pain.

The potential psychosocial effects of unrelieved pain include anxiety, fear, apprehension, depression, and suicide. Pain interrupts sleeping habits, ADLs, and interpersonal relationships, leading to altered quality of life. Chronic pain threatens beliefs about self-control and self-image, which heightens anxiety and the sense of helplessness. Chronic pain can also be associated with guilt-producing behavior (e.g., retribution for prior actions), which further heightens the anxiety level. A person with chronic pain may be socially isolated by the pain or other factors, which in turn exacerbates the pain.

54. What are the economic effects of patient pain?

The patient's length of stay in hospital can be extended by chronic pain, leading to increased health care costs. Sick time, disability claims, and loss of productivity or employment are potential outcomes for patients with chronic pain.

55. What agencies can the nurse contact for further pain management information?

- American Academy of Pain Management (ACPM)
  13947 Mono Way No. A
  Sonora, CA 95370
  (209) 533-9744
  http://www.aapainmanage.org/index.html
- American Academy of Pain Medicine
  4700 W. Lake Avenue
  Glenview, IL 60025
  (847) 375-4731
  http://www.painmed.org
- American Chronic Pain Association
  P.O. Box 850
  Rocklin, CA 95677
  (916) 632-0922

- American Society of Pain Management Nurses
  7794 Grow Drive
  Pensacola, FL 32514
  (888) 342-7766
  http://www.aspmn.org
- Agency for Healthcare Quality and Research
  Publications Clearinghouse
  P.O. Box 8547
  Silver Spring, MD 20907
  1-800-358-9295
- American Pain Society
  4700 West Lake Ave.
  Glenview, IL. 60025-1485
  (847) 375-4715
  http://www.ampainsoc.org

BIBLIOGRAPHY

1. American Society of Anesthesiologists: Practice guidelines for chronic pain management. Anesthesiology 86(4):995–1004, 1997.
2. Anderson C: What's new in pain management? Home Healthcare Nurse 18(10):648–656, 2000.
3. Carns P, et al: Health Care Guideline: Assessment and Management of Acute Pain. Bloomington, IN, Institute for Clinical Systems Improvement, 2002.
4. Dempsey SK: Pain assessment. Adv Nurses 3(2):10–14, 2001.
5. Gunnarsdottir S, Donovan HS, Serlin RC, et al: Patient-related barriers to pain management: The barriers questionnaire II. Pain 99:385–396, 2002.
6. Huether S, McCance K: Understanding Pathophysiology, 2nd ed. St Louis, Mosby, 2000.
7. Kreger C: Spinal anesthesia and analgesia: Getting to the root of the pain. Nursing 2001 31(6): 36–42, 2001.
8. Lewis SM, Heitkemper MM, Dirksen SR: Medical Surgical Nursing: Assessment and Management of Clinical Problems, 5th ed. St Louis, Mosby, 2000.
9. Malloy P, Moran K: Getting ready for the survey: A multidisciplinary approach to addressing the new JCAHO pain standard. Adv Nurses 3(2):21–24, 2001.
10. McCaffery M, Pasero C: Pain: Clinical Manual, 2nd ed. St Louis, Mosby, 1999.
11. McCaffery M, Pasero C: How to choose the best route for an opioid. Nursing 2000 30(12):34–40, 2000.
12. Schoen DC: NAON Core Curriculum for Orthopaedic Nursing, 4th ed. Pittman, NJ, Anthony J. Jannetti, 2001.
13. United States Department of Health and Human Services: Acute Pain Management in Adults: Operative Procedures: Clinical Practice Guideline. Rockville, MD, Agency for Health Care Policy and Research, 1992.
14. United States Department of Health and Human Services: Management of Cancer Pain: Clinical Practice Guideline. Rockville, MD, Agency for Health Care Policy and Research, 1992.

17. ORTHOPEDIC MEDICATIONS

Debra A. Hrelic, RNC, PhD (c)

1. What is inflammation?

Inflammation is the body's response to tissue injury and infection. It can be divided into three different categories: acute inflammation, the immune response, and chronic inflammation. Inflammation is a protective mechanism in which the body attempts to establish tissue repair by accumulating fluid, blood products (in particular, leukocytes), and chemical action at the site of the injury or infection. Prostaglandins released at the site of injury cause vasodilation, relaxation of smooth muscle, increased capillary permeability, and sensitization of nerve cells to pain. Medications that inhibit the action of prostaglandins are called prostaglandin-inhibitors or anti-inflammatory drugs.

2. What are the cardinal signs of inflammation?

Erythema (redness) is present in the initial phase of inflammation. It is caused by the accumulation of blood in the area of the injury. Kinins, neuropeptides, and histamines are chemical mediators (prostaglandins) that are also released at the site, along with leukocytes and platelets. Histamines dilate the arterioles, enabling this response.

Edema (swelling) occurs with the inflammatory process. Plasma leaks from the intravascular fluids into the interstitial space at the site of the injury. In addition, there is an increase in capillary permeability, as kinins dilate the arterioles.

Heat (warmth) at the inflammatory site can be due to the increased blood and fluid accumulation. Pyrogens, which cause fever, may interfere with the body's temperature-regulating system in the hypothalamus, thus causing heat at the site.

Pain at the site of the injury is caused by the swelling of the tissues as a result of increased interstitial fluids and the release of kinins, neuropeptides, and histamines (chemical mediators).

Loss of function is also caused by the increase of fluids into the injured area. In addition, pain can inhibit range of motion and decrease normal functioning ability.

3. What are NSAIDs? What do they do?

Nonsteroidal anti-inflammatory drugs (NSAIDs) are the family of aspirin-like drugs that inhibit the enzyme cyclooxygenase, which is needed for prostaglandin biosynthesis. In addition to anti-inflammatory properties, NSAIDs also provide pain relief (analgesics), reduce elevated body temperature (antipyretics), and inhibit platelet aggregation (anticoagulants). They act by suppressing inflammation, relieving pain, and reducing fever. NSAIDs may be called prostaglandin inhibitors, or nonopioid analgesics, and have varying degrees of analgesic and antipyretic effects. They are used primarily as anti-inflammatory agents to reduce inflammation with mild-to-moderate pain.

4. Which NSAIDs other than aspirin can be purchased over the counter?

Ibuprofen (Motrin, Nuprin, Advil, Medipren) and naproxen (Aleve) can be purchased without prescription. Generic forms of these medications are also available. A health care provider must prescribe all other NSAIDs.

5. Do all NSAIDs work the same?

NSAIDs are used primarily as anti-inflammatory and analgesic agents; their efficacy varies. Aspirin and ibuprofen are the drugs of choice to relieve headache and reduce fever. Ibuprofen and naproxen are more appropriate for reducing swelling, pain, and stiffness in joints.

6. Are NSAIDs appropriate for all clients?

NSAIDs are contraindicated in people with severe renal or hepatic disease, asthma, and peptic ulcers. NSAIDs should not be given to clients who are taking anticoagulants such as heparin or warfarin (Coumadin). They should be used with extreme caution in clients with bleeding disorders, during early pregnancy and lactation, and in patients with systemic lupus erythematosus (SLE). Like many other medications, NSAIDs should be prescribed with caution in elderly and very young patients. Elderly people are at a greater risk for gastrointestinal (GI) complications. Aspirin should not be used in children with fever of unknown origin, influenza, or chickenpox because of the risk of Reye's syndrome.

7. What are the possible side effects of NSAIDs?

Side effects include GI complications (anorexia, nausea, vomiting, diarrhea), edema, rash, purpura, tinnitus, fatigue, dizziness, lightheadedness, anxiety, and confusion. Bleeding, most commonly in patients with peptic ulcer disease, is also an adverse reaction. Life-threatening adverse reactions include blood dyscrasias, cardiac dysrhythmias, renal failure or insufficiency, and anaphylaxis. In some clients with asthma, the administration of aspirin and other NSAIDs can lead to bronchospasm.

8. What are COX-1 and COX-2 inhibitors?

The actions of two enzyme forms of cyclooxygenase (COX-1 and COX-2) are inhibited by NSAIDs. COX-1 protects the stomach lining and regulates blood platelets. When NSAIDs inhibit COX-1, they decrease the protection of the stomach lining. GI symptoms (in particular, stomach ulcers and gastric bleeding) can occur. Other signs of gastric irritation are anorexia, nausea, vomiting, and diarrhea. COX-1 is expressed in the stomach and kidneys. COX-2 is responsible for regulation of the inflammatory response. It triggers inflammation and pain. Inhibition of the COX-2 receptors, as an action of NSAIDs, decreases inflammation and discomfort.

Highly selective COX-2 inhibitors (celecoxib, rofecoxib) have been developed to decrease the unpleasant and potentially dangerous complications of NSAIDs. These medications effect only COX-2 receptor sites and have no effect on COX-1. Therefore, they have no effect on platelet aggregation and bleeding. This selectivity decreases potentially dangerous GI and renal complications, while still decreasing inflammation and pain. COX-2 inhibitors are a preferred option for long-term use of NSAIDs and chronic inflammatory disease. They are better tolerated and less likely to cause GI events.

9. What specific concerns are related to the use of celecoxib or rofecoxib compared with other NSAIDs?

Both celecoxib (Celebrex) and rofecoxib (Vioxx) are selective COX-2 inhibitors. **Celecoxib** is theoretically safe for clients taking warfarin. It is contraindicated for clients with sulfa allergy or hypersensitivity reaction, because it is a member of the sulfonamide family. Celecoxib should not be used in late pregnancy or in patients with kidney or liver problems. Taking celecoxib and aspirin together can increase the risk for developing stomach ulcers.

Rofecoxib takes approximately 5 days to reach a therapeutic level. It is not recommended for clients with severe hepatic insufficiency or advanced kidney disease. Rofecoxib can be taken with or without food. It is currently under evaluation for treating rheumatoid arthritis, inhibiting the progression of Alzheimer's disease, and causing regression of polyps in the colon.

10. What are the nursing implications for clients taking NSAIDs?

The nurse must identify whether the prescribed NSAID is an inhibitor of both COX-1 and COX-2 or COX-2 alone. The nurse also should obtain a drug history, including any over-the-counter medications, and note a history of any allergies or drug reactions. Side effects to watch for include bleeding gums, petechiae, ecchymosis, and black (tarry) stools. Because bleeding time may be prolonged, NSAIDs should be discontinued 1 week before elective surgery or the anticipated date of parturition. The patient should be asked about any GI discomfort and advised to take NSAIDs with meals to prevent GI upset. The nurse should monitor vital signs and check for peripheral edema. In evaluating the effectiveness of the drug therapy, the nurse should ask about and assess for decreases in pain and swelling of joints and an increase in mobility.

11. How do corticosteroids work?

Corticosteroids (prednisone, prednisolone, dexamethasone) suppress inflammation and modify the normal immune response to injury or infection. They are not suitable for use in chronic inflammatory diseases because of the many serious side effects, including adrenal insufficiency. In general, corticosteroids are prescribed for acute episodes of inflammation and arthritis flare-ups, using the lowest possible dose for the shortest period of time.

12. What special concerns apply to the prescription of corticosteroids?

Steroids are potent anti-inflammatory medications that have both systemic and local effects. They decrease the production of prostaglandins, cytokines, and interleukins and, in turn, suppress inflammation. In addition, corticosteroids decrease proliferation and migration of lymphocytes and macrophages, thereby modifying the normal immune response. Health care providers must be extremely cautious in prescribing systemic corticosteroids because they mask the signs and symptoms of infection. Corticosteroids are contraindicated in clients with a hypersensitivity to the drug or with systemic viral or fungal infections. Sensitivity to sulfites or tartrazine is an additional consideration, because some steroid preparations contain these substances. Corticosteroids are not recommended for chronic inflammatory conditions or sustained use. Liver dysfunction may impair the conversion of prednisone into active prednisolone.

13. What side effects and life-threatening reactions may be associated with corticosteroid therapy?

Prednisone significantly interacts with a variety of medications. It can also interfere with accurate laboratory measurement (serum potassium, glucose tolerance tests, urinalysis, and cultures). Complications of corticosteroid therapy may affect any system of the body. Common side effects include euphoria, peptic ulcers, and insomnia. Less common side effects include headaches, hypertension, edema, moon face, buffalo hump, hyperglycemia, weight gain, and depression. Life-threatening side effects include seizures, heart failure, arrhythmias, thromboembolism, and acute adrenal insufficiency.

14. How should corticosteroids be administered?
For the best results, corticosteroids should be administered according to a pre-scribed schedule that preferably follows the normal pattern of cortisol secretion. To reduce or eliminate GI complaints, administer corticosteroids with meals.

15. What factor should be considered when corticosteroids are discontinued?
Before discontinuing the use of corticosteroids, the dosage should be tapered over a period of 5–10 days. Gradually decreasing the dosage prevents adrenal insufficiency or shutdown.

16. What are the nursing implications for clients taking corticosteroids?
Because corticosteroids can affect nearly every body system, the nurse must be alert to the potential for severe side effects. Most adverse effects occur with long-term or high-dose usage. The nurse obtains a drug history, including any over-the-counter medications, because corticosteroids interact with a variety of medications. The nurse notes any history of drug allergies or drug reactions.

Central nervous system (CNS) adverse reactions may include emotional lability, paresthesias, seizures, insomnia, nervousness, and increased intracranial pressure with papilledema. Possible endocrine and metabolic adverse reactions include glucose intol-erance, hyperglycemia, hyperlipidemia, iatrogenic diabetes, obesity, increased serum lipids and serum triglycerides, protein wasting, amenorrhea, and postmenopausal bleeding. The nurse must be alert for cardiovascular problems, including thromboem-bolism, arrhythmias (secondary to potassium alterations), hypertension, and congestive heart failure. GI side effects may include pancreatitis, ulcerative esophagitis, increased appetite, nausea or vomiting, and peptic ulcer perforation or hemorrhage. The patient should be observed for fluid retention or edema. Lab results must be monitored for potassium and sodium loss and negative calcium balance.

Other possibilities include an altered inflammatory response, leukocytosis, and leukopenia; duration of corticosteroid therapy may also correlate directly with oppor-tunistic infections. Growth failure in children, myopathy, and osteoporosis are poten-tial musculoskeletal side effects of corticosteroid usage. Increased intraocular pressure, cataracts, glaucoma and exophthalmia are potential ocular side effects. Integumentary side effects, such as acne, ecchymosis, petechiae, thinning and increased fragility of the skin, striae, purpura and subcutaneous fat atrophy, may develop. If the dose of med-ication is not gradually tapered, withdrawal syndrome may develop. Cushingoid char-acteristics may also develop with long-term usage.

17. What are DMARDs? When are they used?
Disease-modifying antirheumatic drugs (DMARDs) include gold therapy, im-munosuppressive agents, and antimalarials. DMARDs have more toxic side effects than NSAIDS. They are used to control immune-mediated arthritic disease when NSAIDs are not effective. DMARDs are prescribed for rheumatoid arthritis to alter the disease process itself and to slow its progression. It may take from 6 weeks to 6 months to see the effects of DMARDs, which are comparatively slow-acting. The efficacy of long-term therapy with DMARDs is somewhat controversial.

18. What are the nursing implications of DMARDs?

The nurse should obtain a complete health history and a complete medication history. In monitoring lab results, proteinuria and hematuria should be evaluated before initiating and during therapy. Observing the client for adverse or allergic reaction (anaphylaxis) to gold compounds is important. Such reactions usually occur within the first 15 minutes after injection. The nurse should check for side effects, instructing clients to report them immediately. The client should be told that several weeks to several months may elapse before any effect can be seen. To evaluate the effectiveness of DMARD therapy, assess the patient's pain and amount of inflammation.

19. What is gold therapy?

Gold therapy, also called chrysotherapy, is the most frequently used form of DMARD. It is used to relieve the inflammation and pain of rheumatoid arthritis and to arrest disease progression and resulting deformities. Gold therapy inhibits the synthesis of prostaglandins and decreases phagocytosis. It is contraindicated in cases of severe hepatic or renal disease, colitis, systemic lupus erythematosus (SLE), eczema, pregnancy, and blood dyscrasias. It should be prescribed with caution in people with diabetes mellitus and congestive heart failure. Use of gold therapy slightly increases liver enzymes and may interact with anticancer drugs to cause bone marrow depression. Gold compounds are available in parenteral form (aurothiomalate and aurothioglucose) for intramuscular administration and in oral form (auranofin). They also are indicated for use in active rheumatoid arthritis.

20. What are the side effects and life-threatening reactions of gold therapy?

A significant number of clients receiving gold compounds experience some form of toxicity that ultimately results in discontinuation of therapy. The most common side effect is pruritus. Other side effects include GI disturbances (anorexia, nausea, vomiting, diarrhea), stomatitis, abdominal cramping, CNS disturbances (dizziness, headache), metallic taste, peripheral neuropathy, rash, and photosensitivity. Uncommon side effects include corneal gold deposits, urticaria, hematuria, proteinuria, and bradycardia. Life-threatening reactions involve anaphylaxis, angioedema, acute renal failure, thrombocytopenia, aplastic anemia, agranulocytosis, leukopenia, and fatal bone marrow suppression. Side effects may occur at any time during therapy or several months after therapy.

21. When are immunosuppressive agents used?

Immunosuppressive agents are used to treat rheumatoid arthritis that does not respond to other anti-inflammatory medications. Drugs such as azathioprine (Imuran), cyclophosphamide (Cytoxin), and methotrexate (Mexate) are used in low doses to suppress the inflammatory process of rheumatoid arthritis. These drugs are not used unless other treatment options fail.

22. When are antimalarials used?

Like immunosuppressive therapy, antimalarials are used only when other methods of treatment are not effective. The mode of action of antimalarials in suppression of rheumatoid arthritis is not clear. It may take from 4 to 12 weeks for the effects of treatment to become apparent. Antimalarials are usually given in combination with NSAIDs when rheumatoid arthritis is not controlled.

23. What medications are used to treat gout?

Allopurinol (Alloprin, Purinol, Zyloprim, Lopurin) is used to control the primary hyperuricemia that accompanies severe gout and to prevent flare-ups of acute gouty attacks. Allopurinol is administered on a long-term basis to clients with chronic gout and is not used in the treatment of acute gout.

Colchicine, used in acute gout attacks, has anti-inflammatory properties. It is highly effective in treating acute gout but is not an effective analgesic for other types of pain. Colchicine does not affect uric acid clearance by the renal system. Low doses may be used for prophylaxis to reduce the frequency of multiple gout attacks.

Probenecid is used for recurrent attacks of gout. The acute attack of gout must subside before probenecid is used. It inhibits renal tubular reabsorption of uric acid, thereby promoting renal excretion. Caution must be exercised in patients with blood dyscrasias, uric acid kidney stones, and history of uric acid disease. Clients must have adequate fluid intake to avoid crystallization of uric acid in acidic urine.

24. What are the side effects of antigout medications?

Side effects include renal complications (bladder spasms, nephrotoxicity, proteinuria, hematuria, anuria, acute renal failure), integumentary symptoms (angioedema, urticaria, injection site reaction, skin necrosis, tissue necrosis, median nerve neuritis), and endocrine effects (hypothyroidism). GI disturbances are the most common adverse reactions to colchicine. Nausea, vomiting, abdominal pain, and paralytic ileus are often seen. These effects may indicate toxicity; therefore, the medication is generally discontinued until symptoms subside.

25. What are the nursing implications of antigout medications?

As always, the nurse obtains a complete medical history as well as a complete medication history, including over-the-counter drugs. Education and prevention are key components in the treatment of gout. Clients should be advised to take colchicine immediately when symptoms occur. They must also be educated about possible side effects, possible signs of toxicity, and when to notify their health care provider. Clients need to be told to avoid alcohol, which can cause increased uric acid in the blood and thus increase the likelihood of a gouty attack. The nurse should review the patient's diet, identifying foods that are high in purines to decrease dietary intake of uric acid. The nurse also should evaluate the client's response to the antigout drug and monitor lab results, including blood and urine, at least monthly.

26. What medications are available for the treatment of osteoporosis?

Alendronate (Fosamax) is used to treat and prevent osteoporosis in postmenopausal women. It is also used in the treatment of Paget's disease. Alendronate is a highly selective inhibitor of bone resorption. It has been found to increase bone mineral density. For optimal absorption, alendronate needs to be taken on an empty stomach with 8 oz of water, at least 30 minutes before any food, beverage, or other medication is taken. Because esophageal irritation is a concern, clients are advised to sit or stand immediately after taking alendronate.

Calcitonin (Calcimar) is available by injection and is effective for osteoporosis and bone pain after a compressed fracture. Side effects include GI symptoms (nausea, vomiting, diarrhea), flushed feeling, rash, and local reaction at injection site. Miacalcin nasal spray also blocks resorption of bone but is not as effective as alendronate. It is an alternative for patients with esophageal problems. Side effects may include irritation or ulceration of the nostril and GI complications (nausea, vomiting, diarrhea), flushing, or rash.

Conjugated estrogens (Prempro, Premphase, Premarin without progesterone) are an effective treatment for postmenopausal osteoporosis. They should be combined with calcium and vitamin D. Side effects of estrogens include breast pain, vaginal bleeding, weight changes, possible increased risk for uterine or breast cancer, possible increased clotting problems, and deep vein thrombosis. Conjugated estrogens may cause hypercalcemia in clients with metastatic bone lesions.

Raloxifene (Evista) is an oral alternative for women who cannot tolerate estrogens or who have a family history of breast cancer. It acts by binding to estrogen receptors, producing estrogen-like effects on bone, and results in decreased resorption of bone and decreased bone turnover. It should not be used in women with a history of clotting problems. Raloxifene can cause leg cramps, hot flashes, deep vein thrombosis, and pulmonary embolus (if deep vein thrombosis is untreated).

Risedronate (Actonel) is also used in the treatment of osteoporosis. Like alendronate, risedronate improves bone mineral density and helps to prevent fractures. Risedronate may produce esophageal symptoms, including heartburn or reflux, and therefore should be taken with water. Clients are advised not to lie down after administration but to remain sitting or standing. In addition, clients should wait a full 30 minutes before ingesting any other food, beverage, or medication.

27. When are muscle relaxants used?

Muscle relaxants are used in the management of muscle spasms associated with acute musculoskeletal disorders or injuries. They are also used as supportive therapy in clients suffering from tetanus or fibromyalgia. Examples include cyclobenzaprine, carisoprodol, chlorphenesin, chlorzoxazone, metaxalone, methocarbamol, and orphenadrine.

28. Are muscle relaxants safe for all clients?

Muscle relaxants are contraindicated in clients with hyperthyroidism because of an increased risk of developing arrhythmias or tachycardia. Caution should be exercised in clients who have heart failure, cardiac arrhythmias, or atrioventricular block and during the acute recovery phase of myocardial infarction.

Careful monitoring is required for patients with increased intraocular pressure, glaucoma, or urinary retention because of the anticholinergic properties of muscle relaxants. Caution also should be exercised in pregnant or breastfeeding women.

29. What are the potential side effects and adverse reactions of muscle relaxants?

The most common side effects of muscle relaxants are mild CNS depression and anticholinergic activity. Additional effects include fatigue, loss of strength, nausea, vomiting, constipation, dyspepsia, dysgeusia, blurred vision, headache, nervousness, drowsiness, dizziness, dry mouth, and confusion. Life-threatening side effects include seizures and anaphylactic reactions.

30. What drug interactions must the nurse consider when administering skeletal muscle relaxants?

Then nurse must be concerned with possible interactions between muscle relaxants and other CNS depressants or antimuscarinic drugs. Muscle relaxants also react with tramadol, guanethidine, monoamine oxidase inhibitors, H-1 blocking agents, alcohol, and various herbal remedies.

31. What are the nursing implications of muscle relaxants?

The nurse should obtain a complete health history, including any preexisting diseases, as well as a complete medication history, including over-the-counter and herbal remedies. While the patient is taking muscle relaxants, the nurse should observe for CNS depression, monitor for sedation and dizziness, assist in ambulation, and ensure client safety. The effectiveness of the muscle relaxant should be monitored to determine whether the client's muscular pain has decreased or disappeared. The patient should be instructed to avoid use of alcohol or other CNS depressants. Side effects that the nurse should monitor include seizure activity, blood pressure changes, and paralytic ileus. The patient should also be educated about potential side effects and drug interactions and when to notify their health care provider. If the patient's usual dosage has been high or if the medication has been used over a prolonged period, the medication should be tapered gradually when it is discontinued to avoid rebound spasms.

32. What medications are available for the treatment of osteomyelitis?

Osteomyelitis refers to a bone infection, usually caused by bacteria. Bone infection, if left untreated, can result in deterioration of the bone itself. Osteomyelitis may be acute or chronic and can affect any age group. Antibiotic therapy is the treatment of choice for osteomyelitis; up to 2 months of intravenous and oral antibiotics may be required, accompanied by bed-rest and immobilization. Osteomyelitis is difficult to cure and may persist for years.

Specific antibiotic treatment is based on the infecting organism, as determined by culture. Cefazolin, cephalothin, and cephradine are frequently the drugs of choice because of their ability to penetrate into the bone itself, thereby directly attacking the infection. Oral ciprofloxacin has also been successful in the treatment of *Pseudomonas aeruginosa* osteomyelitis.

33. Discuss the side effects and adverse reactions of cephalosporin treatment.

Nausea, diarrhea, and rash are common side effects of cephalosporins. Less common side effects include dizziness, headache, vomiting, anorexia, anemia, and pruritus. Leukopenia, thrombocytopenia, Stevens-Johnson syndrome, and anaphylactic reactions are potential life-threatening reactions. As with any antibiotic, superinfection is also a risk.

34. What are the nursing implications of cephalosporin treatment?

Cephalosporins are contraindicated in patients with hypersensitivity to cephalosporins or with serious hypersensitivity to penicillin. In addition, they should be used with caution in clients with a history of renal impairment or GI disease. The nurse should assess the client for infection before and throughout therapy. Culture and sensitivity tests for infection should be done before initiation of therapy. Observation for allergic reactions, including anaphylaxis (rash, pruritus, laryngeal edema, wheezing), is extremely important. Epinephrine, an antihistamine, and resuscitation equipment should be kept available to treat anaphylactic reaction. The nurse also should be aware of pain at intramuscular site and phlebitis at the intravenous site.

Cephalosporin treatment may cause a positive Coombs' test in clients who receive high doses or in newborns whose mothers were treated with cephalosporins before delivery. Other lab considerations include a possible increase in serum levels of aspartate aminotransferase (AST), alanine aminotransferase (ALT), alkaline phosphatase, bilirubin, lactate dehydrogenase (LDH), blood urea nitrogen (BUN), and creatinine. Rare but serious complications of cephalosporin treatment include leukopenia, neutropenia, agranulocytosis, thrombocytopenia, eosinophilia, lymphocytosis, and thrombocytosis. The nurse should instruct the patient to take the entire course of medication, unless otherwise directed by the health care provider. Clients also should be educated about possible allergic reactions or side effects and told when to notify their health care provider.

35. What considerations apply to the use of nonprescription joint and cartilage supplements?

Herbal/nutritional supplements are common alternatives to prescription medications for joint and cartilage problems. Descriptions of herbal/nutritional supplements differ because of the lack of governmental regulations in regard to specific ingredients. Efficacy also varies according to source and report. Supplements have been used in conjunction with a prescribed regimen and as alternatives to standard therapy. Patients should discuss herbal/nutritional supplements with their health care providers before using them. No scientific body of evidence has established either the effectiveness and or the adverse effects of these supplements.

BIBLIOGRAPHY

1. Arthritis and Pain Medication. Retrieved April 24, 2002, from <http://enotes.tripod.com/painRx.htm>.
2. Aschenbrenner DS, Cleveland SW, Venable SJ: Drug Therapy in Nursing. Philadelphia, Lippincott Williams & Wilkins, 2002.
3. Celebrex Facts: Celebrate Arthritis Pain Relief. Retrieved April 24, 2002, from <http://www.celebrex.com/celebrex_facts.asp>.
4. Celebrex vs. Vioxx: How These New Arthritis Meds Differ. Retrieved April 24, 2002, from <http://www.healthboards.com/arthritis/2006.html>.
5. Deglin JH, Vallerand AH: Davis's Drug Guide for Nurses, 7th ed. Philadelphia, F.A.Davis, 2001.
6. Furst D, Munster T: Nonsteroidal anti-inflammatory drugs, disease modifying, antirheumatic drugs, non-opioid analgesics, and drugs used in gout. In Basic and Clinical Pharmacology, 8th ed. New York, Lange Medical Books/McGraw-Hill, 2000, pp 596–623.
7. LeFever Kee J, Hayes ER: Pharmacology: A Nursing Process Approach, 3rd ed. Philadelphia, W.B.Saunders, 2000.
8. Lehne RA: Aspirin-like drugs: Nonsteroidal anti-inflammatory drugs and acetaminophen. In Pharmacology for Nursing Care. Philadelphia, W.B. Saunders, 1994, pp 777–791.
9. Lew DP: Osteomyelitis. N Engl J Med 336:999, 1977.
10. McCuistion LE, Gutierrez KJ: Real-World Nursing Survival Guide: Pharmacology. Philadelphia, W.B. Saunders, 2002.
11. Nelson JD: Toward simple but safe management of osteomyelitis. Pediatrics 99:883, 1997.
12. Osteoporosis Medications—Arthritis Central. Retrieved April 24, 2002, from <http://www.arthritiscentral.com/html/medsosteo.htm>.
13. Reynolds M: Go With Herbs. Retrieved May 20, 2002, from <http://www.gowithherbs.com/903-4.htm>.
14. Shannon MT, Stang CL, Wilson BA: Nurses Drug Guide 2000. Norwalk, CT, Appleton & Lange, 2000.
15. Wheeless' Textbook of Orthopaedics: Management of Gout. Retrieved April 24, 2002, from <http://www.medmedia.com/o2/86.htm>.
16. Wheeless' Textbook of Orthopaedics: NSAIDS. Retrieved April 24, 2002, from <http://www.medmedia.com/oa2/110.htm>.

18. REHABILITATION

Barbara J. Heckman, MSN, RN, ANP-C

1. Define rehabilitation.

Rehabilitation can be defined as restoring a person to his or her fullest physical, psychological, social, spiritual, educational, and vocational potential after a disabling disease, anatomic impairment, or injury. Under the concept of rehabilitation, the patient works to obtain optimal function despite residual disability, even if an irreversible pathologic process causes the impairment.

2. Discuss the scope of rehabilitation.

Rehabilitation is a holistic and comprehensive approach to medical care that uses an interdisciplinary team approach, including the collaborative efforts of a doctor, nurse, psychologist, social worker, dietician, and physical, occupational, speech, recreational, and vocational therapists, as appropriate. The patient and family as well as the team members set goals and desired outcomes. Rehabilitation can occur in a variety of settings, including the hospital, rehabilitation facility, clinic, private office, and the patient's or family member's home. The scope of rehabilitation nursing encompasses primary prevention through acute and subacute levels of nursing care. Anticipated client outcomes include increased independence, a shortened length of stay, and an improved quality of life.

3. What nursing theories support the rehabilitation concept?

Rehabilitation nursing is built on a foundation of several nursing theories, including the following:

- Martha Rogers' energy fields theory
- Rosemary Parse's man-living-health model
- Virginia Henderson's description of nursing's uniqueness
- Ida Orlando's theory of nurse-patient relationships
- Hildegaarde Peplau's definition of clinical nursing therapeutics
- Imogene King's Open Systems Model
- Sister Calista Roy's Adaptation Model
- Myrna Levine's definition of nursing intervention as a way to help patients conserve energy as well as structural, personal, and social integrity
- Dorothea Orem's definition of the nursing role
- Dorothy Johnson's Behavioral Systems Model
- Betty Neuman's Total Systems Model
- Nancy Roper's Activities of Daily Living Model

Rehabilitation nursing theories range from the use of one theory, such as King's Open Systems Model, which can be used in goal setting, client and family participation, and identifying the client's social system, to Roper's Activities of Daily Living Model, which incorporates the theories of Orlando and Peplau.

4. What are the current disability theories?

Erving Goffman defined the "stigma" that is attached to a person with a disability. He noted that a person with a subtle or nonvisible disability is labeled as passable within the norm, whereas a person with a clearly visible disability is labeled as deviant. The person labeled as deviant is viewed negatively by society and has limited social acceptance. Tamara Dembo's theory builds on Goffman's theory. Dembo theorized that the person with a disability is not only labeled negatively, but also that the disability is "spread" to represent the total perception of that person. Speaking loudly to a person who is blind is an example of Dembo's theory. She also notes that people with disabilities are seen as suffering in society. Beatrice Wright added the theory of a relationship between perception of disability and impressions about attributes of the person with a disability.

5. What are rehabilitation motivational theories?

Rehabilitation motivational theories were proposed by Constantina Safilios-Rothschild and Abram Maslow. Safilios-Rothchild established a social construct of disability that is used when the patient reenters the community. Maslow's theory assists clients in assessing priorities by utilizing a hierarchy of basic needs.

6. What other theories are used in rehabilitation nursing?

Other theories used in rehabilitation nursing include theories of health and wellness, family and ecologic systems theory, cognitive and social learning theories, change theory, psychosocial developmental theories, and role theory. These theories examine relationships within the patient and among the patient, family, and society. These theories assist in explaining the "whys" of rehabilitation nursing. For example, why does a certain phenomenon occur, why do some patients deal with their disabilities better than others, and why does society treat disabled persons as it does?

7. What models are available for theory-based rehabilitation nursing practice?

Models for theory-based rehabilitation nursing practice include client-centered, setting-centered, provider-centered, and collaborative practice models. The client-centered model focuses on the developmental level of the client, type of disability, cultural aspects, and family as client, whereas the setting-centered model focuses on the setting of care, such as acute care, long-term care, community-based settings, and home care. Primary care, case management, nurse-managed care, and independent practice/consultation are included in the provider-centered model. Collaborative practice models involve multidisciplinary teams, interdisciplinary teams, and transdisciplinary teams in their theory on rehabilitation nursing practice.

8. What is CARF?

CARF is the Commission on Accreditation of Rehabilitation Facilities. It is similar to the Joint Commission on Accreditation of Health Organizations (JCAHO) in that it sets minimal standards that the rehabilitation facility must meet to become accredited. Surveys are completed of each rehabilitation facility before accreditation can be given.

9. List the members of the rehabilitation team and their functions.

The rehabilitation team is made up of doctors, nurses, social workers, and therapists. The following list summarizes their functions:

Physiatrist: a physician who specializes in physical medicine and rehabilitation. Physiatrists diagnose and treat disease and disability using physical agents such as heat, cold, light, water, electricity, and mechanical devices.

Prosthetist/orthotist: a specialist responsible for the evaluation, design, fabrication, fit, function, and education of orthoses such as braces and prostheses or artificial limbs.

Psychologist: a mental health professional who tests personality types, problem-solving skills, psychological status, intelligence, memory, and perceptual functioning. Through counseling the psychologist helps patients and their significant others to adjust to the disease or disability and prepares them for rehabilitation participation.

Rehabilitation nurse: a nurse who specializes in the care of patients with physical impairments. Rehabilitation nurses assess the physical and educational needs of patients and their significant others. They also assist patients in setting short- and long-term goals.

Social worker: a professional who interacts with the patient, family, and significant others as well as the rehabilitation team to formulate an adequate discharge plan. Social workers assist in evaluating the patient's living situation, provide information about available resources, and facilitate application to community programs.

Occupational therapist: a therapist who focuses on functional activities that maximize independence. Occupational therapists provide many services, such as evaluation and training in self-care activities (e.g., grooming, bathing, dressing); teaching transfer techniques to and from a wheelchair; evaluation and training in upper extremity function and strength; assistance in the functional use of upper extremity prostheses; driving evaluations, if needed; evaluation and training to maximize function in sensory, perceptual, and cognitive deficits; and home evaluations with suggestions to maximize independence in the home setting.

Physical therapist: a therapist who helps the patient to restore function. Services include restoration and preservation of joint range of motion; evaluation of muscle strength, length, and tone; gait, balance, and transfer evaluations and training; evaluation of the need for assistive devices for mobilization (e.g., walkers, canes, wheelchairs); management of edema; assessment of skin breakdown and pain with mobility; instruction in exercises to restore and preserve function of a joint; and evaluation of the patient's home for discharge preparations.

Recreation therapist: a therapist who uses recreation purposefully as an intervention to produce a physical, social, or emotional change. Recreation therapy may involve one-on-one interactions between patient and therapist or group dynamics.

10. How do these different members work together?

They work together by forming a rehabilitation team that helps patients and families meet their rehabilitation goals.

11. What are the different types of rehabilitation teams?

The three most common teams found in rehabilitation include the multidisciplinary team, the interdisciplinary team, and the transdisciplinary team.

12. What is a multidisciplinary team?

A multidisciplinary team is a combination of different disciplines that provide specific services to the patient. Each member sets discipline-specific goals that work toward goals of the patient and the team as a whole. Communication among team members is imperative for success. The team's outcomes are the sum of each discipline's efforts.

13. How does the interdisciplinary team work?

An interdisciplinary team works with an ideal of collaboration among team members. The team identifies goals, and team members work to prevent duplication or conflict among these goals. Each member works toward attaining the goals within the parameters of his or her discipline. Collaboration among the team members occurs when goals overlap discipline boundaries.

14. What is unique about the transdisciplinary team?
The transdisciplinary team is made up of various disciplines, but the outstanding characteristic of this team is the blurring of boundaries between disciplines. The team members are cross-trained to minimize duplication and maximize efforts in assisting the patient in goal attainment. Because of the blurring of boundaries, the team members must be flexible and receptive to working within wider domains of functioning.

15. What types of goals are set? Who sets them?
According to Mosby, a goal is simply the purpose toward which an endeavor is directed. The patient, family member, and rehabilitation team collaborate to set patient goals. The goals may consist of physical, mental, emotional, and spiritual elements. Both short-term and long-term goals are set at admission and then revised as the patient progresses or if there is a change in patient status or diagnosis.

16. Define orthopedic rehabilitation.
Orthopedic rehabilitation is the concept of restoring patients to their fullest physical, locomotive, and motor potential. It includes achievement of optimal range of motion and optimal use of the skeleton, muscles, joints, and related tissues after injury, trauma, surgery, and disease.

17. What factors influence soft tissue healing?
Trauma, surgery, immobilization, posture, and repeated stress are a few of the factors that influence soft tissue healing. Trauma and immobilization can significantly change the normal mechanics of soft tissues. The biochemical properties of connective tissue are altered during trauma and immobilization. Collagen fibers are laid down in a haphazard "haystack" fashion, which results in a decrease in the extensibility of connective tissues. The goal is remobilization as soon as possible to promote the deposition of new collagen fibers in an orderly fashion.

18. What are the four phases of scar tissue?
Phase I: the inflammatory phase. This phase occurs immediately after trauma or surgery and usually lasts up to 24–48 hours.
Phase II: the granulation phase. This phase is characterized by an increase in the vascularity of tissue and the most extensive remodeling of tissue. Team members need to work closely to determine the extent of movement relative to risk.
Phase III: the fibroplastic phase. This phase, which involves an increase in the number of fibroblasts and rate of production of collagen fibers and ground substance, enables tissue elongation. It can last 3–8 weeks, depending on the histologic makeup and vascularity of the damaged tissue.
Phase IV: the maturation phase. During this phase collagen matures, solidifies, and shrinks. At the end of this phase, tissue remodeling becomes difficult because the tissue reverts to a more mature, inactive, and nonpliable status.

19. What rehabilitation guidelines should be followed in managing scar tissue?
Guidelines include assessing the stage of scar tissue development, beginning light movement as soon as possible to control the direction and length of scar tissue, and stressing scar tissue at the appropriate times to avoid greater tissue injury.

20. What are the goals of mobility work?
The two effects of movement or massage are reflexive and mechanical. Maxey and Magnusson[9] list the following goals of the mechanical changes of mobility work:
- To allow hydration and rehydration of connective tissue
- To promote the breaking and subsequent prevention of cross-links in collagen fibers
- To facilitate the breaking and prevention of macroadhesions
- To allow the plastic deformation and permanent elongation of connective tissues
- To promote the laying down of collagen fibers and scar tissue in the length and direction appropriate for the applied stresses
- To promote the molding and remolding of collagen fibers during the fibroplastic and maturation stages of scar tissue shrinkage
- To prevent scar tissue shrinkage.
- To facilitate the more generalized effects of increased blood flow, increased venous and lymphatic return, and increased cellular metabolism

21. Explain the principle of short and long.
According to the principle of short and long, tissues that are immobilized in a shortened range become more extensible when they are immediately elongated. This principle is useful in examining techniques for massage and mobilization of connective tissue.

22. What techniques are used for mobilization of connective tissue?
- **Muscle slay**: widening or separating longitudinal fibers of muscle or connective tissues that have adhered together. Such adhesions cause fibers to become less efficient in their contracting ability. They also limit the ability of the tissue to lengthen and shorten.
- **Transverse muscle bending**: mobilizing the contractile unit perpendicular to the fibers, thus causing the connective tissue to mobilize and allowing an increase in overall muscle mobility.
- **Bony clearing**: a technique of longitudinal stroking that attempts to clear fascia from a bony surface, thus enhancing mobility along planes of normal movement.
- **Cross-friction**: a type of aggressive massage performed at different angles to access connective tissue fibers in a variety of directions and thus mobilize scar tissue by breaking adhesions. This technique vascularizes nonvascular connective tissue and is particularly effective in the healing of tendons and ligaments.

23. What are the most common injuries that require rehabilitation in athletes?
The most common injuries faced by an athlete that require rehabilitation are injuries to soft tissue, ligaments, tendons, and muscle. Most of these sports-related injuries result from overuse, direct contact, and soft tissue failure. Often repeated use or type of motion causes inflammation due to friction. Examples of overuse are bursal inflammation, plantar fasciitis, and stress fractures. Football players experience direct contact injuries such as acromioclavicular joint separations. Pulled hamstrings and

Achilles tendon ruptures are examples of soft tissue failure most often seen in runners, sprinters, joggers, and jumpers.

24. What is the difference between a sprain and a strain?
Strain is a general term used to indicate damage (usually muscular) resulting from excessive physical force, whereas sprain refers to a more traumatic injury to tendons, muscles, or ligaments around a joint. A sprain is characterized by pain, swelling, and ecchymosis of the skin over the joint. The duration and severity of symptoms vary with the extent of injury to the tissue.

25. How are sprains classified?
Sprains can be classified into three categories. In a **first-degree sprain**, the tissue is slightly torn and the joint is stable with minimal pain and swelling. In a **second-degree sprain**, the injury is more severe; the tissue is significantly torn, but the joint remains stable. A second-degree sprain involves a considerable amount of pain, swelling, and ecchymosis. Usually weight-bearing is difficult. A **third-degree sprain** involves a complete tear of the tissue, and the joint is unstable. Swelling, ecchymosis, pain, and difficulty with weight-bearing are markedly increased.

26. What should the short-term rehabilitative treatment plan for a sprain include?
• Stop or decrease all weight-bearing activities.
• Apply ice for 20 minutes at a time, as many times as possible, throughout the day.
• Prevent swelling by applying compression with an Ace wrap.
• Elevate extremity above heart level to promote return circulation and prevent swelling.
• Prescribe splint, sling, and crutches as necessary.
• Treat pain with a nonsteroidal anti-inflammatory drug (NSAID).

27. What should the long-term rehabilitative treatment plan of a sprain include?
• Alternate heat with cold (i.e., hot water bath for 4–5 minutes alternating with cold water bath for 1–2 minutes). Always end with the cold-water treatment.
• Begin light exercise, with strengthening and stretching exercises progressing to resistive exercises.
• Treat pain, again with NSAIDs.

28. Explain the acronym RICE.
When thinking of short-term interventions for treating a sprain, think of **RICE** therapy:
R = Rest   **C** = Compression
I = Ice   **E** = Elevation

29. Describe the rehabilitation plan for ligament injuries.
The most common injuries to ligaments are tears. Rehabilitation must first take into consideration the degree of the injury as well as the level of activity that the affected area is to undertake. The rehabilitation plan should include initial immobility, NSAIDs, and pain control, followed by a program that includes splinting the affected area with an external device to provide support and stability to the injured ligament. A graded exercise program is suggested for ligament injuries.

Rehabilitation for patients with severe tears may begin only after surgery in which the injured ligament is reconstructed or reconstituted. Maintenance of structural stability and range of motion and strengthening of surrounding musculature are necessary components of the treatment program.

30. What are the primary goals in the treatment and rehabilitation of tendon injuries?

The primary goals in the treatment and rehabilitation of tendon injuries include initial reductions in pain, swelling, and inflammation. Flexibility and strengthening exercises should be well planned according to the activity that the tendon will endure in the future. Maintenance exercises as well as pre- and postactivity flexibility programs are necessary to prevent further injury.

31. What type of muscle injury is most frequently seen in the rehabilitation setting?

The most common muscle injury affects the hamstrings. This muscle group suffers from pulls and tears frequently during sports-related activities because of muscle fatigue and overuse. Muscle strains occur when the muscle is cold, lacks proper circulation, and has not been properly stretched. Muscle strength does not appear to be a factor in the prevention of muscle strain injuries.

32. What type of rehabilitation program is necessary for a muscular injury?

Muscular injury requires a rehabilitation program that educates patients about proper flexibility routines. Initially ice is applied to reduce hemorrhage and decrease inflammation. Once hemorrhaging of the muscle has stopped, anti-inflammatory medication and ultrasound are used to enhance soft tissue extensibility and facilitate stretching.

33 Describe the phases of management and rehabilitation to restore function after a muscle injury.

According to DeLisa et al.,[4] the rehabilitation process can be divided into eight phases, each of which is part of the overall plan to restore function:

- Phase 1: Control the inflammatory process
- Phase 2: Control pain
- Phase 3: Restore joint range of motion and soft tissue extensibility
- Phase 4: Improve muscular strength
- Phase 5: Improve muscular endurance
- Phase 6: Develop specific sport-related biomechanical skill patterns (i.e., coordination and retraining)
- Phase 7: Improve general cardiovascular endurance
- Phase 8: Establish maintenance programs

The maintenance of motivation in the sports-injured patient appears to be the key to success.

34. What are resistive exercises?

Resistive exercises are carefully progressed exercises that must be performed on a regular basis at a minimum of 3 times per week. Active resistant exercise is the movement of a muscle group against a resistive force. Initially, progressive resistance exercise is performed on the muscles that assist in the movement of the injured area. Once the affected area begins to show improvement, the exercises are performed on both the injured extremity and the unaffected extremity to promote strengthening and conditioning for the whole body. The limits of performance must be continuously increased to improve muscle strength.

35. How are isometric exercises performed?

Isometric exercises increase muscle tension by applying pressure against a stable force. The exercise involves contractions of a desired muscle group that are held for 5–6 seconds with 10–20 seconds of rest between each contraction. Contractions can be completed by opposing different muscle groups against each other, as in pressing the hands together. There is no joint movement, and the muscle length remains the same, but muscle strength, tone, and endurance are maintained or improved. The isometric contractions should be carried out frequently each day in sets of 10 or 12 repetitions.

36. How do isotonic exercises differ from isometric exercises?

In isotonic exercises the muscle contracts and causes movement. Because there is no significant change in resistance, the force of the contraction is constant. Isotonic exercise uses free weights, elastic bands, universal exercise machines, or cammed equipment. It is accomplished through repetition of isolated patterns. Isotonic exercise enhances joint mobility and helps to improve muscle strength and tone.

37. What is unique about isokinetic exercise?

In isokinetic exercises, maximum force is exerted by a muscle at each point throughout the active range of motion as the muscle contracts. Isokinetic exercise is progressive, with the first set carried out at a weight allowing 12–15 repetitions. The weight is increased progressively after sets of repetitions until only two or three repetitions can be accomplished at one time. Isokinetic exercise allows the patient to control speed while maintaining force. Progression is marked by measurement of the patient's ability to resist movement.

38. What is the difference between eccentric and concentric contractions?

An **eccentric** muscle contraction involves lengthening of the muscle fibers, as when a weight is lowered through a range of motion. The muscle yields to the resistance, allowing it to be stretched. Eccentric muscle contractions are beneficial in increasing the load ability of a muscle. They are used in the rehabilitation of injuries such as wrist extensor tendinitis, patellar tendinitis, Achilles tendinitis, and rotator cuff tendinitis. **Concentric** muscle contraction, on the other hand, involves a common form of muscle contraction that occurs in rhythmic activities when the muscle fibers shorten as tension develops. Concentric contraction exercise programs are most commonly used in the rehabilitation of injured athletes.

39. Summarize the recommended guidelines for rehabilitation of a rotator cuff repair.

The therapy guidelines for a rotator cuff repair, according to Maxey and Magnusson,[9] involve six phases:

Phase 1 (1–4 weeks after surgery). Goals of rehabilitation include decreasing pain and providing comfort; decreasing inflammation and edema; increasing range of motion of joints; minimizing cervical spine stiffness; protecting the surgical site; maintaining full elbow and wrist range of motion; and maintaining and improving distal muscle strength. Interventions include cryotherapy; electrical stimulation; pendulum exercises with shoulder flexion, external rotation, internal rotation, and abduction; isometric exercises; active range of motion with elbow flexion and extension; active range of motion in all ranges of the cervical spine; progressive resistance exercises; and resistance free joint mobilization.

Phase 2 (5–8 weeks after surgery). Goals of rehabilitation include protecting the surgical site; improving range of motion; increasing strength; decreasing pain and inflammation; maintaining elbow and wrist range of motion; and minimizing cervical stiffness. Interventions include progression of active range of motion; proprioceptive neuromuscular facilitation; shoulder flexion, external rotation, and abduction; soft tissue mobilization; and cardiovascular conditioning.

Phase 3 (9–12 weeks after surgery). Rehabilitation goals include expansion in range of motion; avoidance of impingement problems; gaining full range of motion; increasing strength and function; decreasing soft tissue restrictions and scarring; and alleviation of pain. Interventions include active range of motion using wand exercises; isotonic exercises with shoulder flexion and abduction; scapula exercises with abduction and external rotation; and manual resistive exercises.

Phase 4 (13–16 weeks after surgery). Goals include maintenance of full range of motion, increasing strength and endurance, and improving function. Interventions include progression of exercises performed during phase 3; addition of stretching exercises to the shoulder; isokinetic exercises; trunk and leg strengthening exercises; and joint mobilization exercises for the cervical and thoracic spine, as appropriate.

Phase 5 (17–21 weeks after surgery). Rehabilitation goals include maintenance of full range of motion, increase in strength and endurance, improving neuromuscular control, return to functional activities, and initiation of sport activities. Interventions include the continuation of phase 4 exercises, continuation of joint mobilization efforts as appropriate, and initiation of a throwing program when appropriate.

Phase 6 (22 plus weeks after surgery). Rehabilitation goals include return to everyday activities, maintenance of full range of motion, continued strengthening and endurance, and gradual return to full activities. Athletes usually can return to their sport between 6 and 12 months after surgery. Interventions include maintaining a stretching and strengthening program.

40. What type of setting is best for a patient recovering from a rotator cuff injury?

The rehabilitation program can take place in an inpatient or outpatient setting. The rehabilitation team can create a program that suits the patient's needs and abilities in either setting. In devising a rehabilitation program, it is important to individualize the program and take into consideration factors such as age, condition of the repaired tissues, size of the tear, rate of healing, and the patient's abilities and previous level of function. The key to a successful program is individualizing the program to meet the patient's needs, abilities, and expectations.

41. Outline the postsurgical rehabilitation guidelines for patients with carpal tunnel syndrome.

Maxey and Magnusson[9] describe three phases of a postoperative rehabilitation program for patients with carpal tunnel syndrome:

Phase 1 (weeks 1–4): the inflammatory phase. Rehabilitation goals include decreasing pain; controlling edema; improving active range of motion of the upper extremity; beginning self-management of activities of daily living; educating the patient and significant others about restrictions on activity, exercise, and mobility; increasing strength and gross grasp; decreasing paresthesias and sensitivity; decreasing adhesion formation while increasing scar mobility; prevention of further injury; and maintenance. Rehabilitation interventions include educating the patient about surgical site protection; instructing the patient and significant others to monitor drainage; initial treatment of hand and wrist with elevation and ice; application of hot packs to the area 2 weeks after surgery; beginning active range of motion exercises to the shoulder, elbow, forearm, and fingers; and beginning mobilization of the median nerve.

Phase 2 (weeks 4–6): the proliferation phase. Rehabilitation goals include decreasing pain by 70%; resolution of edema; decreasing sensitivity and adhesion formation of scar; increasing active range of motion of the wrist; increasing tolerance of the upper extremity for reaching away from body; independence with activities of daily living with the use of assistive devices; and beginning to simulate work-related activities. Interventions include continuation of active range of motion exercises to the upper extremity; initiation of stretching exercises of the wrist; beginning wrist isotonic exercises; continuing with scar desensitizing techniques; initiation of scar massage; and providing a work ergonomic evaluation and continuing to simulate work activities in increasing time increments.

Phase 3 (6–12 weeks after surgery): the remodeling and maturation phase. The goals of this phase include decreasing the number of exercises and stretches; acquiring adequate strength to return to work activities on a full-time basis; self-management of symptoms; and education about prevention of future similar injuries. Interventions include progression with upper extremity strengthening exercises, with emphasis on endurance and return-to-work activities; slowly decreasing the number of exercises and stretches; providing an evaluation of functional capacity; and continuing work simulation activities.

42. What is the difference between complete and incomplete spinal cord injuries?

A **complete** spinal cord injury involves complete or total severance of the spinal cord. Such injuries stop all neural transmission at the level of the injury. An **incomplete** injury does not completely sever the spinal cord, allowing some transmission of motor and/or sensory information transmission.

43. What is the Frankel Classification System? How is it used in rehabilitation?

The Frankel Classification System was devised to allow better communication about the degrees of completeness of spinal cord injuries. Sine et al.[12] describe five classes:

Class A indicates that the extent of injury is severe and that neurologically the patient has no motor or sensory function below the level of the injury.

Class B indicates that the patient has some sensation below the level of the injury but no motor control.

Class C indicates that the patient has sensation below the level of injury as well as useless motor function.

Class D indicates that the patient is capable of standing or doing limited walking with an assistive device or walker. The patient may also have some volitional control of bowel and bladder.

Class E indicates recovery.

The Frankel Classification System helps to provide an individualized rehabilitation program. It is used in realistic goal setting, progressing expectations, and discharge planning. The team members can refer to the class system when determining patient outcomes.

44. What types of impairment result from injury at the different levels of the cervical spine?

Patients with a C3 injury lose the use of the diaphragm and require continuous respiratory assistance. Patients with a C4 injury can lift and bend their arms only, and most require some assistance to perform such movements. Patients with a C5 injury lose wrist extension, and patients with a C6 injury lose the use of their fingers, resulting in the inability to grasp items. Patients with C7 injury lose use of the small muscles of the hand, decreasing its functional capacity.

45. What types of impairment result from injury at the different levels of the thoracic and lumbar spine?

A patient with a spinal cord injury from T1 to L2 requires trunk and abdominal support; rarely is functional ambulation possible. Patients injured at L2–L3 have leg paralysis and require leg braces. They have a "swing-through" crutch gait with decreased trunk stability and increased energy cost. Patients with an L4 injury demonstrate foot drop. They require leg braces and may require crutches for ambulation. Patients experiencing an injury at L5 experience loss of bowel, bladder, and sexual function. They may have a "waddle" type of gait but can ambulate without the use of aids.

46. What types of spinal injuries are most often seen in rehabilitation?

The two most common spinal injuries requiring rehabilitation are lumbar microdiscectomy and lumbar spinal fusion. These injuries are due to poor use of body mechanics as well as sports-related injuries.

47. What types of rehabilitation techniques should be used to treat a spinal injury such as a lumbar microdiscectomy?

Rehabilitation techniques include decreasing inflammation through the use of cold packs and anti-inflammatory medications. Patients must also avoid all loaded lumbar flexion activities during the first 6 weeks. Skin integrity and surgical site healing must be assessed on a frequent basis. Pain control during the first several weeks is imperative for a successful rehabilitation program.

The rehabilitation team begins with educating the patient about proper body mechanics for sitting, sleeping, standing, walking, lifting, and bending. A progressive exercise program includes treadmill walking, pelvic rocking in several different positions, abdominal bracing, and partial squats. These exercises progress to active range of motion exercises that include isometrics and self-nerve mobilization through stretching.

48. What types of rehabilitation techniques should be used to treat a spinal injury such as a lumbar fusion?

There are two types of recovery from spinal fusion surgeries. The simple type requires no rehabilitation; the complex type involves complications such as muscle weakness, stiffness, and poor movement habits that necessitate a rehabilitation program. One of the most important rehabilitation techniques is education about proper body mechanics for getting in and out of bed (log roll), in and out of a chair (keeping back straight), up and down from the floor (kneeling and lowering to arms), lying down (support with pillows), sitting (neutral spine positioning), standing, dressing (which may require use of aids), bending (hips flexed), reaching, pushing and pulling, lifting (bent knees, with spine straight not necessarily vertical), and carrying objects (knees slightly flexed with the object close to center of body).

After the patient progresses through the first 6 weeks, the rehabilitation team institutes an exercise program that begins with passive range of motion exercises and stretches and then progresses to isometrics, a walking program, and soft tissue massage to promote soft tissue mobilization after the incision line is closed.

49. Distinguish among non–weight-bearing, toe-touch/touch-down weight-bearing, and partial weight-bearing.

The non–weight-bearing patient may not apply any weight to the affected extremity. Toe-touch or touch-down weight-bearing requires the patient to place the toes of the affected leg on the ground without applying significant weight to the extremity. Partial weight-bearing is a percentage of weight that the leg can bear, as determined by the rehabilitation team (usually 50% or less).

50. How can patients be taught how much weight to apply during toe-touch weight bearing?

To ensure that the patient is not applying too much pressure during toe-touch or touchdown weight-bearing, tape a cracker to the bottom of the affected foot. The patient should not apply pressure that will "crack the cracker." A small scale may also be used to assist patients in knowing how much weight to bear during partial weight-bearing.

51. What are the types of mobilization assistive devices?

There are several different types of mobilization devices. The first is the wheelchair. It is important to obtain a wheelchair that not only fits the patient's size but also his or her needs. One needs to take into consideration the length of time that the patient will spend in the chair, whether it should have specialized cushions, and whether the chair needs motorization or the patient has the ability to self-propel. There are also many different types of wheelchair accessories, such as footrests that are fixed and footrests that elevate.

Other mobility devices include canes (e.g., straight canes, quad canes), different types of walkers (walkers with wheels, rolling walkers, walkers without wheels), and crutches. It is important that the crutches be at the appropriate height for the patient. The top of the crutch should lie comfortably under the arm in the axilla. The patient should be able to swing the affected leg through without difficulty or loss of balance.

52. What are the rehabilitation goals for patients with total hip replacement?

Rehabilitation goals include avoidance of peripheral nerve damage; prevention of heel ulcers; prevention of dislocation of the replacement; minimizing leg edema; avoiding postoperative pneumonias; increased voluntary movement of the involved leg; mobility training; total hip precautions; transfer and gait training; and an active range of motion exercise program. Each patient is different and progresses at his or her own rate, according to health status and age. The average rehabilitation length of stay for patients with total hip replacement is 10–14 days.

53. What are total hip precautions?
Total hip precautions are mobility precautions to help prevent dislocation of the new hip. These precautions include the prevention of hip flexion past 90°, adduction past the body's midline, and internal rotation of the hip. Often leg abductor wedges are used to assist in maintaining hip precautions.

54. What rehabilitation techniques are used for rehabilitating patients with total knee replacement?
Rehabilitation includes the initial use of a continuous passive movement (CPM) machine, beginning at 0°–40° and progressing 5°–10°, as tolerated by the patient, for 5–20 hours per day. Deep breathing exercises are important in the prevention of pneumonia. The patient should be taught how to do ankle pumps to decrease edema and prevent an embolus or thrombosis. Range of motion exercises should begin with knee extension and flexion, then progress to isometrics and active range of motion exercises. The patient should be taught transfer and gait techniques. Pain control is necessary to ensure a successful rehabilitation program.

55. What is the average length of the rehabilitation program in an anterior cruciate ligament reconstruction? What are the goals?
The average rehabilitation program is 1–4 weeks. The goals of the program are to decrease and control edema, provide education about gait, and increase mobility and strength. Active range of motion initially should be 0°–10° of extension and 130° of flexion. The patient should be able to bear 75–100% of body weight by the end of the fourth week. Exercise begins as stretching and progresses to active range of motion exercises. The patient can often return to a sport by 8–12 months after surgery.

56. What are the outcomes of a rehabilitation program for patients with a meniscal repair?
Rehabilitation outcomes include full range of motion and return of 90–100% of strength by 11 weeks after surgery. The patient should be able to return to full activity or sport by 12–18 weeks after surgery.

57. Are outpatient rehabilitation settings as effective as inpatient settings for patients with a lower extremity injury?
The setting should be individualized according to the patient's needs. Many elderly patients progress better in an inpatient setting, where training and education can be reinforced on a continuous basis.

BIBLIOGRAPHY

1. Anderson LE (ed): Mosby's Medical, Nursing, and Allied Health Dictionary. St. Louis, Mosby, 1998.
2. Beers MH, Berkow R (eds): The Merck Manual, 17th ed. West Point, NY, Merck & Co., 1999.
3. Black JM, Matassarin-Jacobs E: Medical-Surgical Nursing: Clinical Management for Continuity of Care. Philadelphia, W.B. Saunders. 1997.
4. DeLisa JA (ed): Rehabilitation Medicine: Principles and Practice. Philadelphia, J. B. Lippincot, 1993.
5. Goroll AH, May LA, Mulley AG: Primary Care Medicine: Office Evaluation and Management of the Adult Patient. Philadelphia, Lippincott Williams & Wilkins, 1995.
6. Guyton AC, Hall JE: Textbook of Medical Physiology, 9th ed. Philadelphia, W. B. Saunders, 1996.

7. Dunphy LM: Management Guidelines for Adult Nurse Practitioners. Philadelphia, F. A. Davis, 1999.
8. Hoeman SP: Rehabilitation Nursing: Process and Application. St. Louis, Mosby, 1996.
9. Maxey L, Magnusson J: Rehabilitation for the Postsurgical Orthopedic Patient. St. Louis, Mosby, 2001.
10. McCance KL, Huether SE: Pathophysiology: The Biologic Basis for Disease in Adults and Children. St. Louis, Mosby, 1998.
11. Mladenovic J (ed): Primary Care Secrets, 2nd ed. Philadelphia, Hanley & Belfus, 1999.
12. Sine RD, Liss SE, Rouch RE, et al: Basic Rehabilitation Techniques: A Self-instructional Guide. Gaithersburg, MD, Aspen Publishers, 1988.
13. United States Department of Health and Human Services: Acute Low Back Problems in Adults: Clinical Practice Guideline. Rockville, MD, Agency for Health Care Policy and Research, 1994.
14. Uphold CR, Graham MV: Clinical Guidelines in Adult Health. Gainesville, FL, Barmarrae Books, 1999.

INDEX